Pierfrancesco Fusco
Rafael Blanco
De Q. Tran
Franco Marinangeli

ULTRASOUND GUIDED NERVE BLOCKS OF THE TRUNK AND ABDOMINAL WALL

edra

ULTRASOUND GUIDED NERVE BLOCKS OF THE TRUNK AND ABDOMINAL WALL
Pierfrancesco Fusco, Rafael Blanco, De Q. Tran, Franco Marinangeli

2022 – Reprint

ISBN: 978-88-214-5489-9
eISBN: 978-88-214-5490-5

Book Publishing Manager: Costanza Smeraldi
Paper, Printing and Binding Manager: Paolo Ficicchia
Cover: Gaetano Altamura
Layout and copyediting: ALTER EDOM s.r.l., Noventa Padovana (PD), Italy

Edra S.p.A.
Via G. Spadolini 7,
20141 Milano (Italy)
Tel. 02 881841
www.edizioniedra.it

Printed by "*Rotomail Italia*" S.p.A., Vignate (MI), Italy, May 2022

(*) Edra S.p.A. is a part of LSWR GROUP

To all those brave enough to improve themselves
by making mistakes.

To all the parents who make sacrifices to empower
their children in fulfilling their dreams.

Pierfrancesco Fusco

Preface

Regional anesthesia has undergone a process of evolution and revolution over the last decade, mainly due to the introduction of ultrasound, the acquisition of new anatomy and sonoanatomy knowledge, as well as recent discoveries on the role of the fascia.

This process has led to regional anesthesia playing a key role in surgery and postoperative pain management, cutting down on the use of opioids or avoiding their use altogether, in line with the ERAS pathway.

This progress is supported by recent scientific evidence showing that fascia and nerve blocks offer a good level of safety and are effective with a reduced incidence of serious side effects.

Together this has contributed to the growth of our discipline along with a renewed enthusiasm for a modern approach to regional anesthesia and pain therapy, which are most effective when correctly included in clinical paths.

In 2016 these innovations led to the birth of our editorial project, with the first Italian book entirely dedicated to chest and abdominal wall blocks. Subsequently, in 2018 the same text was translated into Spanish for the South American market and, more recently in 2021-22 this same editorial project led to not just an English version of the existing text, but an entirely new book which coming five years after the publication of the original includes important updates and has undergone a full redesign.

The most significant additions to this new version are the contributions from the most prominent experts in the field, who have made their scientific skills and clinical experience available to everyone, allowing the traditional methods of teaching to be transformed into a practical training path.

This new work is also a milestone for all professionals in anesthesiology and pain therapy, with drawings, tables, flow charts, detailed anatomical and sonoanatomic pictures, videos taken by the authors and real clinical cases included in each chapter.

The volume opens with a chapter dedicated to the anatomy and function of fascia. There is a section dedicated to paraneuraxial blocks, which outlines the multitude of applications for paravertebral and ESP blocks, according to the emerging vision of regional anesthesia for the treatment of both acute and chronic pain.

The text continues with chapters dedicated to the anterior thoracic blocks with applications in surgical contexts such as breast surgery, cardiac surgery, thoracic surgery or thoracic trauma management.

The chapters dedicated to blocks of the anterior and posterior abdominal wall underline the importance of applying these techniques not only in open abdominal surgery but above all in laparoscopic surgery and robotic surgery, adding value to the ERAS pathway.

In the last part of the book there is an important chapter on pediatric wall blocks and their applications.

The book ends with a series of chapters ranging from neck band blocks, through the application and indication of the LIA and wound infusion, to the modern simulation applied to fascial blocks.

We conclude with an innovative chapter on the application of RA techniques in the COVID-19 era.

Our intention was to combine our passion and scientific skills to provide a useful tool for daily clinical activities, improving clinical treatment paths and the perioperative outcome of our patients, particularly at a time when all these techniques are an essential knowledge base for modern anesthesia.

Finally, our sincere thanks go to all the authors and co-authors who made valuable contributions.

Pierfrancesco Fusco

Rafael Blanco
De Q. Tran
Franco Marinangeli

Authors

Pierfrancesco Fusco
Department of Anesthesia and Intensive Care Unit, San Salvatore Academic Hospital of L'Aquila, L'Aquila, Italy

Rafael Blanco
Anaesthesia & Critical Care, King's College Hospital Dubai, United Arab Emirates

De Q. Tran
Department of Anesthesia Montreal St. Mary's Hospital McGill University, Montreal, Quebec, Canada

Franco Marinangeli
Department of Anesthesiology, Pain Treatment and Palliative Care, University of L'Aquila, L'Aquila, Italy

Contributors

Andrea Luigi Ambrosoli
Day Surgery Unit, Azienda Ospedaliera Ospedale di Circolo e Fondazione Macchi, Polo Universitario, Varese, Italy

Francesca Angelucci
Department of Anestesia and Intensive Care, San Salvatore Academy Hospital, L'Aquila, Italy

Claude Thierry Bagaphou
Section of Anesthesia, Intensive Care and Pain Medicine, Department of Emergency Medicine, Città di Castello Hospital, Città di Castello, Perugia, Italy

Astrid U. Behr
Anesthesia and Intensive Care Unit, Camposampiero Hospital, Padua, Italy

Dario Bugada
Department of Emergency and Intensive Care, ASST Papa Giovanni XXIII, Bergamo, Italy

Danilo Canzio
Department of Anestesia Intensive Care and Pain Medicine, Policlinico P. Giaccone, Palermo, Italy

Gianluca Cappelleri
Anesthesia, Intensive Care and Pain Therapy Policlinico di Monza, Monza, Italy

Walter Ciaschi
Intensive Care Unit, Department of Anesthesia and Pain Therapy, Fabrizio Spaziani Hospital, Frosinone, Italy

Fabio Costa
Unit of Anesthesia, Intensive Care and Pain Management, Policlinico Campus Bio-Medico Foundation, Campus Bio-Medico University, Rome, Italy

Fausto D'Agostino
Unit of Anaesthesia, Intensive Care and Pain Management, Policlinico Campus Bio-Medico Foundation, Campus Bio Medico University and Teaching Hospital, Rome, Italy

Francesca De Sanctis
Department of Critical Care Medicine and Anesthesiology, St. Maria Hospital, Terni, Italy

Cristiano D'Errico
Department of Postoperative Intensive Care Unit and Hyperbaric Oxygen Therapy, U.O.C., O.T.I., A.O.R.N. Cardarelli, Naples, Italy

Stefano Di Carlo
Department of Anesthesia and Cardiac Surgery Intensive Care, Giuseppe Mazzini Hospital, Teramo, Italy

Fabrizio Fattorini
Department of Anaesthesiology, Critical Care Medicine and Pain Therapy, Sapienza University of Rome, Rome, Italy

Giuseppe Gazzerro
Pain Department AO "Ospedali dei Colli", Monaldi Hospital, Naples, Italy

Antonio Giorgi
Department of Medicine and Surgery, University of Milano Bicocca, Monza, Italy

Fabio Gobbi
Department of Anesthesiology and Intensive Care, Humanitas Gradenigo, Torino, Italy

Vittorio Lucchetta
Department of Anesthesia and Intensive Care, Padua Hospital, Padua, Italy

Alberto Manassero
Department of Anesthesiology and Intensive Care, S. Croce e Carle Hospital, Cuneo, Italy

Roberta Monzani
Department of Anaesthesia and Intensive Care Units, IRCCS Humanitas Research Hospital, Rozzano, Milan, Italy

Giuseppe Paladini
Anesthesia and Intensive Care Unit, Department of Pediatrics, "Vittore Buzzi" Children's Hospital, Milan, Italy

Giuseppe Pascarella
Unit of Anesthesia, Intensive Care and Pain Management, Policlinico Campus Bio-Medico Foundation, Campus Bio-Medico University, Rome, Italy

Gianmarco Petroni
Department of Anesthesia and Intensive Care Unit, San Salvatore Academic Hospital of L'Aquila, L'Aquila, Italy

Emiliano Petrucci
Department of Anesthesia and Intensive Care, San Salvatore Academic Hospital of L'Aquila, L'Aquila, Italy

Raffaele Perna
Department of Anesthesia and Intensive Care Unit, San Salvatore Academic Hospital of L'Aquila, L'Aquila, Italy

Carmine Pullano
Villa Pia Clinic, Rome, Italy

Gianluca Russo
Department of Anesthesia, Intensive Care and Pain Medicine, Lodi Hospital, Lodi, Italy.

Paolo Scimia
Department of Anesthesia and Intensive Care Unit, Giuseppe Mazzini Hospital Teramo, Teramo. Italy

Giuseppe Sepolvere
Department of Anesthesiology and Cardiac Surgery Intensive Care Unit, San Michele Hospital, Maddaloni, Caserta, Italy

Roberto Starnari
Italian National Research Center on Aging, Department of Anesthesiology, INRCA Hospital, Ancona, Italy

Carla Stecco
Department of Neuroscience, Institute of Human Anatomy, University of Padova, Italy

Mario Tedesco
Department of Anesthesia and Intensive Care Unit and Pain Therapy, Mater Dei Hospital, Bari, Italy

Andrea Tognù
Anesthesia, Intensive Care and Pain Therapy, IRCCS Istituto Ortopedico Rizzoli, Bologna, Italy

Gilda Tornatore
Department of Anesthesia, Intensive Care and Pain Medicine, Lodi Hospital, Lodi, Italy

Vito Torrano
Department of Emergency and Urgency, Anesthesia and Intensive care Unit 1, ASST Grande Ospedale Metropolitano Niguarda, Milan, Italy

Luigi Tritapepe
Anaesthesia and Intensive Care Division, San Camillo-Forlanini Hospital Rome, Italy

Francesco Vasques
Anesthesia and Intensive Care Unit, Camposampiero Hospital, Padua, Italy

Nicola Zadra
Pediatric Anesthesia Unit, Department of Pediatrics, Padua Hospital, Padua, Italy

Contents

Chapter 1 • Myofascial planes of the trunk 1
C. Stecco

Chapter 2 • Thoracic paravertebral block (TVB) 13
G. Cappelleri, D. Bugada

Chapter 3 • Erector spinae plane block (ESP block) 27
P. Scimia, E. Petrucci, A. Manassero, S. Di Carlo

Chapter 4 • Deep and superficial serratus plane block and intercostal nerve block 39
V. Torrano, G. Russo, A. Giorgi, P. Scimia, G. Sepolvere, P. Fusco

Chapter 5 • Interpectoral plane block (IPP) and Pectoserratus plane block (PSP) (PECS 1 and PECS 2 blocks) 61
P. Fusco, S. Di Carlo, E. Petrucci, G. Sepolvere, R. Blanco

Chapter 6 • Superficial parasternal intercostal plane block (PIP) 81
P. Fusco, G. Paladini, P. Scimia, L. Tritapepe, G. Sepolvere

Chapter 7 • Trasversus abominis plane block (TAP) 91
P. Fusco, R. Perna, F. Gobbi, P. Scimia, W. Ciaschi, A.L. Ambrosoli, F. Fattorini

Chapter 8 • Iliohypogastric (IH), Ilioinguinal (II), and Genitofemoral (GF) nerve block 111
P. Scimia, C.T. Bagaphou, R. Monzani, P. Fusco

Chapter 9 • Rectus sheath block 127
G. Russo, V. Torrano, G. Gazzerro, G. Tornatore

Chapter 10 • Transversalis Fascia Plane (TFP) block 141
A.U. Behr

Chapter 11 • Quadratus lumborum block (QLB) 153
A.U. Behr, F. Vasques

Chapter 12 • Ultrasound-guided trunk and abdominal wall blocks in children 165
V. Lucchetta, G. Paladini, N. Zadra

Chapter 13 • Fascial plane blocks of the neck: superficial and intermediate cervical plexus block 183
G. Sepolvere, C. D'Errico, M. Tedesco

Chapter 14 • Local infiltration analgesia (LIA) and continuous wound infusion (CWI) 193
F. Costa, G. Pascarella, D. Canzio, F. D'Agostino, A. Tognù

Chapter 15 • Fascial plane blocks and neuraxial blocks: two planets not so far apart 205
R. Starnari, C. Pullano

Appendix 1 • Ultrasound-guided regional anesthesia simulation 217
P. Fusco, G. Petroni, F. Angelucci

Appendix 2 • Regional anesthesia in the COVID-19 era 219
F. De Sanctis, P. Fusco

Subject Index 229

Video

Video 1.1 • Dissection of the thoracic region to show the pectoral fasciae involved in the PECS block 6

Video 1.2 • Dissection of the back to show the thoracolumbar fascia and the area involved in the erector spinae block 7

Video 2.1 • Paravertebral block 19

Video 3.1 • Technique to correctly perform US-guided ESP block 32

Video 3.2 • Ultrasound visualization of the correct diffusion of the injected solution in the target fascial plane (ESP) 32

Video 3.3 • Technique to correctly perform a continuous US-guided ESP block 32

Video 4.1 • Deep serratus plane block 45

Video 4.2 • SAPB: chest tube insertion for pneumothorax 61

Video 5.1 • PECS 1 71

Video 5.2 • PECS 2 74

Video 6.1 • Parasternal block 84

Video 6.2 • Superficial PIP: cardiac surgery 89

Video 7.1 • TAP 97

Video 7.2 • Mid-axillary approach 97

Video 7.3 • Subcostal approach 101

Video 8.1 • US-guided Ilioinguinal and Iliohypogastric nerve block. Note “double V sign” 117

Video 9.1 • Block of the sheath of the rectus abdominis muscle 133

Video 9.2 • Lateromedial approach 133

Video 11.1 • Performance of QLB II 158

Video 11.2 • Transmuscular QLB by Børglum 160

VIDEO

Video 12.1 • Thoracic paravertebral block 168

Video 12.2 • Ilioinguinal and iliohypogastric nerve block 174

Video 13.1 • Thyroidectomy 186

Video 13.2 • Carotid endarterectomy 186

Video 14.1 • Preperitoneal wound catheter placement 198

Video 14.2 • Spinal anesthesia + CWI 204

Video 15.1 • Continuous Spinal Anesthesia 207

Myofascial planes of the trunk

Carla Stecco

The purpose of this chapter is to illustrate the anatomy of the trunk not as a list of distinct elements, but considering the role of fasciae in connecting muscles, vessels, and nerves.
Particularly, in the trunk it is possible to identify three myofascial planes (superficial, intermediate, and deep) and a superficial fascia, organized like the layers of an onion (**Figure 1.1**). Between two planes lays the loose connective tissue (**Figure 1.2**), which makes sure that each muscle group can autonomously slide and move. Furthermore, the nerves use these layers of loose connective tissue to spread to the various parts of the body, thus becoming one of the targets of locoregional anesthesia.

For anesthesiologists, it is important to know the anatomical organization of these myofascial planes because it determines the space for the diffusion of anesthetics and, therefore, must be considered as one of the key elements to understand the quantity of anesthetic to be injected and the modalities for its distribution. Besides, the various myofascial layers fuse in some specific areas, creating well defined compartments, that may limit local anesthetic spread. However, these lines of fusions have not been fully described and are subject to significant variability. Besides, adhesion formation after surgery or trauma may cause new lines of fusion that can produce pathological compartmentalization of a fascial space, further restricting local anesthetic diffusion.

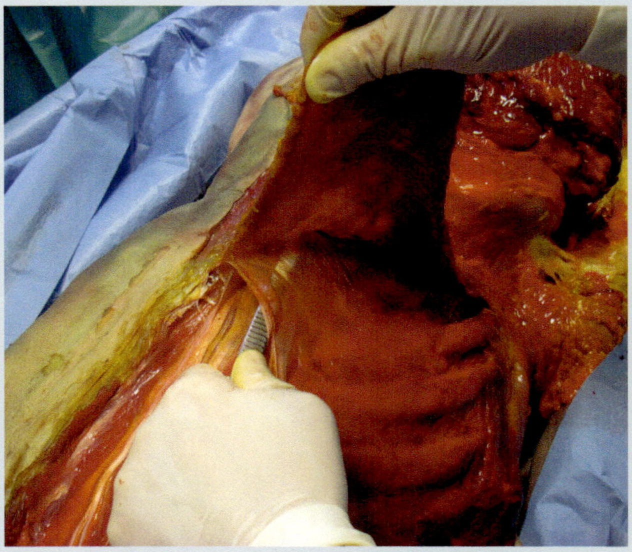

Figure 1.1 Dissection of the trunk: it is possible to note the three myofascial planes. The hand lifts the latissimus dorsi, with the serratus posterior inferior muscles, to show the cavity of the erector spinae muscles.

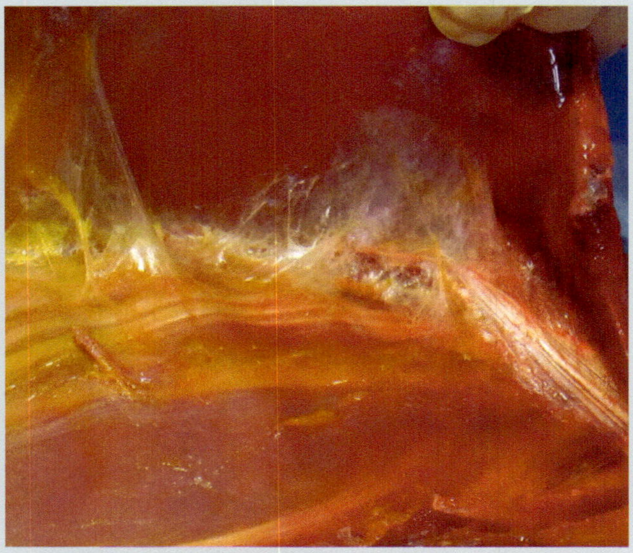

Figure 1.2 Loose connective tissue between myofascial planes. This tissue is highly hydrated and makes sure that adjacent myofascial planes move autonomously. The nerves take advantage of these spaces to move from the exit of the spinal canal to the end of the innervation.

A separate paragraph will be dedicated to the microscopic aspects of the fasciae, considering the fibrous and loose components of the deep fasciae. The fibrous component defines the barrier that keeps the anesthetic in a given space. If the fibrous component increases or creates adhesions, the anesthetic diffusion compartment may vary. For example, a thicker fascial plane with multiple fascial layers may mean a potentially greater barrier to local anesthetic diffusion and a thinner might make this easier. Alternatively, a thicker layer may provide a more distinct sonographic and tactile endpoint than a thin layer for needle puncture as well as keeping the local anesthetic within the interfascial plane thus allow for greater extent of spread to reach target nerves within. Conceivably, it may be more difficult to inject local anesthetic with precision within a fascial plane that is bordered by thin fasciae and it may be less likely that the drug stays within the fascial plane because it can easily penetrate the fascia to enter the muscle, especially with high injection pressure. The loose connective tissue defines the environment where the anesthetic drug will diffuse, consequently the viscosity and hydratation of this tissue can define the ability of the drugs to spread far away. Finally, special focus will be made to the innervation and vascularization of the fasciae. Indeed it is possible that the nerve network inside fasciae could be a direct target of the regional anesthesia and that the wall blocks can even interrupt the pain signal originated from the deep fascia itself. Lastly, due to the rich vascularization of the fasciae, fasciae could play a role in systemic toxicity.

SUPERFICIAL FASCIA

In the chest and abdomen, the superficial fascia is always easily recognizable, but it becomes very thick and visible especially in the distal part of the abdomen, where it is named in a specific way: Scarpa's fascia. The superficial fascia consists of a continuous fibroelastic layer that divides the subcutaneous tissue into two layers: the superficial adipose tissue (SAT) and the deep adipose tissue (DAT) (**Figure 1.3**). The superficial fascia is the homologous of the panniculus carnosus in mammals. For this reason, it is frequent to find some striated muscular fibers inside the superficial fascia, and in some areas such as neck, face, and scrotum, they become well organized to form muscles such as the platysma, the mimic muscles, and the dartos muscle. Furthermore, the superficial fascia splits to wrap superficial vessels and cutaneous nerves. In particular, Caggiati (1999) showed how the superficial fascia is an excellent support for the walls of saphenous veins. Indeed many fibrous septa connect the tunica adventitia of the superficial veins to the superficial fascia, acting like bicycle spokes. Moreover, the superficial fascia supports and organizes the lymphatic vessels in the hypodermis and also the cutaneous nerves, protecting them from the traumas caused by excessive stretching. The superficial fascia is richly innervated and contains both free nerve endings and corpuscular receptors such as Pacini and Ruffini corpuscles. These nerve elements are tightly connected to the collagen fibers inside the fascia, and for this reason they can perceive the mechanical stimuli applied to the superficial fascia itself. It is also possible to assume that their position in relation to the skin can permit to distinguish between light and heavy pressure, thus collaborating with the skin receptors involved in exteroception.

The superficial fascia is connected through fibrous septae both to the derma (retinacula cutis superficialis or skin ligaments) and to the deep fascia (retinacula cutis profundis), and the features of this septae determine both the motility of the skin in relation to the deep

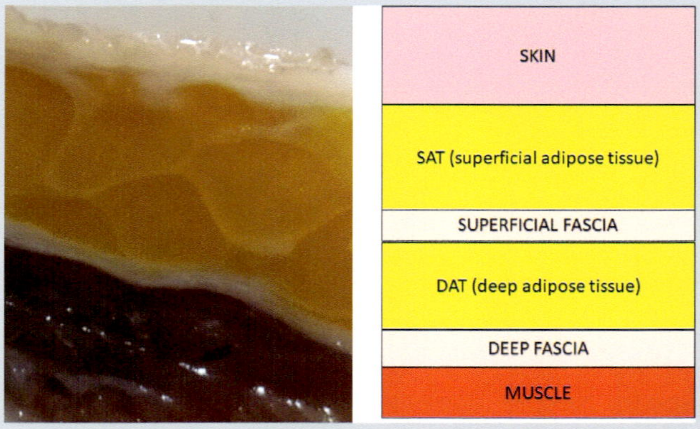

Figure 1.3 Organization of the subcutaneous tissue.

TABLE 14.1 MYOFASCIAL PLANES OF THE TRUNK

	MUSCLES	FASCIAE
SUPERFICIAL MYOFASCIAL PLANE	Pectoralis major muscle Trapezius and latissimus dorsi muscle Deltoid muscle Gluteus maximus muscle External oblique muscle	Pectoral fascia Thoracolumbar fascia (posterior layer) Deltoid fascia Fascia of the gluteus maximus muscle Fascia of Rizk
INTERMEDIATE MYOFASCIAL PLANE	Subclavius and pectoralis minor muscle Serratus anterior and posterior muscles Rhomboid, infraspinatus, supraspinatus muscle External oblique muscle	Clavipectoral fascia Serratus fasciae Fascia of rhomboid muscles, infraspinatus and supraspinatus fascia Fascia of the external oblique muscle
DEEP MYOFASCIAL PLANE	Intercostal muscle Internal oblique muscle and Transversus abdominis muscle	Fascia of intercostal muscles and periosteum Fasciae of the IO muscle and of the transversus muscle, anterior layer of the TLF

planes and the organization of adipose lobules of the subcutis. Usually, these septa are thick and almost perpendicular in the SAT, where they firmly anchor the superficial fascia to the skin and create well-defined compartments for the adipose lobules, whereas the septa are usually oblique and thin in the DAT, guarantying in such a way a good level of autonomy of the superficial fascia in relation to the deep one. In the trunk, the superficial fascia adheres to the deep fascia along the sternum, the linea alba, the entire spine, along the spine of the scapula and the clavicle, at the level of the sixth rib and over the inguinal ligament. These adhesions allow to divide the subcutis in several compartments, which might organize the lymphatic drainage and the superficial venous return.

DEEP FASCIA

The organization of the deep fascia in the trunk is more complex compared to that of limbs. In fact, in the limbs there is only a single aponeurotic fascia which wraps all the muscles and divides them in compartments, whereas in the trunk there are three muscle planes delimited by three different fascial layers.

Between each myofascial layers, there is some loose connective tissue that guarantees the autonomy of the various muscle planes. These myofascial planes fuse together at some points and create specific lines towards which all the muscle forces converge. In particular, the most important fusion lines are the linea alba and the lateral raphe on the sides of the erector spinae. Furthermore, in the trunk there are a few deep fasciae with aponeurotic features (thoracolumbar fascia and the rectus sheath), whereas the others show epimysial features, in other words, usually the fasciae of the trunk are thin and adherent to the underlying muscles. Therefore, it makes no sense to study the fasciae and muscles of the trunk as separate units, but it is much better to talk about myofascial units (**Table 14.1**). This myofascial organization is due to the embryological development of the trunk muscles. In particular, the muscles of the most superficial plane of the trunk originate from the somites of the limbs and progressively develop in the trunk up to the midline, guided by the most superficial lamina of the trunk itself, which is penetrated by the muscular component. The result is a myofascial plane characterized by large muscles intricately connected to the investing fascia, which works as a bridge maintaining anatomical continuity.

First myofascial plane of the trunk

The first myofascial plane is formed by large flat muscles that connect the trunk to the limbs, such as trapezius, pectoralis major, latissimus dorsi, gluteus maximus and the external oblique, connected by a thin fascia closely adhering to various muscles. This deep fascia originates in the neck, wraps the sternocleidomastoid and the trapezius muscle, passes over the clavicle by partly adhering to it, and finally splits in two layers to include the pectoralis major muscle. This fascia literally continues with the deltoid and axillary fascia (**Figures 1.4** and **1.5**), giving rise to a fibrous expansion in the branchial fascia. The two layers of the pectoral fascia adhere to each other over the serratus anterior to form a single fascial lamina, which some authors call anterolateral thoracic fascia. Posteriorly, this single layer splits again to wrap the latissimus dorsi (**Figure 1.6**). Medially, the fascia partly adheres to the sternum, thus becoming its periosteum, and partly goes beyond it to continue with the contralateral pectoral fascia (**Figure 1.7**). Distally, this fascia continues with the fascia of Rizk, that is the fascial layer that covers the external oblique muscle. Numerous fibers get over the midline along the linea alba and continue with the fascia of the opposite side. In this way, an anatomical and functional continuity among the muscles of the thorax and abdomen is established, while the rectus sheath plays the role of harmonizing the action of all these muscles. Posteriorly, the Rizk fascia takes part in the formation of the superficial layer of the thoracolumbar fascia. Distally, the fascia of the external oblique muscle thickens to form the inguinal and the lacunar ligament, while the most superficial fasciae continue with the fascia lata.

Second myofascial plane of the trunk

The second myofascial plane in the trunk is represented by the clavipectoral fascia, which wraps and connects the subclavius, pectoralis minor, and anterior serratus. There is a large cleavage plane between the

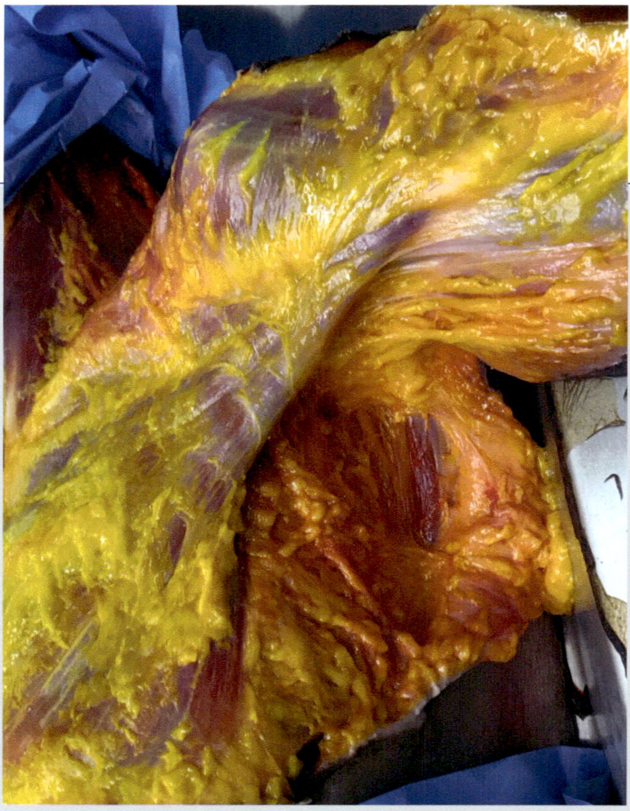

Figure 1.4 Dissection of the anterior part of trunk and shoulder. Note that the fascia wrapping the pectoralis major muscle is the one that also wraps the deltoid muscle, and both continue with the brachial fascia. This myofascial plane also forms the floor of the axillary cavity, and posteriorly continues with the fascia of the latissimus dorsi and the trapezius.

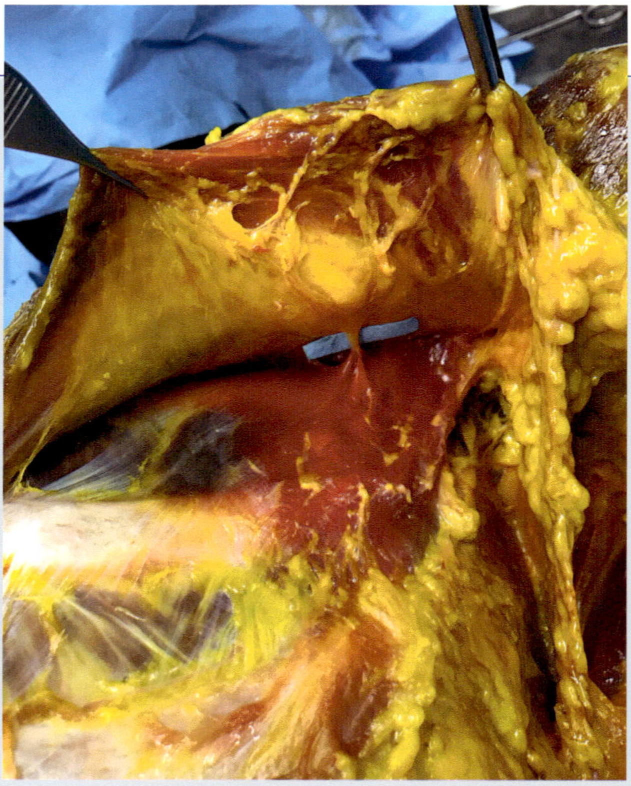

Figure 1.5 Dissection of the thoracic wall: the pectoralis major muscle is lifted to show the pectoralis minor muscle and the medial pectoral nerve.

pectoralis major and this fascia due to the presence of some loose connective tissue, where it is also possible to find the two pectoral nerves (**Figure 1.8**). Posteriorly, the clavipectoral fascia continues with the fascia of the rhomboid muscles and of the levator scapulae muscle, thus forming the so-called "serrato-romboid complex", described in 1987 by Nguyen to emphasize the continuity between the anterior serratus muscle and the rhomboid muscles. Laterally, this fascia forms the suspensory ligament of the armpit and continues with the fascia of the coracobrachialis muscle.

At the axillary level, a large anatomical space between this myofascial plane and the superficial one is created, filled by adipose tissue, where the long thoracic and thoracodorsal nerves are found (**Figure 1.9**). The first one innervates the serratus anterior, while the second one the latissimus dorsi and the teres major. Distally, the clavipectoral fascia continues with the fascia of the external oblique muscle. The fascia of the external

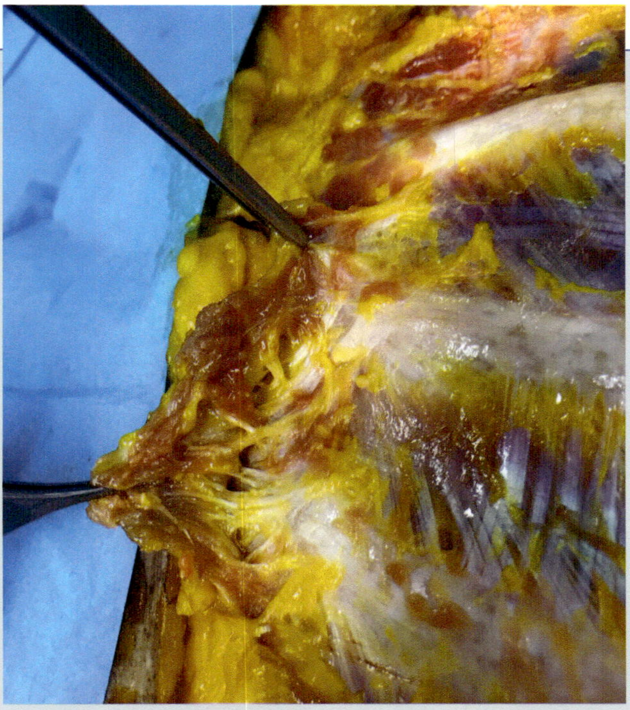

Figura 1.7 Dissection of the parasternal region. The pectoralis major muscle has been removed and its sternal insertions lifted with forceps to show the anterior cutaneous branches of the intercostal nerves.

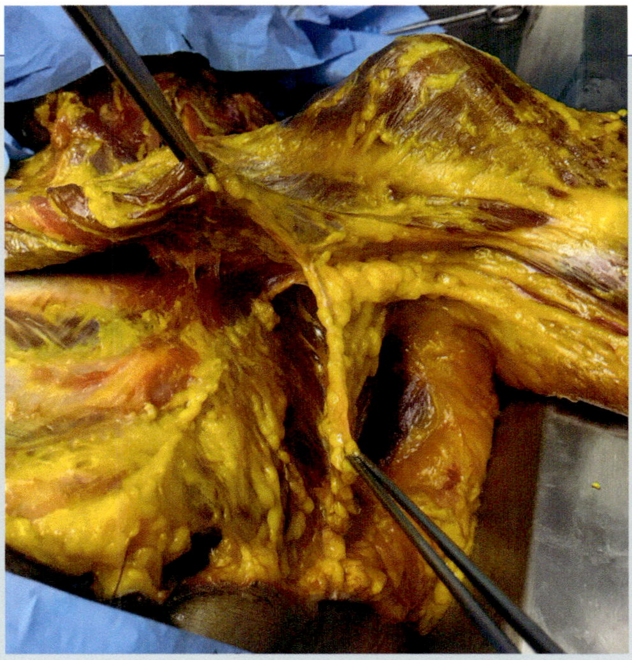

Figure 1.6 Myofascial planes at the level of the trunk and axillary cavity. Note the fascia of the pectoralis major which continues with the fascia of the latissimus dorsi, whereas deep in the fascia of the serratus major muscle it forms a second myofascial plane. This space is usually wide and filled with adipose tissue. At this level, it is possible to find the long thoracic nerve and the thoracodorsal nerve.

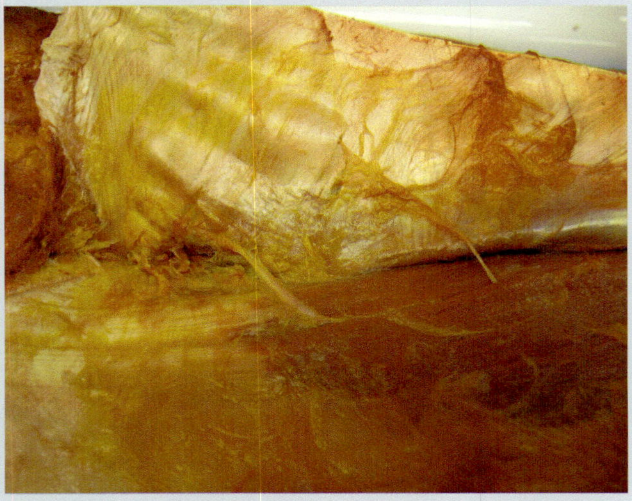

Figure 1.8 Dissection of the lumbar region. The posterior sheet of the thoracolumbar fascia has been lifted to show the erector spinae muscles and the dorsal branches of the spinal nerves. The posterior sheet of the FTL inserts itself into the spinous processes and delimits, together with the anterior sheet that inserts itself into the transverse processes, the compartment of the erector spinae muscles. Laterally, the two sheets fuse together in the lateral raphe, which also represents the posterior fusion line of the fasciae of the large abdominal muscles, in a symmetrical manner compared to what is highlighted anteriorly on the sides of the rectus muscle.

oblique muscle is a very thin fibrous layer that wraps the muscles at both sides and is separated from the fascia of the internal oblique muscle by a thin layer of loose connective tissue, whilst it is adherent to the Riszk fascia externally. In such a way, the fascia covering the outer layer of the external oblique muscle is always much more thicker respect to the deep one (**Figure 1.10**, **Video 1.1**).

Third myofascial plane of the trunk

The third myofascial plane in the trunk is formed by the intercostal fascia, that wraps the intercostal muscles and continues as periosteum over the ribs. From the inner side, this fascia adheres to the parietal pleura to form the endothoracic fascia. This adhesion allows the parietal pleura to follow the movements of the ribcage, thus guaranteeing lung expansion. On the contrary, there is a neat separation between the parietal peritoneum and the muscular fasciae in the abdomen, to prevent the contraction of abdominal muscles from interfering with the peristaltic movements of the intestine. The endothoracic fascia divides the paravertebral space

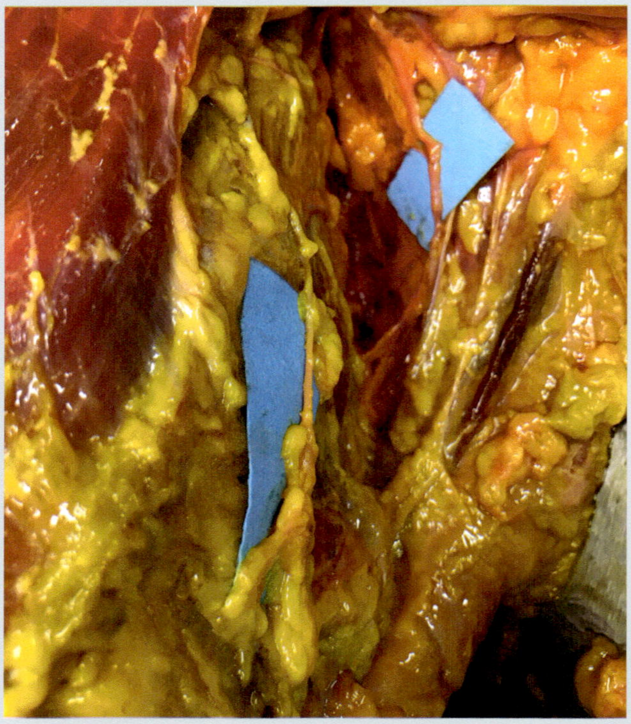

Figure 1.9 Dissection of the axillary cavity to show the long thoracic nerve and the thoracodorsal nerve.

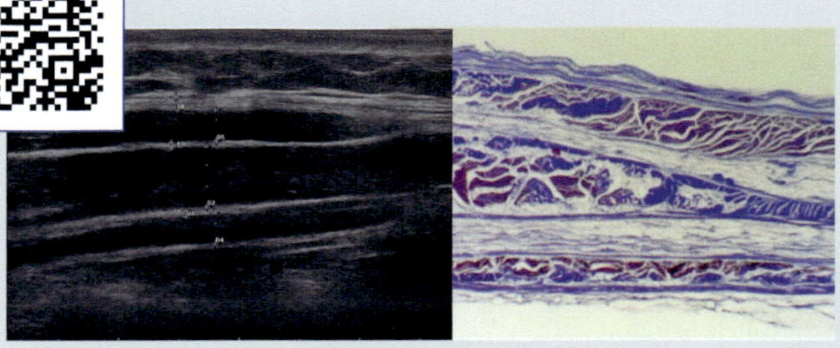

Figure 1.10 Ultrasound and histological evaluation of the abdominal wall. Note the thin fibrous layers that wrap the three abdominal muscles and the loose connective tissue between them that allows the autonomous gliding of the various myofascial layers. Note also the fasciae of the external oblique muscle: the outer layer is thicker respect to the inner one due to the presence of the Rizk fascia that reinforces and adheres the EO fascia.

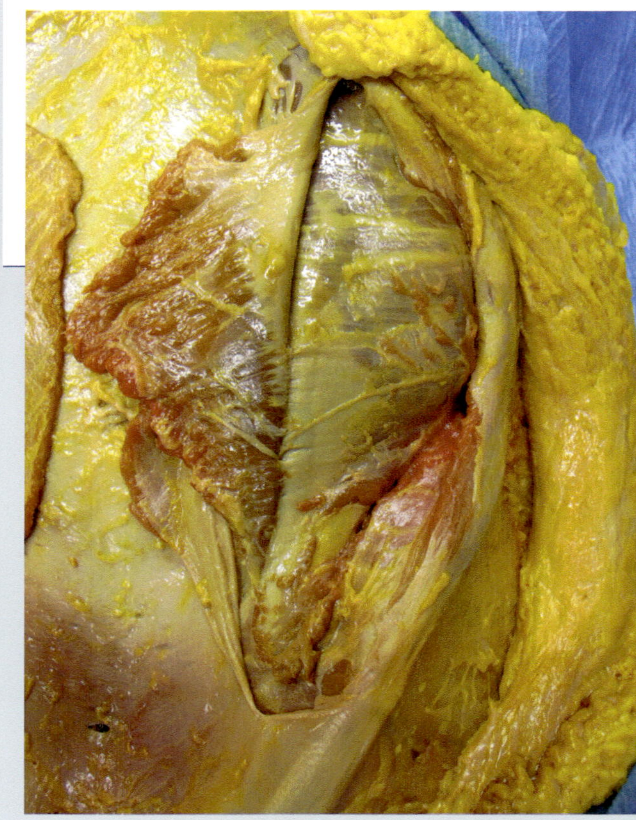

Figure 1.11 Dissection of the anterior abdominal wall; the internal oblique muscle has been lifted to show the transverse muscle and the subcostal nerves that run in the transversus abdominis plane (TAP).

in two compartments: the extrapleural compartment, containing the sympathetic ganglia, and the subendothoracic compartment, containing the spinal nerves with their ganglia. The extrapleural plane is widely used as cleavage plane in thoracic surgery. The endothoracic fascia continues in the diaphragmatic fascia and joins the transverse fascia at the level of the esophageal hiatus, forming the phrenic-esophageal ligament.

At the abdominal level, this myofascial plane is represented by the internal oblique muscle and the transversus abdominis muscle with their fasciae (**Figure 1.11**). These two muscles have a common embryological development, and only later they will be divided by a fascial layer and loose connective tissue. This new myofascial layer corresponds to the TAP (transversus abdominis plane), inside which run the nerves that spread to the anterior wall of the abdomen (**Figures 1.13**, **1.14**).

Medially, the aponeurosis of the transversus muscle goes beyond the midline for its entire extension, continuing with the contralateral muscle and forming a digastric muscle between the two sides. Posteriorly, the fascia of the transversus abdominis muscle collaborates with the internal oblique muscle to form the anterior layer of the thoracolumbar fascia, which will constitute, together with the transverse processes, the anterior wall of the erector spinae cavity. Internally, the fascia of the transversus abdominis muscle is in relation with the transversalis (or preperitoneal) fascia. This fascia appears evident especially in the distal part of the abdomen, where it thickens and continues with the parietal pelvic fascia, the vesico-umbilical fascia, and with the innermost layer of the spermatic cord, whereas in the rest of the abdomen it adheres to the inner side of the

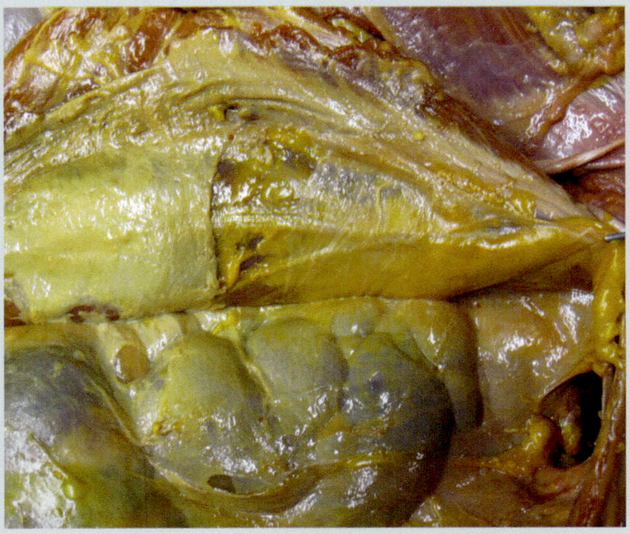

Figure 1.12 Dissection of the anterior abdominal region; the rectus muscle has been lifted to show the line of Douglas and the transverse fascia that covers the inferior epigastric vessels.

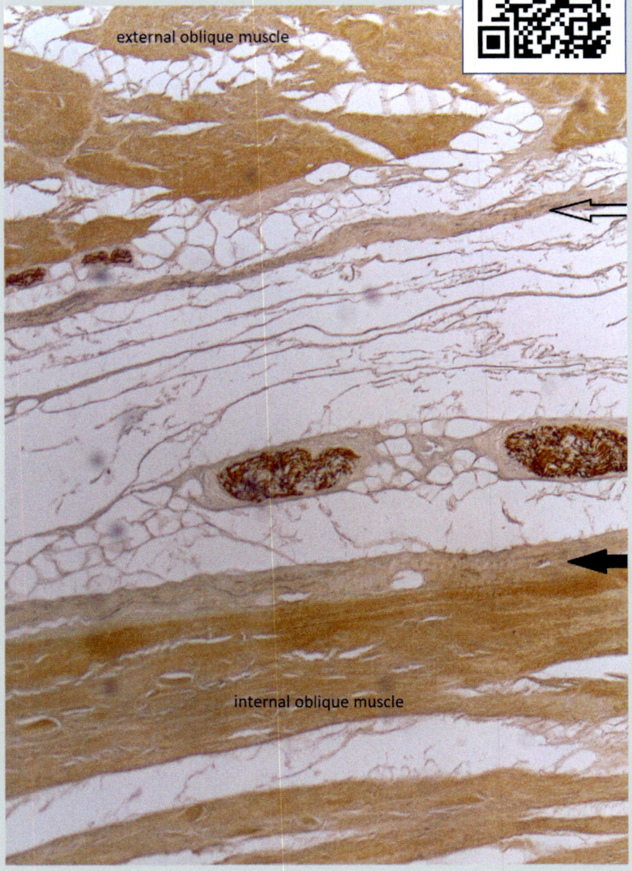

Figure 1.13 The S100 immunohistochemical staining allows to show two large nerves that run along the loose connective tissue placed between the internal fascia of the external oblique muscle (transparent arrow) and the external fascia of the internal oblique muscle (black arrow). Furthermore, it is possible to identify 2 little nerves placed between the fascia of the external oblique muscle and the muscle tissue. It is possible to note how the abdominal muscles are wrapped by one of their thin and fibrous fasciae, while the loose connective tissue between two fasciae guarantees the presence of a sliding surface and a diffusion area for anesthetics.

Myofascial planes of the trunk

transversus abdominis muscle, thus becoming recognizable only by microscopic examination. Cranially, it continues with the diaphragmatic fascia. Posteriorly, this fascia detaches from the inner wall of the transversus abdominis muscle to cover the iliopsoas muscle and the quadratus lumborum muscle. Therefore, a triangular space on the side of the quadratus lumborum muscle is created, in which the subcostal, iliohypogastric, and ilioinguinal nerves are found. This space is the ideal target of the TFP (transversalis fascia plane) block, thus allowing the compartmentalization of the anesthetic within a limited space inside the nerve. Unfortunately, the fasciae that delimit this space are difficult to visualize by ultrasound (**Figure 1.13**, **Video 1.2**).

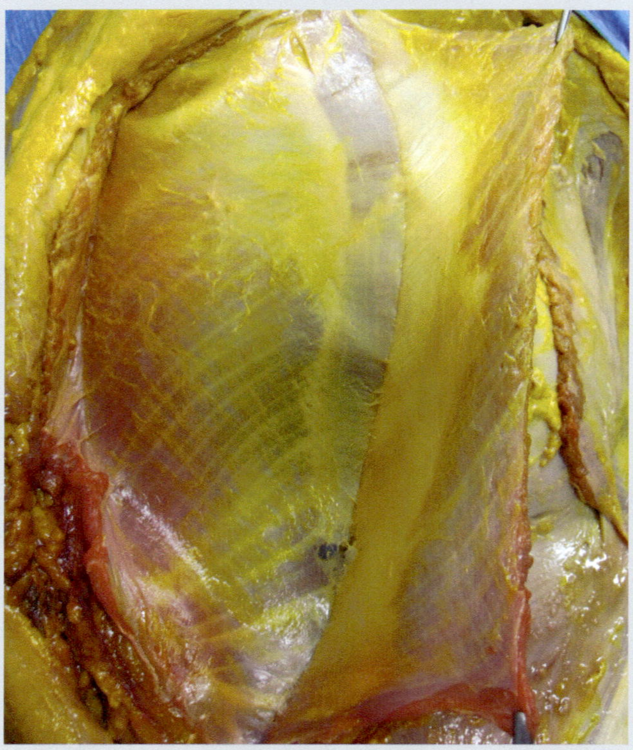

Figure 1.14 Dissection of the abdomen. The external oblique muscle has been laterally sectioned and lifted towards the midline using the sliding plane between this muscle and the internal oblique muscle. Both muscles are wrapped by one of their epimysial fasciae and there is a thin layer of loose connective tissue between them. At the level of the rectus sheath, the aponeuroses of the internal and external oblique muscle fuse together.

MICROSCOPIC ASPECTS OF THE FASCIAE

It is well known that the spread of anesthetic drugs can vary among the various patients, and currently there is no way to preliminarily understand the effectiveness and extension of a wall block. Really, a better understanding of the microscopic aspects of fasciae and how they change with various chemical, physical and metabolic inputs could help optimize anesthetic outcomes. The fascia represents a complex connective tissue structure composed of various kinds of cells embedded in abundant extracellular matrix and rich in nervous fibers: each single component plays a key and specific role in fascial tissue and answers in different ways to the various stimuli. The nervous components define the sensitive role of the fascial tissue, whereas the cellular components adapt the fascia to varying conditions, defining the metabolic properties, and synthesize the extracellular matrix. The ECM is made up of two components: the fibers, essentially collagen type I, with some fibers of collagen type III and elastic fibers, which give support and organization to the structure; and the water component, or rather the ground substance, a water-rich gelatinous substance rich in glycosaminoglycans, which confers turgor and flexibility to the tissue, permits the gliding and transports metabolic material.

The cells of fascial tissue

The dominant cells of the fascial tissue are the fibroblasts (Langevin et al., 2004; Benjamin, 2009): their principal role is to maintain the structural integrity and organization of the tissue, being involved in the mechanotransduction and secreting precursors of collagen and elastic fibers. Recently, Correa-Gallegos et al. demonstrated that are the fascial fibroblasts of superficial fascia, coordinating their action with the coagulation cascade, drive and produce the temporary matrix into wounds. For these Authors, fasciae are a sort of deposit with an efficient mechanism to speedily seal large open wounds. Wan et al, using live imaging of fascia fibroblasts and fate tracing of the fascia extracellular matrix (ECM), showed that Connexin 43 expression is substantially upregulated in specialized fibroblasts of the fascia deep beneath the skin that are responsible for scar formation, and the disruptions of these mechanisms have wide clinical implications in treating fibrosis, aggravated scarring and impaired wound healing.

Especially along the surface of each fascial layers are present the fasciacytes, in small clusters of rounded cells, specialized in the synthesis of the hyaluronan of the ground substance (Stecco et al., 2018). They are fibroblast like cells specialized for hyaluronan synthesis, which allows fascial gliding among the various fascial sublayers. In normal healthy fascia, about 30% of the fibroblasts are fasciacytes, although this percentage may vary, according to the stimuli to which the fascial tissue is subjected.

The fascia also present cells with contractile activity, named myofibroblasts, which regulate the basal tone of the tissue. These cells show contractile activity, via the adherens junctions, which open mechanosensitive ion channels in adjacent cells (Follonier et al., 2008). Myofibroblasts are well known and characterized in some pathological fibrotic contractures that affect the fascia: they can present an abnormal proliferation, which conduce to a pathological contractures as the Dupuytren and Ledderhose diseases, or the frozen shoulder. Nevertheless, some works have recently well described and documented their role also in normal fascial tissues (Schleip and Klingler, 2019; Schleip et al., 2019).

Lastly, fascial structures have recently been described as containing telocytes, specialized connective tissue cells provided with long thin extensions called telopodes (Dawidowicz et al., 2015; Dawidowicz et al., 2016). These cells communicate each other by means of cell junctions or extracellular vesicles, creating a network system in the interstitial extracellular matrix.

The fibers of the extracellular matrix

The principal fibers are the collagen fibers (especially collagen type I and III), which provide a supporting framework of tissues and cells, and elastic fibers (elastin and fibrillin). The amount of these fibers varies according to the various fasciae, for example the aponeurotic fasciae are not elastic in the "stretchy" sense because they usually contain less than 1% of elastic fibers (Stecco C. et al., 2008), whilst the superficial fasciae has around 13% of elastic fibers (Pirri et al., 2021). The amount of elastic fibers seems vary with aging, as happens in all the subcutaneous tissues. Rodrigues Junior et al. (1990) demonstrated that in the transversalis fascia of the human inguinal triangle there is a decrease in the oxytalan fibres and an increase in the amorphous substance of the elastic fibres with aging, and these changes may be responsible for alteration in the resistance of the transversalis fascia. Besides, Hirata et al. (2011) showed that the fasciae of pelvic floor of multiparous women have less elastic fibers and more disarranged respect to the nulliparous ones. Also the collagen fibers change according to various hormonal, mechanical and chemical inputs. Recently it was demonstrated that different levels of estrogenic and relaxin hormones can modulate the production of collagen I, collagen III and fibrillin (Fede et al., 2019). It seems that the postmenopausal fasciae have more collagen type I (8.4% versus 5.2% in control) and less collagen III (1.5% versus 2.4%), explaining why the fasciae becomes more rigid with aging. On the contrary, during pregnancy the fasciae becomes more elastic, with increased amounts of collagen-III (6.7%) and fibrillin (3.6%, compared to 0.5% of the control) and a corresponding decrease of collagen I (1.9%). Also in diabetes there is a chronic alteration of the connective tissue, with a thickening of collagen fibers and a fragmentation of the elastic fibers, leading to a fascial stiffness. Arkkila et al. (2001) demonstrated that in diabetic subjects the synthesis of the collagen type III fibers increases whereas the synthesis of collagen type I fibers decreases. Besides, in diabetes patients, the ECM turnover is affected by chronic hyperglycemia, determining accumulation of larger collagen quantity resulting in ECM thickening. Finally, also the formation of advanced glycation end product (AGEs) directly boost the ECM components production. AGEs can dramatically affect collagen tissue viscoelasticity and molecular deformation (Fessel et al., 2014).

The extracellular matrix

The water component of fasciae is composed of a complex mixture of glycosaminoglycans (GAGs), among which the hyaluronan is the most important one (Stecco et al., 2011; Fede et al., 2018). Many factors can influence the production of the various and the viscosity of the loose connective tissue. For example it is well known that prolonged immobilization increases its viscosity, and consequently it reduces the ability of the anesthetic drugs to spread in that fascial compartment. Data from Cleland (1979) and Fouissac et al. (1993) show that the intrinsic viscosity of hyaluronan is decreased by about 25% as the temperature is increased from 25° to 65° C. According to Pigman et al. (1960), the viscosity of HA is also strongly dependent on the pH, whilst for Gatej et al. (2005) the behavior of HA in aqueous solution depends on the pH only for extreme values. Recently Fede et al. (2020) documented that the human fascial fibroblasts are able to in vitro produce HA-rich vesicles only a few hours after treatment with an agonist of CB_2 receptor: the HA-rich vesicles were quickly released into the extracellular environment, leading to a greater tissue fluidity. This work showed that fascial cells respond to the endocannabinoid system by regulating and remodeling the formation of the ECM and it constitutes the first demonstration of how therapeutic applications of cannabinoids to treat myofascial pain syndromes may have a direct peripheral effect of remodeling of the tissue and its properties, and not only a central nervous system effect in pain perception.

Innervation

Recent studies showed that the muscular fascia is richly innervated and that it can play an active role in proprioception and pain perception (**Figure 1.15**). The nerve fibers in the fascia can be both peptidergic and non-peptidergic. Taguchi et al. (2013) highlighted both Type Aδ and Type C free endings. Type Aδ fibers seem to be sensitive especially to mechanical stimuli, such as impingement, whereas most of the Type C fibers are polymodal (nociceptors), in other words, sensitive to both mechanical and chemical stimuli (for example, bradykinin) as well as heat. Furthermore, Type C fibers seem to have an extremely high mechanical activation threshold (1854 mN), about two times higher than the skin and the muscle.

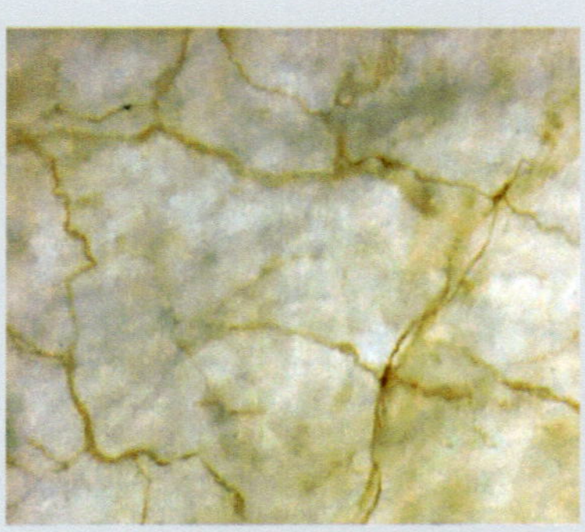

Figure 1.15 Neural plexus inside the deep fascia.

The electrical stimulation of the deep fascia generates a dull and annoying pain, whereas the same stimulation at the level of the hypodermis and superficial fascia generates a well-localized acute pain (Itoh et al., 2004), and this suggests that the two fasciae have different roles: the deep fascia seems to have a proprioceptive function, whereas the superficial fascia collaborates with the skin in exteroception. The adipose layer interposed between the two fasciae (DAT) probably plays a role as insulator, allowing the two fasciae to run and stretch in an independent manner.

In the case of scars, the adhesion between the superficial and deep fascia might lead to an alteration of perception (both proprioceptive and exteroceptive), and to an overstimulation of the receptors found at the level of the scar itself, which might be activated both by muscular contraction and cutaneous stimulation.

Schilder et al. (2014) showed that in healthy volunteers the stimulation of the thoracolumbar fascia with hypersaline solution can generate pain, which is more intense and affects an area larger than the same injection made inside the muscle mass of the erector spinae. Similar results have also been obtained by Deising et al. (2012) with the NGF injection in the thoracolumbar fascia. Furthermore, these authors observed long-lasting sensitization of the nociceptors in the deep fascia to mechanical pressure and chemical stimulation with acid solution. This mechanism can help explain the chronic musculoskeletal pain. In addition, the same authors showed that the free nerve endings are stimulated in a more effective manner when the fascia is "prestretched" by muscular contraction.

In a more recent study, Hoheisel (2015) also highlighted an increase of the SP-positive (nociceptive) fibers in the chronically inflamed thoracolumbar fascia, proving that the fascia itself can undergo pathological changes which in turn can lead to the chronicity/worsening of symptoms. In the past, similar data were published by Sanchis-Alfonso and Rosello-Sastre (2000) at the level of the lateral retinaculum of the knee, highlighting a growth of the nociceptive fibers, immunoreactive to the substance P, in patients with patellofemoral pain syndrome. A chronic irritation of the muscular fascia can also induce sensitization at the level of the spine. In fact, Hoheisel et al. (2011) showed that in the rats where a chronic inflammation of the thoracolumbar fascia had been created, the metamers affected by the nociceptive afferent increased, whereas Taguchi et al. (2013) showed that repeated mechanical stimuli can stimulate the expression of c-Fos in the spinal metamers connected to the sensitive fibers.

Vascularization

Fasciae presents a rich vascular plexus inside and in its surface (**Figure 1.16**). According to Bhattacharya et al. (2010), these vascular networks are supplied by the musculocutaneous and septocutaneous perforators. While piercing the deep fascia, they form subfascial vascular plexus. After coming out on the superficial surface, they form suprafascial vascular plexus. Besides, also inside the deep fascia many small vessels could be recognized, forming another intrafascial plexus that maintains the continuity of the horizontal and vertical vascular network which enhances the vascularity and provides a communication with the subcutaneous and subdermal plexus. This rich vascularization of the various fasciae has to be kept in mind because it could represent a way for adsorption of the anesthetic drugs and consequently can explain the systemic toxicity that could be described also after regional anesthesia.

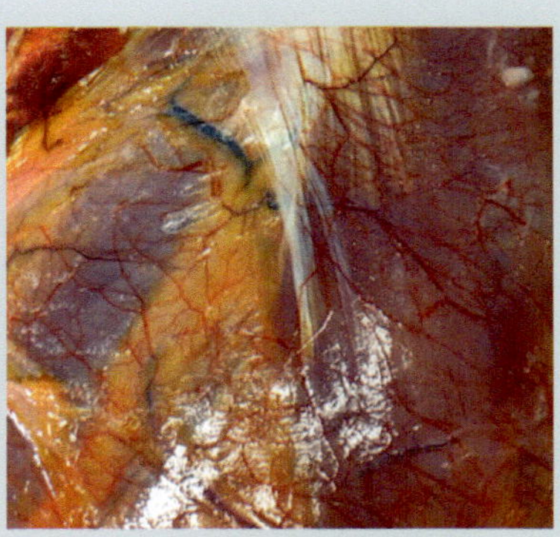

Figure 1.16 Vascular plexus inside the deep fascia.

Conclusions

A number of characteristics of fascia may influence the clinical effectiveness of fascial plane blocks. Firstly, fascial planes are in continuity with each other in a similar manner of the vascular system, where the name of a vessel changes at defined anatomical boundaries, without any change in the vessel itself. Without a clear anatomical boundary, the anesthetic drugs can diffuse far away from the site of injection. Really, if a patient presents a scar around the area of injection, it can create an adhesion between two fascial layers, hindering the spread of the drug.

Secondly, the spread of anesthetic drug is permitted by the loose connective tissue, that creates a gliding surface between two adjacent fascial layers. The purpose of gliding is to reduce the friction associated with movement and the ease of gliding is influenced by interfascial hyaluronan (HA), a lubricating glycosaminoglycan secreted by fasciacytes. The loose connective tissue can vary its viscosity according to various chemical and physical inputs. HA is sensitive to temperature and pH, in particular two degrees Celsius are sufficient to change the viscosity of HA, which means viscosity of loose connective tissue. Moreover HA tolerates alkalosis well, while badly acidosis and it is sufficient a pH of 6.6 for increasing viscosity about 20%. This would be an important limit for local anesthetic or dye diffusion.

Thirdly, fascia is itself a sensitive organ. It is richly innervated with sympathetic and nociceptive fibers and thus may contribute to both acute and chronic myofascial pain syndromes and it could be itself target of anesthetic drugs.

Fourthly, the fasciae have a judge vascular network inside, that could adsorb the anesthetic drugs, collaborating to the systemic toxicity.

RECOMMENDED READING

- Apaydin N, Uz A, Evirgen O, Loukas M, Tubbs RS, Elhan A. The phrenico-esophageal ligament: an anatomical study. Surg Radiol Anat. 2008;30:29-36.
- Arkkila PE, Rönnemaa T, Koskinen PJ, Kantola IM, Seppänen E, Viikari JS. Biochemical markers of type III and I collagen: association with retinopathy and neuropathy in type 1 diabetic subjects. Diabet Med. 2001 Oct;18(10):816-21.G.
- Bhattacharya V, Barooah PS, Nag TC, Chaudhuri G et al. Detail microscopic analysis of deep fascia of lower limb and its surgical implication. Indian Journal of Plastic Surgery (2010) 43(2):135-40
- Caggiati A. The saphenous venous compartments. Surg Radiol Anat. 1999;21:29-34.
- Cleland RL (1979) Effect of Temperature on the Limiting Viscosity Number of Hyaluronic Acid and Chondroitin 4-Sulfate.Biopolymers. 18(7): 1821–1828.
- Cowman MK, Lee HG, Schwertfeger KL, McCarthy JB, Turley EA (2015) The Content and Size of Hyaluronan in Biological Fluids and Tissues. Front. Immunol. 6, 261.
- Dawidowicz J, Matysiak N, Szotek S, Maksymowicz K (2016) Telocytes of Fascial Structures. Adv. Exp. Med. Biol. 913, 403– 424.
- Deising S, Weinkauf B, Blunk J, Obreja O, Schmelz M, Rukwied R. NGF-evoked sensitization of muscle fascia nociceptors in humans. Pain. 2012;153:1673-9.
- Fede C, Angelini A, Stern R, Macchi V, Porzionato A, Ruggieri P, De Caro R, Stecco C (2018) Quantification of hyaluronan in human fasciae: Variations with function and anatomical site. J. Anat. 233, 552–556.
- Fede C, Pirri C, Petrelli L, Guidolin D, Fan C, De Caro R, Stecco C (2020) Sensitivity of the Fasciae to the Endocannabinoid System: Production of Hyaluronan-Rich Vesicles and Potential Peripheral Effects of Cannabinoids in Fascial Tissue. Int. J. Mol. Sci. 21, 2936.
- Fede C, Pirri C, Fan C, Petrelli L, Guidolin D, De Caro R, Stecco C (2021) A Closer Look at the Cellular and Molecular Components of the Deep/Muscular Fasciae. Int J Mol Sci. 30;22(3):1411.
- Fessel, Y.F. Li, V. Diederich, M. Guizar-Sicairos, P.Schneider, D.R. Sell, V.M. Monnier, J.G. Snedeker, Advanced glycation end-products reduce collagen molecular sliding to affect collagen fibril damage mechanisms but not stiffness, PLoSOne. 2014; 9 (11).
- Fouissac E, Milas M, Rinaudo M: Shear-rate, Concentration, Molecular Weight, and Temperature Viscosity Dependencies of Hyaluronate, a Wormlike Polyelectrolyte.Macromolecules. 1993; 26(25): 6945–6951
- Gatej I, Popa M, Rinaudo M: Role of the pH on hyaluronan behavior in aqueous solution. Biomacromolecules. 2005; 6(1): 61–7
- Gibson W, Arendt-Nielsen L, Taguchi T, Mizumura K, Graven-Nielsen T. Increased pain from muscle fascia following eccentric exercise: animal and human findings. Exp Brain Res. 2009;194:299-308.
- Hirata E, Koyama M, Murakami G, Ohtsuka A et al. Comparative histological study of levels 1-3 supportive tissues using pelvic floor semiserial sections from elderly nulliparous and multiparous women. J Obstet Gynaecol Res. 2011 Jan;37(1):13-23.
- Hoheisel U, Taguchi T, Treede RD, Mense S. Nociceptive input from the rat thoracolumbar fascia to lumbar dorsal horn neurones. Eur J Pain.2011;15:810-5.
- Hoheisel U, Rosner J, Mense S. Innervation changes induced by inflammation of the rat thoracolumbar fascia. Neuroscience.2015;6: 351-9.
- Nguyen HV, Nguyen H. Anatomical basis of modern thoracotomies: the latissimus dorsi and the "serratus anterior-rhomboid" complex. Surg Radiol Anat. 1987;9:85-93.
- Pigman W, Hawkins W, Gramling E, et al (1960) Factors affecting the viscosity of hyaluronic acid and synovial fluid. Arch Biochem Biophys. 89: 184–93.
- Rizk NN. A new description of the anterior abdominal wall in man and mammals. J Anat. 1980;131:373-85.
- Rodrigues AJ, De Tolosa EM, De Carvalho CA (1990) Electron microscopic study on the elastic and elastic related fibres in the human fascia transversalis at different ages Gegenbaurs Morphol Jahrb. 136(6):645-52
- Sanchis-Alfonso V, Rosellò-Sastre E. Immunohistochemical analysis for neural markers of the lateral retinaculum in patients with isolated symptomatic patellofemoral malalignment. A neuroanatomic basis for anterior knee pain in the active young patient. Am J Sports Med.2000;28:725-31.
- Sato T, Hashimoto M. Morphological analysis of the fascial lamination of the trunk. Bull Tokyo Med Dent Univ. 1984; 31:21-32.
- Schilder A, Hoheisel U, Magerl W, Benrath J, Klein T, Treede RD. Sensory findings after stimulation of the thoracolumbar fascia with hypertonic saline suggest its contribution to low back pain. Pain. 2014;155:222-31.
- Schleip R, Gabbiani G, Wilke J, Naylor I, Hinz B, Zorn A, Jäger H, Breul R, Schreiner S, Klingler W (2019) Fascia Is Able to Actively Contract and May Thereby Influence Musculoskeletal Dynamics: A Histochemical and Mechanographic Investi-gation. Front. Physiol. 10, 336.
- Sebastien C, Regnier M, Lantieri L, Pétoin S, Guérin-Surville H. Anterolateral thoracic fascia: an anatomic and surgical entity. Surg Radiol Anat. 1993;15:79-83.
- Singer E. Fasciae of the human body and their relations to the organs they envelop. Williams & Wilkinns Company, Baltimore, 1935.
- Stecco C, Stern R, Porzionato A, Macchi V, Masiero S, Stecco A, De Caro R (2011) Hyaluronan within fascia in the etiology of myofascial pain. Surg. Radiol. Anat. 33, 891–896.
- Stecco C. Functional Atlas of the Human Fascial System. Elsevier Health Sciences UK, 2015.
- Stecco C, Fede C, Macchi V, Petrelli L, Biz C, Stern R, De Caro R (2018) The fasciacytes: A new cell devoted to fascial gliding regulation. Clin. Anat. 31, 667–676.
- Sterzi G. Il tessuto sottocutaneo (tela subcutanea). Luigi Niccolai, Firenze, 1910.
- Taguchi T, Yasui M, Kubo A, et al. Nociception originating from the crural fascia in rats. Pain. 2013;154:1103-14.
- Tesarz J, Hoheisel U, Wiedenhofer B, Mense S. Sensory innervation of the thoracolumbar fascia in rats and humans. Neuroscience. 2011;194:302-8.
- Vannucchi MG (2020) The Telocytes: Ten Years after Their Introduction in the Scientific Literature. An Update on Their Morphology, Distribution, and Potential Roles in the Gut. Int. J. Mol. Sci. 21, 4478

Thoracic paravertebral block (PVB)

Gianluca Cappelleri, Dario Bugada

The paravertebral block (PVB), first described by Eason in 1979, allows, with a single injection, to block the dorsal and ventral branches, as well as the sympathetic fibers (the only case outside the neuraxis), producing an ipsilateral, segmental motor, sensory and sympathetic block of contiguous thoracic dermatomes (multilevel block). Blockade of the communicating branches and sympathetic chain results in a block comparable to the peridural block, but, unlike the latter, it is ipsilateral, with minimal hemodynamic changes, which are equivalent to those of a peripheral block. PVBs can be monolateral or bilateral, with single injection in one or more metameres, or continuous, which is made possible by the placement of a perinervous catheter. The mechanism of action of the PVB is the result of direct penetration of the local anesthetic into the spinal nerves, including the dorsal rami, communicating rami, and sympathetic chain.

ANATOMY

The thoracic paravertebral space (TPVS) is a virtual space, described as triangular in shape, located laterally to the thoracic spine, bounded in the lower margin by the insertion of the psoas muscle at the level of T12. The paravertebral space consists of adipose tissue; immersed in it there are the intercostal nerves, arterial and venous vessels, and the sympathetic trunk. Anteriorly, the space is bounded by the parietal pleura from T2 to T10-11, or by the diaphragm from T10-11 to T12 (**Figure 2.1**). Medially, it is bounded by the vertebral bodies, intervertebral discs, and intervertebral foramina where it connects with the peridural space. Laterally, it continues into the intercostal space at the level of the costotransverse joint (**Figure 2.2**). Superiorly and inferiorly, the TPS is partially separated from the adjacent levels by the ribs and transverse processes.

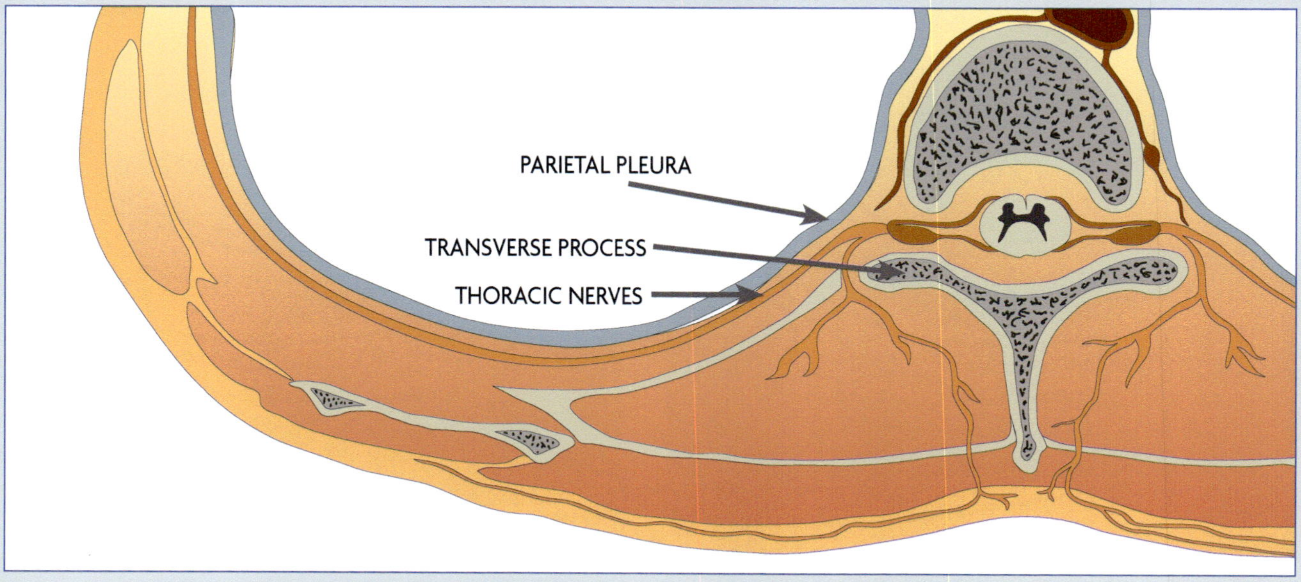

Figure 2.1 Transverse section of the thoracic spine.

The adipose tissue present in the anteromedial portion of the paravertebral space provides the continuity between the superior and inferior levels, generating a connection that extends along all thoracic levels.

Posteriorly, the space is bounded by the transverse process, the rib, and the superior costotransverse ligament. Posterior to the space are located the deep multifidus and rotator muscles of the back, and a layer of adipose tissue that frequently interposes between the muscles and ligaments.

Laterally, the ligament makes contact with the internal intercostal membrane, the aponeurosis of the internal intercostal muscle that gradually takes shape into the actual muscle approximately 4-6 cm lateral to the midline.

The TPVS is bisected by the endothoracic fascia, a thin sheet of connective tissue about 250 microns thick that lies directly behind the pleura and connects it with the chest wall; it participates in delineation of the space and medially fuses with the prevertebral fascia. Cranially, the thoracic paravertebral space lies in close proximity to the adipose tissue of the brachial plexus, phrenic nerve, and cervical sympathetic trunk. This anatomic proximity influences the spread of local anesthetic injected at this site, which can reach the brachial plexus, the stellate ganglion, and the perivascular nerve plexus.

Caudally, the boundary of the space is a matter of debate. At the level of T12, the space is effectively closed by the emergence of the psoas muscle placing this level as the lower boundary; however, other studies have shown a spread to the paravertebral space even when LA (Local Anesthetic) is injected into the lumbar plexus or celiac ganglion, through the medial and lateral arcuate ligaments of the diaphragm.

The intercostal nerve penetrates the space medially and gradually disposes along the inferior border of the rib laterally (**Figure 2.3**).

Alongside the thoracic nerves, the sympathetic nerve fibers of the thoracic chain also run in the paravertebral space: the thoracic paravertebral nerve gives fibers to the sympathetic nervous system and the thoracic sympathetic chain through the preganglionic myelinated fibers of the white communicating rami and the postganglionic unmyelinated fibers of the gray communicating rami (**Figure 2.4**).

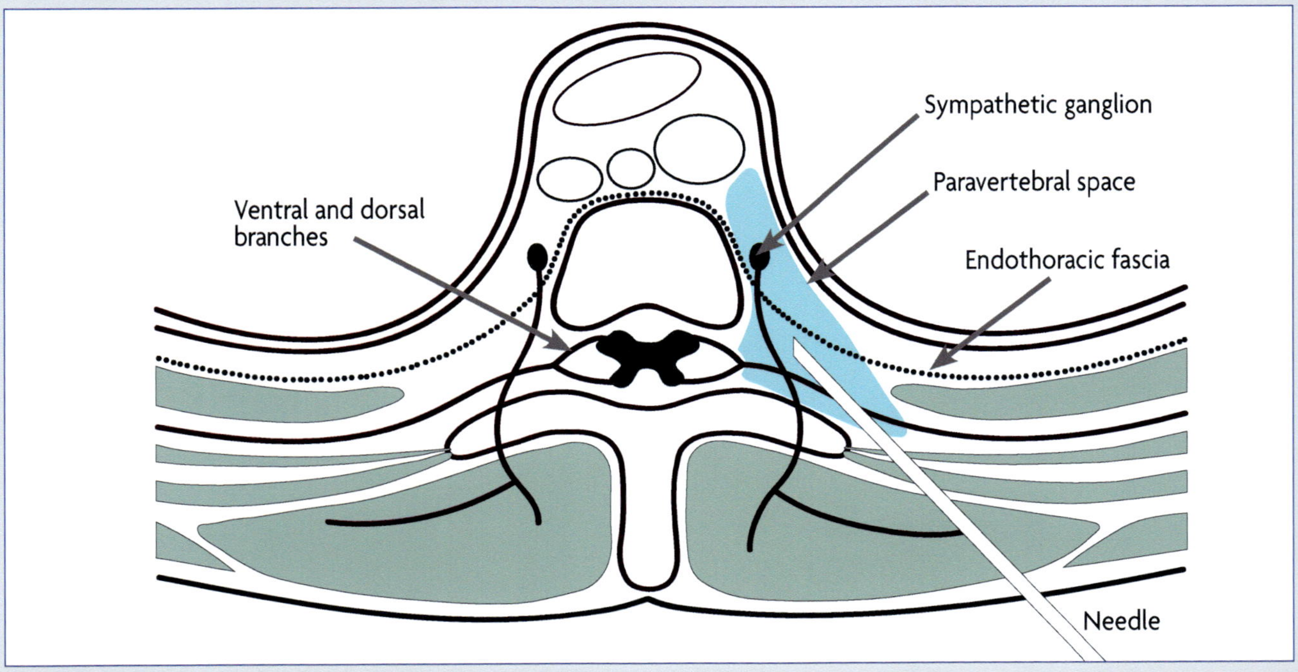

Figure 2.2 The paravertebral space and adjacent structures seen in transverse section.

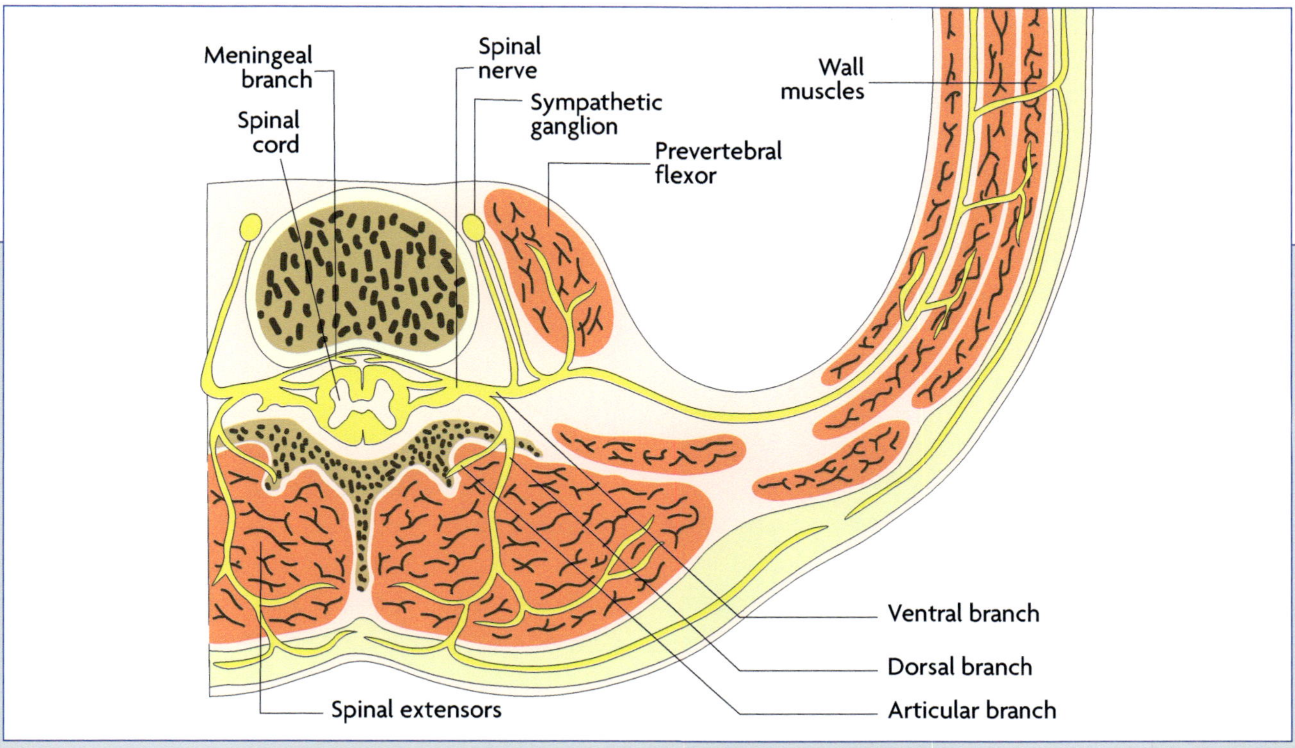

Figure 2.3 Course of nerve branches originating from the paravertebral space. Note the presence within the space of branches originating from the sympathetic nervous system.

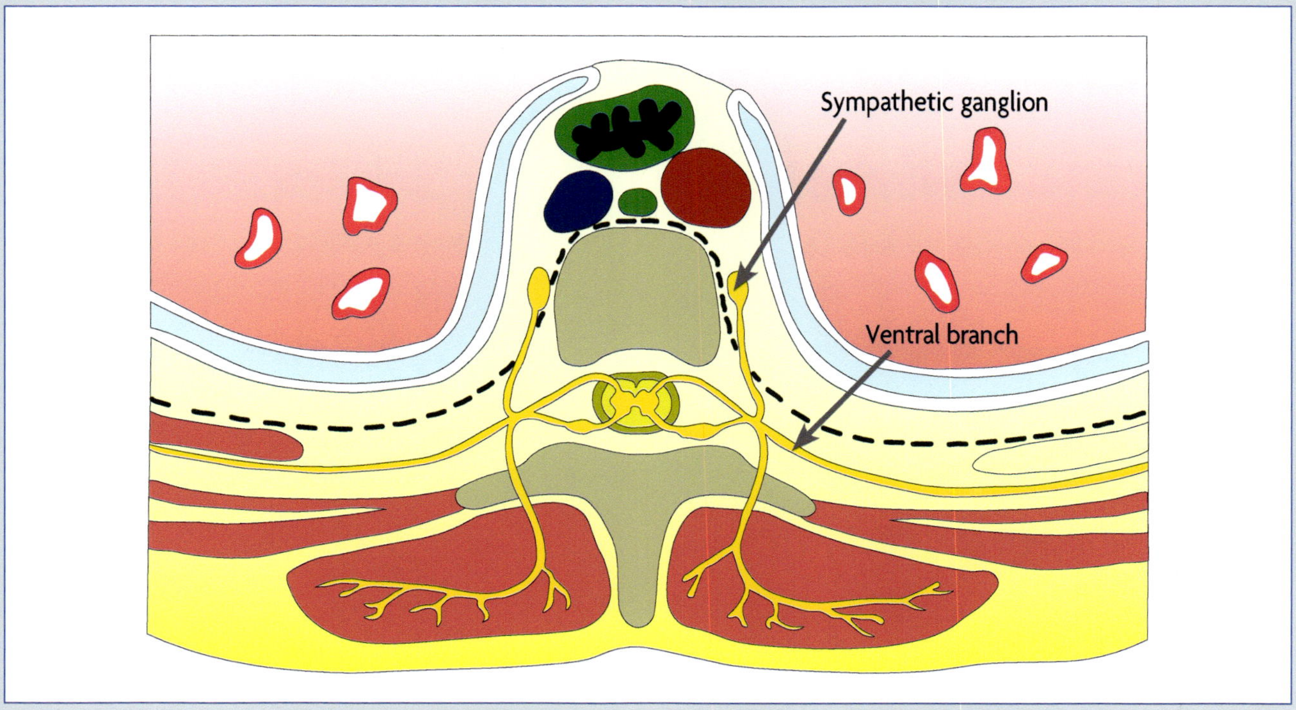

Figure 2.4 Arrangement of the nerves of the sympathetic chain within the paravertebral space.

The nerves originating from the TPS give rise to an anterior and a posterior primary division; the posterior branch innervates the facet joints, the muscles, and skin of the back; the anterior branch, on the other hand, runs laterally and heads into the subcostal groove, becoming the intercostal nerve.
The intercostal and subcostal nerves are responsible for innervation of the skin, muscles, ribs, visceral pleura, and peritoneum.

Sonoanatomy

All the ultrasound techniques rely on the recognition of some fixed landmarks that, in the case of the TPS, are bony structures such as the transverse process, the ribs and the inferior articular process.
The pleura is always visible due to its marked hyperechogenicity, while the costotransverse ligament is not always easy to visualize.
The paravertebral space can be identified by placing the transducer in both transverse and longitudinal positions.

Transverse approach

The probe is positioned laterally to the spinous process starting at a distance of about 3-4 cm from the midline in a transverse position (**Figure 2.5**); proceeding in depth, the first image obtained is the rib articulating with the transverse process. Together they form a large acoustic shadow due to the projection of the rib, where it is possible to see only a thin strip of adipose tissue anterior to the head of the rib that contains the sympathetic trunk. With a slightly lower scan, one can see the "thumb" outline of the transverse process: the paravertebral space is located in front but is obscured by the acoustic shadow created by the transverse process.
What can be seen at this level is the lateral continuation, i.e., the intercostal space (**Figure 2.6**).
By sliding the probe below the transverse process, the paravertebral space is no longer obscured by bony structures and can, therefore, be visualized.
The inferior articular process is visible in a more medial position than the tip of the transverse process. Its

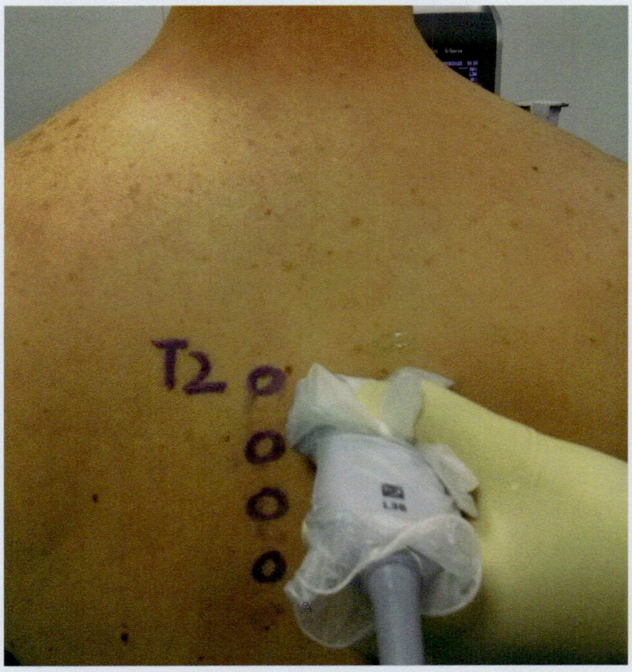

Figure 2.5 Position of the ultrasonographic probe in the transverse approach.

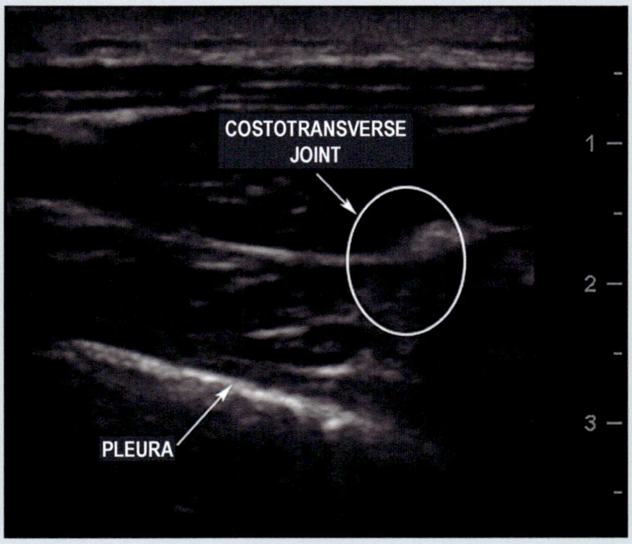

Figure 2.6 Ultrasound visualization of the continuation of the paravertebral space into the intercostal space.

contour and acoustic shadow mark the medial boundary of the paravertebral space (**Figure 2.7**). The pleura appears as a thin hyperechogenic band anteriorly that is highly visible medially but tends to fade toward the center of the image, where the pleura curves reaching at an acute angle to the mediastinum. At this level, the superior costotransverse ligament forms the posterior boundary of the space.

Identification of ultrasonographic anatomic landmarks in the longitudinal approach

The probe is positioned 2-3 cm lateral to the midline in a longitudinal position (**Figure 2.8**).

We will have a view of two adjacent ribs and the space included therein (**Figure 2.9**). At this level, the external intercostal muscle and the internal intercostal membrane form the posterior border of the paravertebral space, visible just laterally to the costotransverse joint. The internal intercostal muscle and the pleura limit the space anteriorly. The high echogenicity of the pleura and the characteristic gliding movements of the lung make the anatomy easily recognizable. With small tilting of the probe, it is possible to identify the costotransverse joint, the image characterized by the cone of shadow generated by the transverse process (posterocaudal) and the rib (ventrocranial) (**Figure 2.10**).

The reflectivity of the pleura decreases as one approaches the midline, being replaced by the image generated by the mediastinal and column structures, thus being less visible.

DESCRIPTION OF TECHNIQUES

The patient can be positioned in lateral decubitus or in a sitting position. Paravertebral blocking can be performed with both a high-resolution linear probe, or with a low-resolution curvilinear probe (however, it allows a larger field of view) (**Figure 2.11**).

The distance between the transverse process and the skin varies as a function of the BMI, but, in general, the depth of the paravertebral space shows constant characteristics. In particular, the central segments of the thoracic tract (T4-T8) are significantly shal-

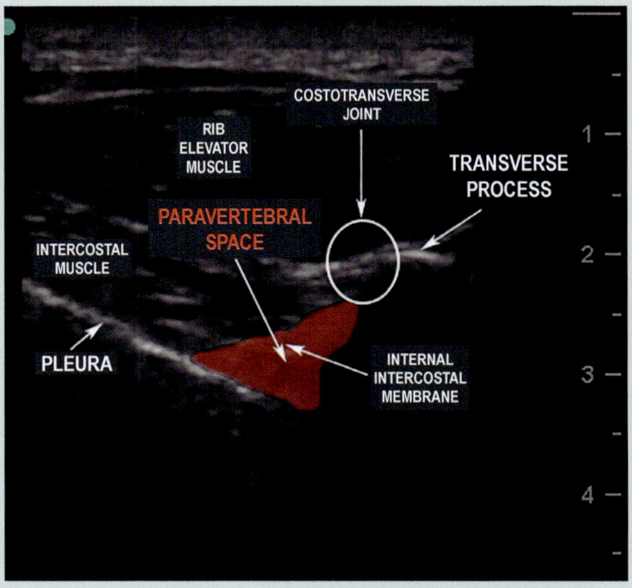

Figure 2.7 Ultrasound visualization of the paravertebral space.

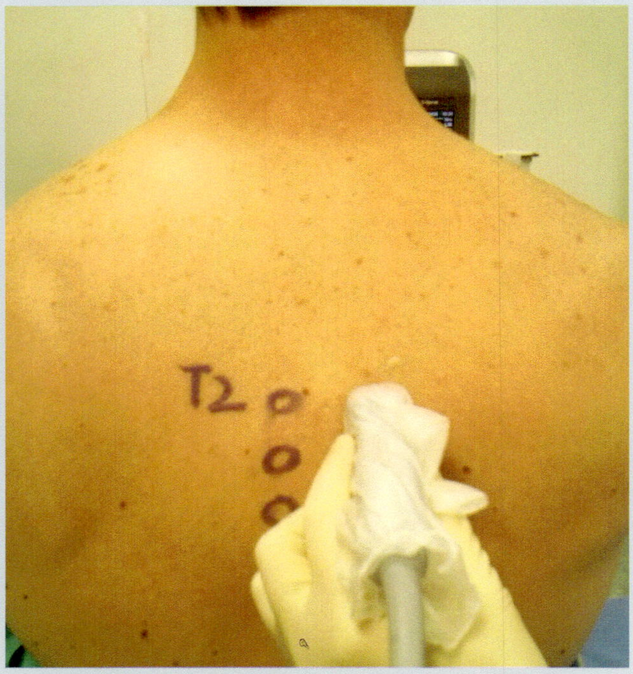

Figure 2.8 Position of the ultrasonographic probe in the longitudinal approach.

Thoracic paravertebral block (PVB)

lower than the distal and proximal segments. With both longitudinal and transverse scanning, the needle (SonoPlex stim Pajunk®) can be introduced either "in-plane" or "out of plane", which are equivalent for this type of block and may depend on the operator's experience.

With the transducer in the longitudinal position, the probe is positioned approximately 2 cm lateral to the vertebral column. The midpoint of the transducer should be aligned between two contiguous transverse processes, so our target will be exactly in the center. With the "in-plane" technique, the needle (SonoPlex stim Pajunk®) is inserted along the lower edge of the transducer and directed cranially (**Figure 2.12**). The target is the costotransverse ligament.

The crossing of this ligament may be accompanied by a slight loss of resistance that can be used as a signal of the tip's entry into the paravertebral space.

At this point, keeping the tip of the needle in view, one can begin the injection of local anesthetic, which will result in a dislocation of the pleura anteriorly, thus confirming the correct placement of the needle (**Figure 2.13**, **Video 2.1**).

The maneuver can be difficult because of the narrow space between the two transverse processes, which forces the needle to be angled a lot. In this case it is possible to proceed "out of plane": the needle (SonoPlex stim Pajunk®) trajectory is direct and, following the distortion of the tissues, the costotransverse ligament can be reached. At this point, it is advisable to proceed slowly with the hydro localization technique, until the dislocation of the pleura anteriorly will confirm the achievement of the target. Either with an in-plane or an out-of-plane techniques, the needle is not directed toward the epidural space, so reducing the likelihood of an anesthetic spread in that space.

With the probe in a transverse position, the first step is the visualization of the transverse process; then, with an adequate tilting of the probe, the cone of shadow projected by the rib will no longer be visible and the anterior pleura will be highlighted with its characteristic brilliance. The in-plane technique requires a needle direction from lateral to medial, up to penetrate in the triangular area delimited by the internal intercostal membrane and by the intercostal muscle posteriorly and by the parietal pleura anteriorly.

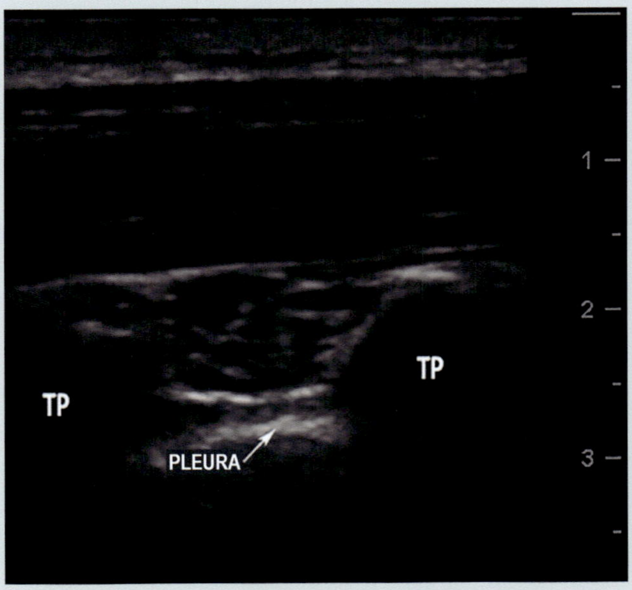

Figure 2.9 Ultrasound visualization of the paravertebral space in the longitudinal approach.

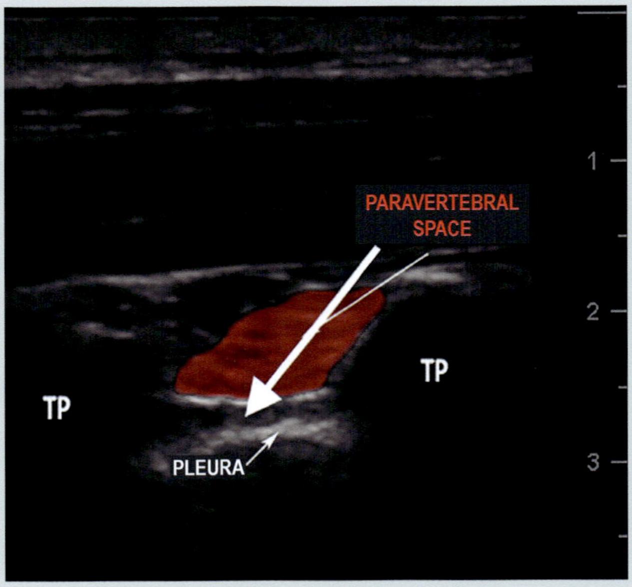

Figure 2.10 Paravertebral space: large white arrow indicates paravertebral space.

The final position of the needle will be in the transition zone between the intercostal and paravertebral space. This type of approach provides supervision of the entire needle path, although it exposes to a greater risk of diffusion into the epidural space through the lateral recess (**Flow charts 2.1**, **2.2 online**).

Continuous blocks and perinervous catheter

The continuous thoracic paravertebral block (PVBc) can be performed with different approaches. A first approach involves placement of the probe (either linear or curve) with a slightly oblique axis lateral to the column. Both the costotransverse ligament and the pleura are visualized. After obtaining a sterile field, the needle (E-Cath®), is inserted with the in-plane technique and a lateral-medial direction until the costotransverse ligament is crossed. Once the anterior displacement of the pleura resulting from the injection of 2 ml of saline solution is visualized, the catheter will be inserted up to a depth of 5 cm beyond the tip. Similarly, the classic transverse approach to the column can be used. With this scan, the costotransverse ligament does not always appear visible; for this reason, some Authors have proposed the association of the loss-of-resistance (LOR) technique to localize the ligament and then proceed with catheter placement after controlling the anterior slip of the pleura by injecting fluid. Without LOR,

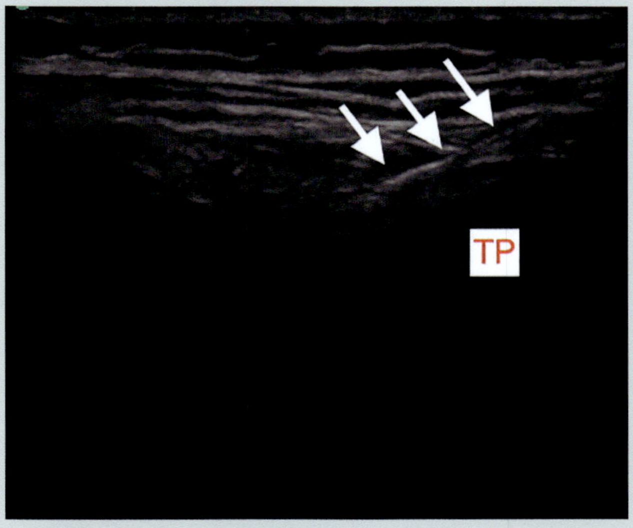

Figure 2.12 Ultrasound visualization of the paravertebral space: the three white arrows indicate the needle (SonoPlex stim Pajunk®) directed toward the paravertebral space.

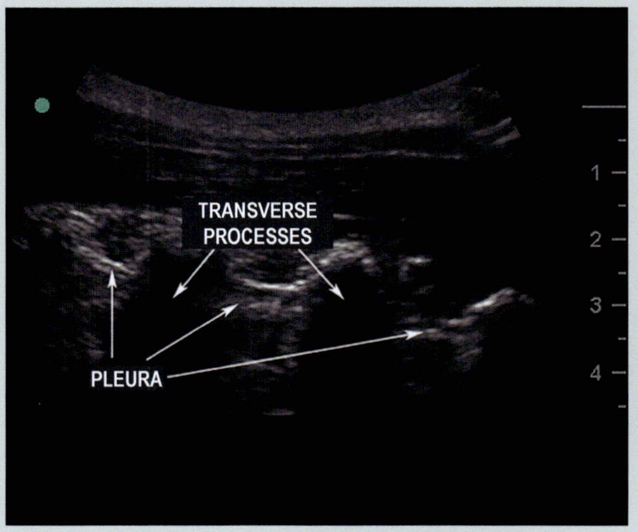

Figure 2.11 Ultrasound visualization of the paravertebral space with a convex probe.

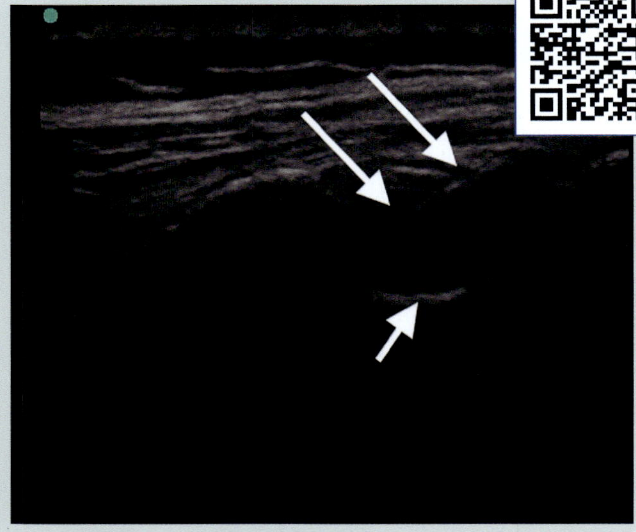

Figure 2.13 The upper white arrows indicate the needle (SonoPlex stim Pajunk®) directed toward the paravertebral space, and the lower arrow indicates the pleura. Note the anterior dislocation of the pleura with characteristic curvilinear shape due to the injection of local anesthetic into the paravertebral space.

the ultrasound technique provides to use the posterolateral border of the inferior articular process as a target using the out-of-plane approach. After the bony contact, the needle is directed laterally to override the bone and, advanced a few millimeters under ultrasound vision. The correct placement of the needle is checked with liquid injections to cause anterior displacement of the pleura and proceed with catheter insertion. Both of these techniques result in a correct needle placement but are burdened by a 30% failure rate in catheter placement.

INDICATIONS

Thoracic surgery: the PVB has been proposed for the treatment of postoperative pain both in case of thoracotomy and thoracoscopy. In the first case, the placement of a catheter is recommended to prolong analgesia beyond the first 12-24h, while in the second case a single block may be sufficient. Although PVB has been found to be as effective as epidural blockade in controlling postoperative pain, it is burdened by a high percentage of failures that partially limit its use. In contrast, nearly 30% of patients undergoing thoracopulmonary surgery are not eligible for peridural anesthesia because of comorbidities or ongoing drug treatments, thus remaining PVB an excellent alternative.

Minimally invasive cardiac surgery: PVB has been successfully used for both minimally invasive mitral valve surgery and mini-thoracotomy procedures. Other areas of application may be pectus excavatum in the pediatric population, or in sternal remodeling.

Breast surgery: this is the primary indication for single-shot PVB. It is commonly used in both oncologic and reconstructive/esthetic surgery. A retrospective study has shown that PVB can reduce the incidence of recurrence after mastectomy, while several publications have shown that PVB is able to reduce the onset of chronic pain after demolitive breast surgery.

It can also be used in case of chronic chest wall pain or postherpetic neuralgia; a single block performed early in the onset of thoracic shingles has been shown to be effective in reducing the duration of pain and the course of the rash, promoting early healing of the skin.

The blockage should not be performed in

- Patients with allergies to the LAs used
- Patients with bleeding diathesis
- Patients with severe scoliosis (relative contraindication)
- Infections in the site of the injection

VOLUMES AND DRUG DOSAGES

PVB can be performed in a single space or multilevel. Although the paravertebral space results in contiguity with adjacent metameres, it is difficult to reproduce a true longitudinal spread of local anesthetic with a single injection (**Table 2.1**).

In any case, a linear correlation between injected volume and block spread has been demonstrated. For antalgic purposes, a volume of 0.07 ml/kg of anesthetic solution per segment should be considered with a single injection. In case of surgical anesthesia, it is advisable to consider a multilevel block of 3-4 metameres depending on the surgery (**Table 2.2**).

Recommended anesthetics are long-acting anesthetics such as ropivacaine or levobupivacaine, with one of the most advantageous systemic toxicity profiles, at concentrations ranging from 0.37-0.75%. Each dermatome requires approximately 3-5 ml. The maximum dose should be considered especially in case of bilateral blocks.

The use of adjuvants added to prolong the analgesic effect of PVB with single-shot technique is questionable: there is not enough evidence in the literature to recommend their use, being those reported in the infusion schemes taken from various studies, dictated mainly by the experience of the author. For this reason, the volumes, and doses of LA reported in this chapter do not consider the possible addition of adjuvants.

TABLE 2.1 RESULTS OF THE MAIN STUDIES THAT EVALUATED THE PARAVERTEBRAL SPREAD OF A LOCAL ANESTHETIC SOLUTION (LA), COMPARING SINGLE INJECTION WITH MULTIPLE INJECTIONS, USING DIFFERENT ANESTHETIC TECHNIQUES

Study (year)	Patients # (pt/group)	Technique	Type of surgery	Methods	Enpoint	Drug and dose	Results
Naja 2006	69 (23)	Bilateral ENS	Mastectomy-thoracotomy-open cholecystectomy-umbilical hernia	3 groups: - 4 vs 1 injection - 4 vs 2 injections - 4 vs 3 injections	Sensory and radiographic spread	0.26 ml/kg LA + 0,10 ml/kg CM	Multiple injections > radiographic spread and clinical spread compared to single injection
Uppal 2017	70 (38-32)	Unilateral US	Mastectomy	2 groups: - T1-T5 = 5 injections - T3-T4 single injection	Sensory block	- Ropivacaine 0.5% 5 ml/ metamere - Ropivacaine 0.5% 25 ml	No difference in sensory spread between single and multiple
Marhofer 2013	10	Bilateral US	Healthy volunteers	Block at T6 on both sides after 2 days	MRI Spread plus pinprick	Mepivacaine 1% 20 ml	Single injection = 4 dermatomes covered but sensory spread unpredictable
Cheema 2003	29	Real-time fluoroscopy	Chronic pain	Repeated injections at a distance of 2 weeks (max 4 times)	Factors determining the LA spread	Bupivacaine 0.5% 10-15 ml + cortisone	Single injection = block, onset, and extension unpredictable

TABLE 2.2 PARAVERTEBRAL BLOCK; METAMERES INVOLVED IN MAJOR SURGERIES AND NUMBER OF RECOMMENDED INJECTIONS

Type of surgery	Concerned metameres	Number of recommended injections
Mastectomy	T1-T5	1 to 5
Quadrantectomy	T1-T5	1 to 3
Laparoscopic cholecystectomy	T6-T9	1 to 2
Laparotomic cholecystectomy	T6-T9	1 to 3
Thoracotomy	T2-T6	1 to 4
Thoracoscopy	T3-T6	1 to 2
Ventral hernias	T8-T11	1 to 3

CONTRAINDICATIONS AND COMPLICATIONS

The complications described in the literature after PVB have a very low incidence, which is considered acceptable in terms of risk/benefit ratio.

Among these, pleural puncture (1%), resulting in pneumothorax (0.5%), is the most feared. With the use of ultrasound, the safety profile of PVB improves, but the risk related to the lack of vision of the needle tip remains. Other complications may be the systemic toxicity of LA, especially in case of multiple injections or bilateral blocks and the spread of LA in the epidural space. In this case, the cause must be sought in the direction of the needle from latero-medial, or from a high injection pressure.

To avoid pressures >15 PSI, it is advisable to perform the block using monitoring coupled with larger capacity syringes (e.g., 20 ml) to decrease downstream injection pressure.

Contraindications to paravertebral block do not differ from those generally applicable to peripheral nerve blocks. Considering the proximity of anatomical structures defined as "noble", inexperience can be considered the first contraindication.

Relative contraindications are a higher BMI or a severe scoliosis and difficulty in correctly recognizing the structures. Although the PVB must be considered in all respects a "peripheral" block, the particular anatomy and the high depth found in the most distal thoracic segments, make the paravertebral space "non-compressible" in case of bleeding. For this reason, in the international guidelines, it is considered a "deep" block and as such subject to the restrictions of central blocks in case of concomitant anticoagulant/antiaggregant therapy or thromboprophylaxis.

Complications

- Pneumothorax
- Hematomas
- Accidental peridural administration of LA
- Accidental subarachnoid administration of LA
- LA toxicity

CHRONIC PAIN

The control of persistent postsurgical pain (PPSP) is an important issue in analgesic strategies after thoracotomy and mastectomy operations, having an incidence varying between 30% and 70%, depending on the Authors.

Paravertebral block should be considered as a valid therapeutic approach also in patients with chronic pain originating from chest wall structures. An injection of 20 ml of LA allows a drug distribution capable of covering about four dermatomes, reducing the need for multiple injections required when blocking intercostal nerves. In addition, in more cranial segments where the scapula may interfere with the performance of intercostal nerve block, paravertebral block can be performed more easily. PPSP after thoracotomy, in most cases, is related to the formation of neurinomas of the intercostal nerves due to entrapment of these in the scar tissue formed at the level of the surgical incision or stretching due to the formation of adhesions. PVB is effective in reducing pain symptoms by deafferentating nerve transmission from the dorsal and ventral branches. Less effective is the use of PVB in controlling postmastectomy PPSP.

Mastectomy is a complex operation with different surgical approaches. In addition, intercostobrachial nerve injury is thought to be the most common cause of chronic postmastectomy pain, and its damage is often manifested by pain in the axillary cavity and upper and medial arm. In this case, the block should be made in the most cranial metamers of the paravertebral space (T1-T2). Another important aspect to consider in chronic postmastectomy pain is breast implantation, probably because of the compression that the periprosthetic capsule determines on the nervous structures of the chest wall. An indication for the use of continuous PVB is the prevention of phantom breast syndrome (incidence up to 40%). Preoperative deafferentation, combined with continuous postoperative infusion, is able to significantly reduce its occurrence (**Flow chart 2.1 online**).

RECOMMENDED READING

- Abdallah FW, Brull R. Off side! A simple modification to the parasagittal in-plane approach for paravertebral block. RegAnesth Pain Med. 2014; 39:240-2.
- Bernard A, Rivera C, Pages PB, et al. Risk model of in-hospital mortality after pulmonary resection for cancer: a national database of the French Society of Thoracic and Cardiovascular Surgery (Epithor). J Thorac Cardiovasc Surg. 2011; 141:449-58.
- Boretsky K, Visoiu M, Bigeleisen P. Ultrasound-guided approach to the paravertebral space for catheter insertion in infants and children. Pediatric Anesthesia. 2013; 23:1193-8.
- Cheema S, Richardson J, McGurgan P. Factors affecting the spread of bupivacaine in the adult thoracic paravertebral space. Anaesthesia. 2003; 58:684-7.
- Dahl JB, Rosenberg J, Lund C, Kehlet H. Effect of thoracic epidural bupivacaine 0,75 on somatosensory evoked potentials after dermatomal stimulation. Reg Anesth. 1990; 15: 73-5.
- Davies RG, Myles PS, Graham JM. A comparison of the analgesic efficacy and side-effects of paravertebral vs epidural blockade for thoracotomy - a systematic review and meta-analysis of randomized trials. British Journal of Anaesthesia. 2006; 96: 418- 26.
- Eason MJ, Wyatt R. Paravertebral thoracic block-a reappraisal. Anaesthesia. 1979; 34: 638-42.
- Exadaktylos AK, Buggy DJ, Moriarty DC, Mascha E, Sessler DI. Can anesthetic technique for primary breast cancer surgery affect recurrence or metastasis? Anesthesiology. 2006; 105: 660-4.
- Gadsden JC, Lindenmuth DM, Hadzic A, et al. Lumbar plexus block using high-pressure injection leads to contralateral and epidural spread. Anesthesiology. 2008; 109: 683-8.
- Hall Burton DM, Boretsky KR. A comparison of paravertebral nerve block catheters and thoracic epidural catheters for postoperative analgesia following the Nuss procedure for pectus excavatum repair. Paediatr Anaesth. 2014; 24:516-20.
- Horlocker TT, Wedel DJ, Rowlingson JC, et al. Regional anesthesia in the patient receiving antithrombotic or thrombolytic therapy: American Society of Regional Anesthesia and Pain Medicine Evidence-Based Guidelines (Third Edition). Reg Anesth Pain Med. 2010; 35:64-101.
- Ilfeld B M, Madison SJ, Suresh PJ, et al. Persistent Postmastectomy Pain and Pain-Related Physical and Emotional Functioning With and Without a Continuous Paravertebral Nerve Block: A Prospective 1-Year Follow-Up Assessment of a Randomized, Triple-Masked, Placebo-Controlled Study. Ann Surg Oncol. 2015; 22:2017-25.
- Joshi GP, Bonnet F, Shah R, et al. A systematic review of randomized trials evaluating regional techniques for post-thoracotomy analgesia. Anesth Analg. 2008; 107:1026-40.
- Lönnqvist PA, Hildingsson U. The caudal boundary of the thoracic paravertebral space. A study in human cadavers. Anaesthesia. 1992; 47:1051-2.
- Luyet C, Eichenberger U, Greif R, et al. Ultrasound-guided paravertebral puncture and placement of catheters in human cadavers: an imaging study. Br J Anaesth. 2009; 102: 534-9.
- Luyet C, Herrmann G, Ross S, Vogt A, Greif R, Moriggl B, Eichenberger U. Ultrasound-guided thoracic paravertebral puncture and placement of catheters in human cadavers: where do catheters go? British Journal of Anaesthesia. 2011; 106: 246-54.
- Makharita MJ, Amr YM, El-Bayoumy Y. Single Paravertebral Injection for AcuteThoracic Herpes Zoster: A Randomized Controlled Trial. Pain Practice. 2015; 15: 229-35.
- Marhofer D, Marhofer D, Kettner SC, et al. Magnetic Resonance Imaging Analysis of the Spread of Local Anesthetic Solution after Ultrasound-guided Lateral Thoracic Paravertebral Blockade: A Volunteer Study. Anesthesiology. 2013; 118:1106-12.
- Naja MZ, Ziade MF, El Rajab M, et al. Varying anatomical injection points within the thoracic paravertebral space: effect on spread of solution and nerve blockade. Anaesthesia. 2004; 59: 459-63.
- Naja MZ. Distance between the skin and the thoracic paravertebral space. Anaesthesia. 2005; 60:680-4.
- Naja ZM, El-Rajab M, Al-Tannir MA, et al. Thoracic Paravertebral Block: Influence of the Number of Injections. Regional Anesthesia and Pain Medicine. 2006; 31: 196-201.
- Ning MC, Karmakar MK. Right thoracic paravertebral anaesthesia for percutaneous radiofrequency ablation of liver tumours. The British Journal of Radiology. 2011; 84:785-9.
- Pintaric TS, Veranic P, Hadzic A, Karmakar M, Cvetko E. Electron-Microscopic Imaging of Endothoracic Fascia in the Thoracic Paravertebral Space in Rats. Regional Anesthesia and Pain Medicine. 2012; 37:215-8.
- Richardson J, Lönnqvist PA, Naja MZ. Bilateral thoracic paravertebral block: potential and practice. British Journal of Anaesthesia. 2011; 106:164-71.
- Saito T, Den S, Tanuma K, Tanuma Y, Carney E, Carlsson C. Anatomical bases for paravertebral anesthetic block: Fluid communication between the thoracic and lumbar paravertebral regions. Surg Radiol Anat. 1999; 21:359-63.
- Saito T, Tanuma K, Den S, Tanuma Y, Miyakawa K, Carney E, Carlsson C. Pathways of anesthetic from the thoracic paravertebral region to the celiac ganglion. Clin Anat 2002; 15:340-4.
- Soto RG, Fu ES. Acute pain management for patients undergoing thoracotomy. Ann Thorac Surg. 2003; 75:1349-57.
- Uppal V, Sondekoppam RV, Sodhi P, Johnston D, Ganapathy S. Single-Injection Versus Multiple-Injection Technique of Ultrasound-Guided Paravertebral Blocks: A Randomized Controlled Study Comparing Dermatomal Spread. Reg Anesth Pain Med. 2017; 42: 575-81.
- Vecchione T, Zurakowski D, Boretsky K. Thoracic Paravertebral Nerve Blocks in Pediatric Patients: Safety and Clinical Experience. Anesth Analg. 2016; 123:1588-90.
- Wallace MS, Wallace AM, Lee J, Dobke MK. Pain after breast surgery: a survey of 282 women. Pain. 1996; 66:195-205.
- Wardhan R. Update on paravertebral blocks. Curr Opin Anesthesiol. 2015; 28:588-92.

CLINICAL CASE 1 – THE ULTRASOUND-GUIDED UNILATERAL PARAVERTEBRAL BLOCK: A SUITABLE ALTERNATIVE FOR HERNIA REPAIR SURGERY

Clinical history and anamnesis Surgical treatment for inguinal hernia is the most commonly general surgical procedure performed in clinical practice.

Despite high frequency of this procedure, perioperative complications can occur, including several that often depend on the clinical condition of the patient.

The anesthetic technique must be appropriate to the clinical characteristics of the patient and for the needs of the surgeon. The ultrasound-guided unilateral paravertebral block (US-guided UPB) can be a viable alternative, due to hemodynamic stability that it provides.

Technique description After IRB approval and written patient consent statement, we visited a 62-year-old male (80 kg, 175 cm, BMI 26, 12), for a large inguinal hernia in the Academic Hospital of L'Aquila. He was suffering from severe coronary artery disease (CAD), not controlled hypertension, insulin-dependent diabetes mellitus and chronic obstructive pulmonary disease.

Before surgical procedure, a multi-segmental (from T9-T10 to T11) unilateral US-guided UPB was performed, associated with sedation by propofol in continuous intravenous infusion (3 mg/kg/h) (**Figure 2.14**).

Results Throughout the peri-operative period there were no related complications. The patient had an excellent control of postoperative pain (NRS 3) and after 12 hours he was discharged from the hospital.

Conclusions The combination of US-guide UPB with a sedation, allows to ensure a good analgo-sedation, with the possibility for the surgeon to also operate on deeper levels. The hemodynamic stability provided is important to prevent the break of a clinical precarious balance, especially in the patient with severe CAD, with a better analgesia compared to the other standard techniques, as demonstrated by Wassef et al.

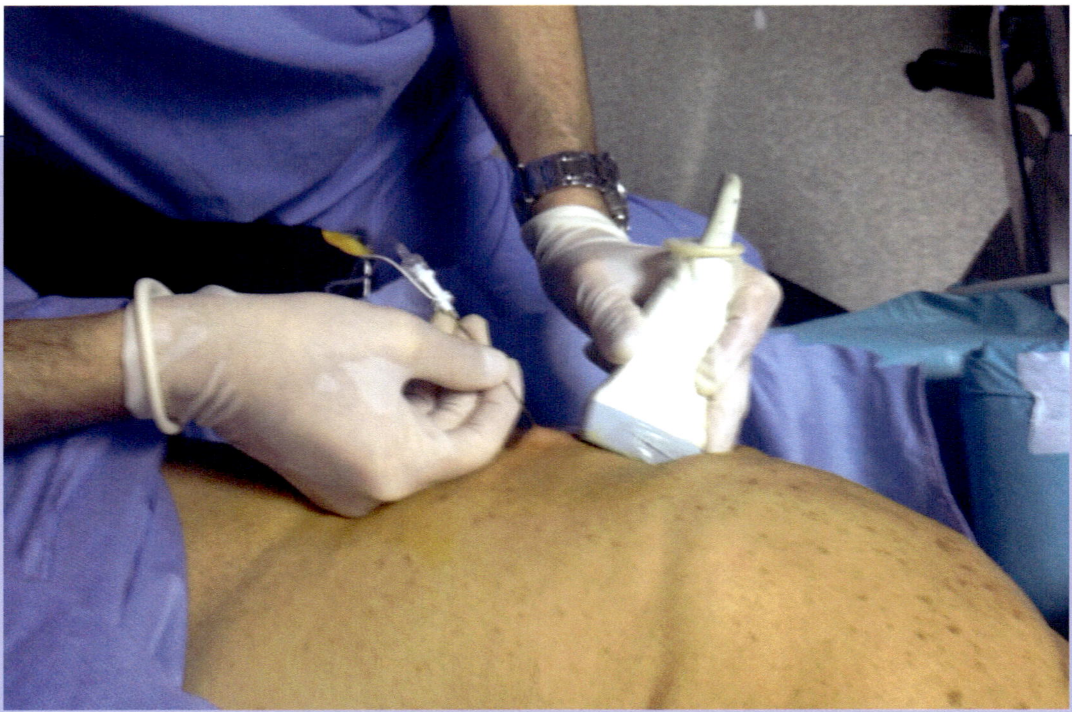

Figure 2.14 Paravertebral block at T10 Level.

CLINICAL CASE 2 – THE ULTRASOUND-GUIDED PARAVERTEBRAL BLOCK: AN APPROPRIATE ALTERNATIVE FOR A PATIENT WITH A HIGH ANESTHETIC RISK TO UNDERGO BREAST SURGERY

Clinical history and anamnesis Breast cancer is the most common malignancy in women around the world, and breast cancer surgery is one of the most frequent procedures conducted in hospitals.

Thoracic paravertebral nerve block (TPVB) is an effective regional anesthetic technique that can provide significant analgesia in breast surgery. This block is a reasonable option to the classic analgesia, in fact it is associated with a superior control of the pain, a reduction in opioids consumption after surgery, a decrease the incidence of postoperative nausea and vomiting and an overall decrease in length of hospital stay.

But the technique is not devoid of potential adverse effects. An accurate anatomic knowledge and adequate technique may help decrease the risk of these effects.

Technique description The patient underwent a right quadrantectomy with sentinel lymph node biopsy. She was in therapy with cardio aspirin for previous TIA and allergy to NSAIDs and codeine.

In the operating room she was premeditated with 2 mg of midazolam.

Subsequently the ultrasound-guided TPVB was performed. Under constant visualization of the needle tip and in complete asepsis, 20 ml of levobupivacaine was injected at the T5 level and 10 ml at the T3 level, unilaterally and observing the collapse of the pleura (**Figure 2.15**).

After 20 min, the dermatomes extension was verified by ice-test. Before proceeding to the surgical incision a sedation with propofol was performed at 4 ml/kg/h in continuous infusion and nasal goggles inserted at 4 l/min.

Results A TPVB provides effective intraoperative anesthesia and postoperative analgesia for patients undergoing breast surgeries, avoiding the administration of opioids and NSAIDs

Conclusions TPVB represents a valid alternative to general anesthesia or epidural block; in fact, unlike the epidural block, it minimizes hypotension ensuring better hemodynamic stability.

A multimodal approach to analgesia includes regional techniques for breast surgery that may reduce the possibility of the development of postoperative complications and chronic pain.

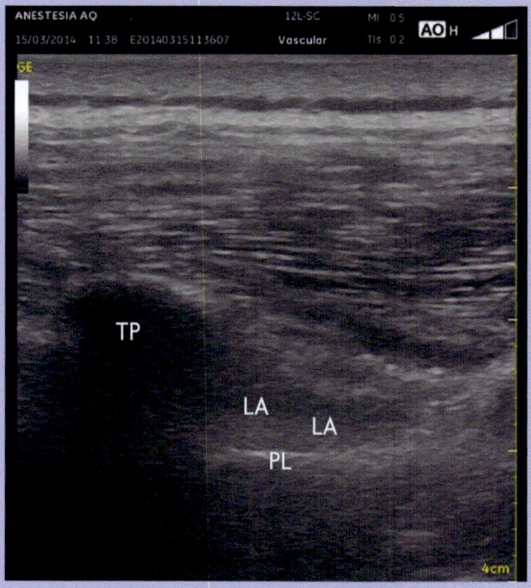

Figure 2.15 Paravertebral block after LA injection with collapse of the pleura: LA: local anesthetic; PL: pleura; TP: transverse process.

CHAPTER

3

Erector spinae plane block (ESP block)

Paolo Scimia, Emiliano Petrucci, Alberto Manassero, Stefano Di Carlo

Erector spinae plane block (ESP block) is a recently introduced locoregional anesthesia/analgesia (LRA) technique which was initially applied in the management of thoracic neuropathic pain, secondary to various conditions such as postoperative pain following thoracic surgery, metastasis, and malunion of the rib. This technique has gained popularity in recent years as a novel ultrasound (US)-guided interfascial plane block by proving to be effective for the treatment of both acute postoperative pain and chronic debilitating pain syndromes affecting the thoracic and abdominal region that are often unresponsive to standard therapies.

The mechanism of action of ESP block has been investigated through clinical and cadaveric studies. Recent evidence from the literature suggests that the clinical efficacy of this technique seems to be linked to a multimodal mechanism of action. First described by Forero et al. in 2016, ESP block performed between erector spinae muscle and transverse process at T5 was able to provide a multi-dermatomal sensory analgesia of the thoracic region with T2-T9 extension. In particular, following a single injection of 20 ml of local anesthetic (LA), the injectate seems to spread through anatomical gaps in the intertransverse connective soft tissues towards the paravertebral space (PVS) in multiple spinal segments over an average of 8 dermatomes, reaching the ventral and dorsal ramus of the thoracic spinal nerve along with the sympathetic ramus communicans at the intervertebral foramen level (**Figure 3.1**).

There has been a long-held dogma that the superior costotransverse ligament (SCTL) needs to be traversed by the needle tip in order to allow the anesthetic solution to reach the PVS.

In the past, anatomists believed that SCTL was a barrier to spread of the anesthetic solution towards the PVS because of the presence of the deep muscles of the column and their complex relationship with the transverse processes.

Based on this assumption, current descriptions of thoracic paravertebral block (PVB) require the needle tip to be anterior and deep SCTL to achieve a successful block.

However, recent cadaver and clinical studies suggest that the SCTL may not be a "barrier" to diffusion of injected solutions and that the PVS is not a clearly delineated anatomical compartment.

The SCTL has a thickness of approximately 1 mm and runs in an oblique fashion from the anterior and inferior surface of the transverse process above, to the upper border of the neck of the rib below. It is possible that an injection posterior to the SCTL will result in solution passing through gaps and fenestrations in the intertransverse connective tissue and reaching the nerve root in the PVS. Based on this hypothesis Cornish defined the ESP technique as a "happily accidental" PVB.

The ESP block is a candidate as a safer PVB variant which allows to block thoracic spinal nerves using injections posterior to the SCTL and outside of the conventional PVS. This technique involves a more superficial and close to the pleura needle placement providing an effective block with a lower risk of complications.

Other authors have also hypothesised an involvement of the lateral cutaneous branches of the intercostal nerves lateral to the angle of the ribs as a possible alternative mechanism to explain clinical efficacy of ESP block, thanks to the extensive medio-lateral spread of the injected solutions in both the superficial and deep erector spinae planes as shown by cadaver studies.

More recent evidence based on magnetic resonance imaging studies provide additional anatomical information on the potential mechanism of the ESP block demonstrating that the visceral and somatic analgesic effects of this technique likely result from both transforaminal and epidural spread of LA.

Some reports showed the efficacy of ESP block in abdominal cavity procedure suggesting the potential mechanism of visceral blockade in addition to the somatic blockade.

Most of the literature findings suggest that ESP block has characteristics of differential blockade determining analgesia without motor block along discernable cutaneous sensory block. In fact, it seems that the small amount of LA reaching the PVS through the foramen provides a block of small A delta and non-myelinated C fibers (pain and sympathetic fibers) but is not able to block large myelinated sensory and motor fibers.

Currently the idea that the ESP technique is only an alternative or simplified variant of PVB has been abandoned, taking into account that recent literature findings seem to suggest a fascinating multimodal mechanism of action of this novel US-guided interfascial plane block.

Anatomy and sonoanatomy

The erector spinae is not just one muscle, but it's also known as the sacrospinalis group of muscles that are primarily responsible for supporting and extending the vertebral column to maintain erect posture. These muscles extend from the sacrum to the skull and mainly develop in the dorsal direction with in-

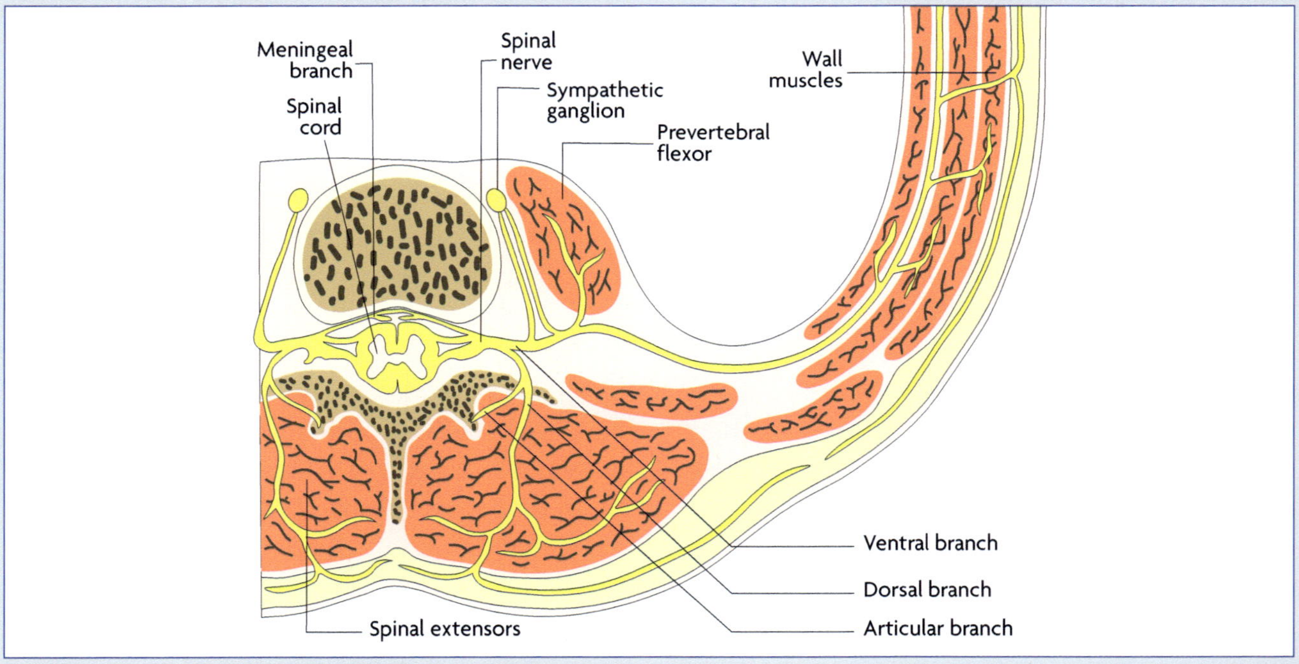

Figure 3.1 Course of the nerve rami originating from the paravertebral space. Note the presence within the space of rami originating from the sympathetic nervous system.

sertion on the spinous and transverse processes of the vertebrae. The architecture of the erector spinae muscle is complex, with three muscle layers distributing in the lumbar, thoracic, and cervical area. The erector spinae is made up of 3 muscles which play an important role in the spinal stability: Spinalis (medially), Longissimus (centrally), Illiocostalis (laterally). The erector spinae belongs to the intrinsic muscles of the spine and extends along the length of the spinal column, allowing it to extend; it is called an erector muscle because it counteracts gravity, allowing the upright position. It lies in the groove to the side of the vertebral column and it's surrounded in the lumbar and thoracic regions by the thoracolumbar fascia, and in the cervical region by the nuchal ligament.

To perform ESP block correctly, the use of US-guidance and a solid understanding of the essential sonoanatomy are required. In particular, it is recommended to place the US-probe longitudinally at 3 cm from the median line of the spine (**Figure 3.2**), in order to identify the trapezius, rhomboid, and erector spinae muscles with their respective fasciae.

The erector spinae plane lies superficial to the transverse processes which appear as finger-like acoustic shadows. Lateral to the transverse process, by increasing the scanning depth, it will be possible to detect the SCTL which delimits the virtual anatomical compartment of the PVS, and the pleura that appears as a regular echogenic line with its "lung sliding", a typical movement synchronous to the respiratory acts, determined by the sliding of the two parietal and visceral pleural leaflets on each other (**Figure 3.3**).

Another aspect that we consider fundamental to achieve a successful block is the knowledge of sonoanatomy of the spine in order to distinguish the target from neighboring anatomical structures. US-guidance plays an important role in helping practitioners more accurately identify intervertebral levels and locate an appropriate site for needle insertion. In particular, it

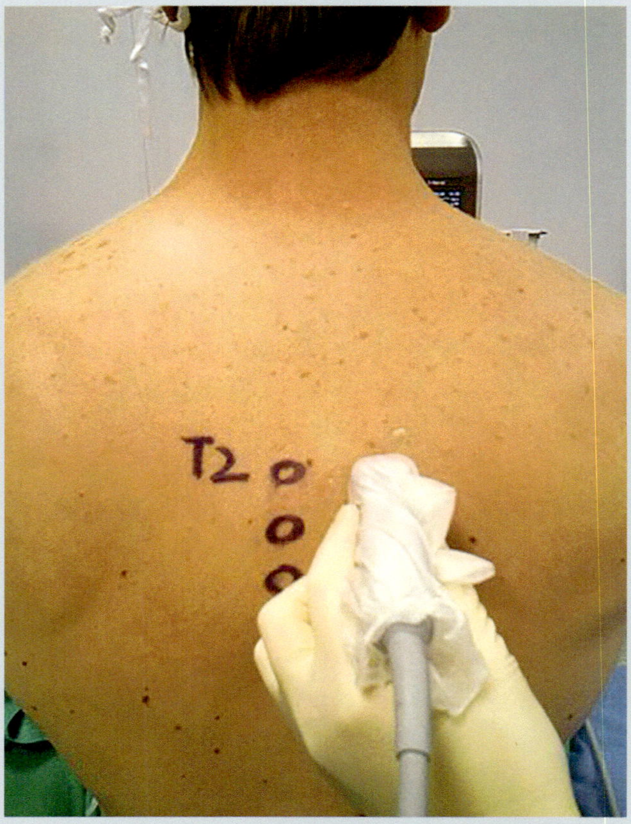

Figure 3.2 Correct position of the probe to perform ESP block. US-probe is placed longitudinally at 3 cm from the interspinous line.

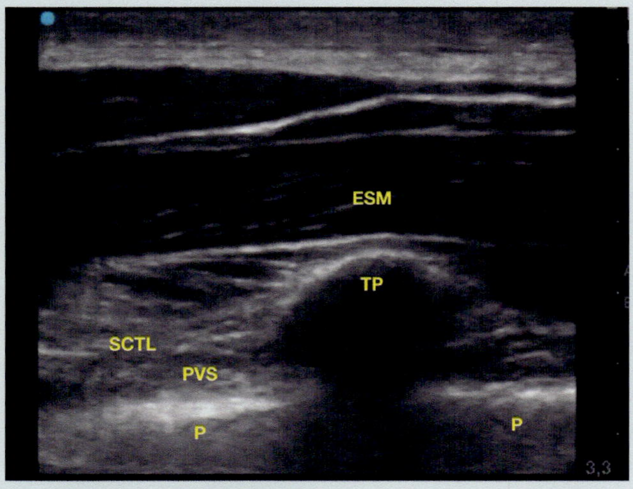

Figure 3.3 Essential sonoanatomy to perform ESP block. It is important to note erector spinae muscle (ESM) superficially to the "finger like" acoustic shadow of the transverse process (TP). In evidence the virtual anatomical compartment of the paravertebral space (PVS) delimited by the superior costotransverse ligament (SCTL) and the underlying pleural line (P).

is important to note that a paramedian sagittal sonogram of the lumbar and thoracic spine allows to identify characteristic sonographic patterns. A sagittal US image of midline spinous process appears as a typical crescent shape with posterior acoustic shadowing that looks like a "mountains sign". By moving the US-probe sideways it is possible to distinguish in medial to lateral direction the laminae which appear discontinuous as a "horse head sign" or sawtooth sign", the articular processes which appear continuous as "camel's humps", and the transverse processes (ESP block target) which appear as hyperechoic structures with finger-like acoustic shadowing beneath showing a "trident sign" (**Figure 3.4**). In order to avoid technical errors it is advisable to observe the transition from the discontinuous pattern of the transverse process view to the continuous hyperechoic line formed by the articular processes, and the transition from the rounded "humps" of the articular processes to the sawtooth-like acoustic shadows of the laminae, with the hyperechoic posterior and anterior complexes visible in between. Moreover, it is important to remember that the thoracic transverse processes arise posterior to the articular processes and articulate with the corresponding ribs that appear as repeating curvilinear structures with deeper, hypoechoic, posterior acoustic shadow. The presence of a rib is also an identifying marker of the transition between L1 and T12 vertebra and can be used to determine the intervertebral level. US is a useful and relatively easy to perform technique but adequate training and clinical experience are required to realize its full potential. The utility of the US-guided approach is most evident in patients in whom technical difficulty is expected because of poor surface anatomic landmarks (e.g., in obesity or after spinal surgery) or distorted spinal anatomy (e.g., scoliosis).

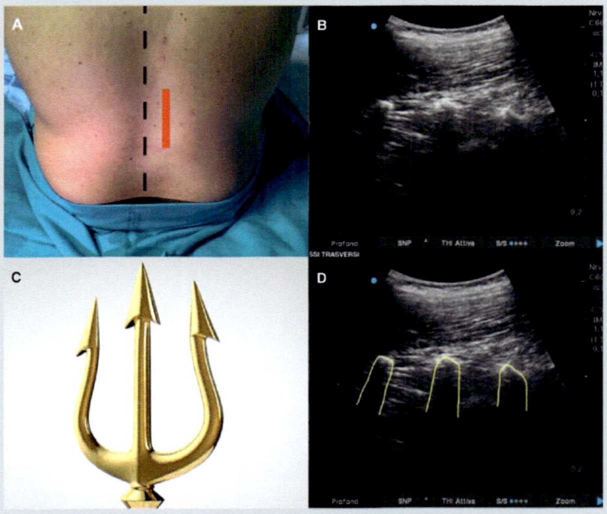

Figure 3.4 **A** In evidence US-probe position longitudinally at 3 cm from the midline to perform ESP block at lumbar level. **B** Paramedian sagittal scan at level of transverse processes. **C** Trident sign. **D** US imaging of transverse processes with their finger like acoustic shadow.

Description of technique

The block has been reported to be performed before surgery with the patient under mild sedation and also right after general anesthesia induction, either before surgical incision, or at the end of the surgery. Preferred patient positioning after general anesthesia induction are lateral decubitus and prone. Before general anesthesia induction, most of the authors suggest a sitting position when performing ESP block in the upper thoracic and prone when performing it at the lower thoracic level, mostly related to the patient and operator comfort.

Although a blind technique based only on anatomical landmarks is theoretically possible, the use of US-guidance is highly recommended to perform this block.

As for the "blind" technique, after careful skin disinfection, a 22 G 50-90 mm needle (SonoPlex stim Pajunk®) is inserted at a distance of about 3 cm from the interspinous line, seeking contact with the transverse process, which acts as a backstop avoiding for further advancement of the needle tip. The anesthetic solution is then injected by slightly withdrawing the needle, after a negative aspiration test for blood and air. For the US-guided technique, usually a high-frequency (12-15 MHz) linear probe is positioned longitudinally 3 cm lateral to the midline of the spine. It is possible to identify from the surface to the depth the trapezius, rhomboid, and erector spinae muscles, which appear superficially in the acoustic shadow of the selected transverse process. For high BMI patients a curvilinear probe (2-6 MHz) is advised. Two different approaches have been described to perform the block: superficial (superficial-ESP block) and deep (deep-ESP block).

The needle insertion point is usually 1 cm away from the US-probe to avoid steep needle entry angle. In-plane approach is recommended either from cranial to caudal or caudal to cranial (**Figure 3.5**). Hydrolocation and tissue movement help to visualize the needle when target deeper than 3 cm. The success of ESP block fully depends on the appropriate spread of the anesthetic solution during the injection. Careful and detailed hydrolocation must ensure that the injectable is located in the target fascial plane. Usually, after appropriate hydrolocation with volume as low as 5 ml of normal saline, the spread will be seen in cranial and caudal directions in at least 3 spinal levels. After confirmation of appropriate spread, the total of injectable can be delivered in aliquots of 3 cc following safety maneuver during injection to avoid intravascular depositions.

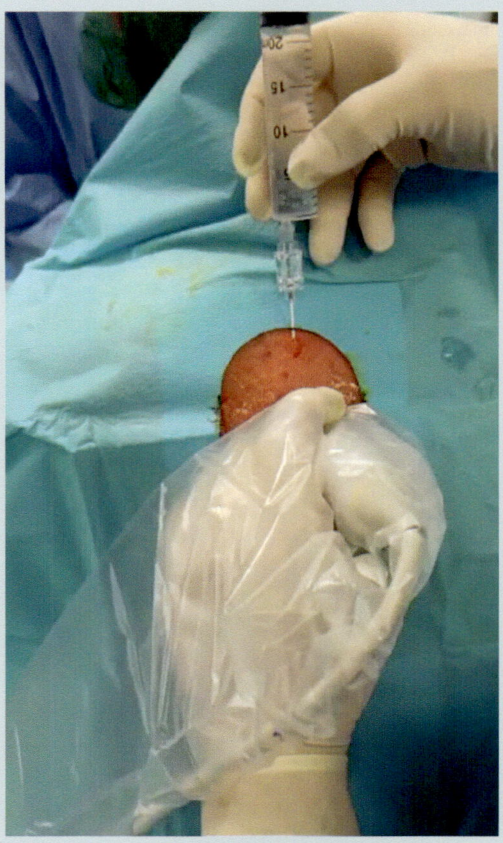

Figure 3.5 In plane approach to perform ESP block. Note the needle insertion point 1 cm away from the US-probe from cranial to caudal direction.

In the superficial approach, a 22 G 50-90 mm echo-reflecting needle (SonoPlex stim Pajunk®) is inserted "in-plane" to the US-beam, preferably in a cranio-caudal direction, until the tip is positioned in the interfascial plane between the rhomboid and erector spinae muscles. At this point, only after performing an aspiration test and a hydrolocation by injection of 2-3 ml of saline solution to confirm the correct positioning of the needle tip, 20 ml of LA will be injected within the target plane. It's useful to emphasize that an adequate spread of LA normally determines the opening of the target plane and the separation of the two fasciae of this amarker first described by Fusco et al. known as the "Double V sign" which allow to exclude a peri-fascial injection.

For deep approach, the needle is inserted in the same way and, after having positioned the tip in the deep plane of the erector spinae muscle, a similar volume of LA is injected, taking care to verify by US the linear diffusion of the injected solution, superficially to the acoustic window of the transverse process (**Figure 3.6**, **Videos 3.1**, **3.2**). Before injecting LA it's important to confirm the spread anterior to the anterior fascia of the erector spinae muscle and posterior to the tip of the transverse process by hydrolocation of normal saline. The aim of the deep ESP block is to penetrate the most anterior layer of the erector spinae muscle and deposit the injectate between this layer and the tip of the transverse process in order to obtain cranial-caudal spread of LA in multiple spinal segments (**Figure 3.7**). The injection of LA in close relation to the intertransverse connective soft tissue allows spread to the PVS, through its porous surfaces or through the foramen where the dorsal ramus of the spinal nerve leaves the intervertebral foramen to innervate back structures. In order to correctly identify the target (tip of the transverse process) when performing thoracic ESP block it's recommendable to move the US-probe either from medial to lateral (lamina to target) or from lateral to

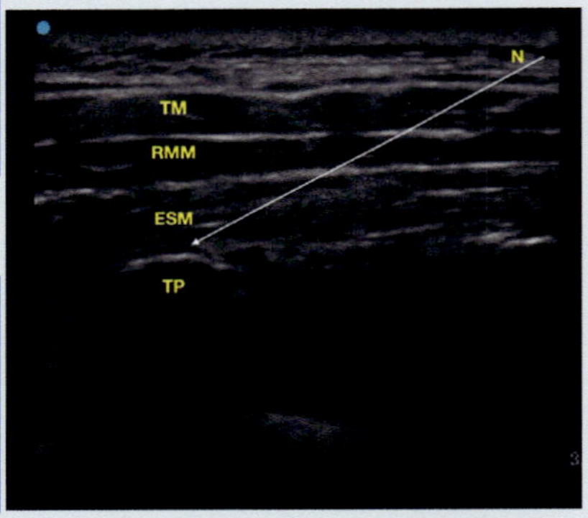

Figure 3.6 Deep-ESP block. In evidence is the tip of the needle deeply to the erector spinae muscle and superficially to the acoustic window of the transverse process. The spread of LA within the fascial plane between the anterior layer of erector spinae muscle and the tip of transverse process is required for a successful block. ESM: erector spinae muscle; N: needle; RMM: rhomboid major muscle; TM: trapezius muscle; TP: transverse process.

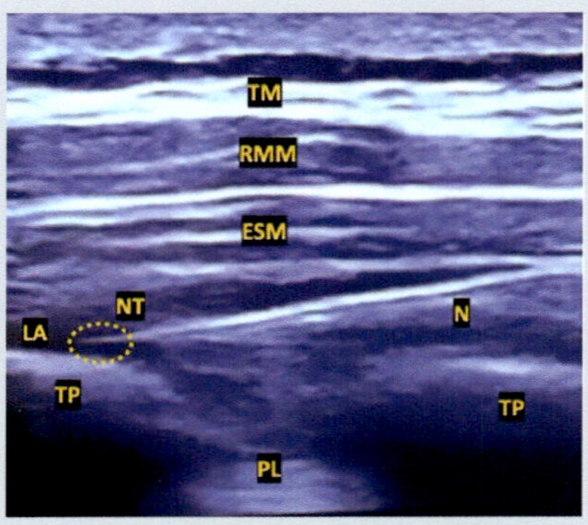

Figure 3.7 Target of Deep-ESP block. The needle tip should be positioned within the fascial plane between the anterior layer of erector spinae muscle and the "roof" of transverse process. Note the spread of local anesthetic ESM: erector spinae muscle; N: needle; RMM: rhomboid major muscle; TM: trapezius muscle; TP: transverse process.

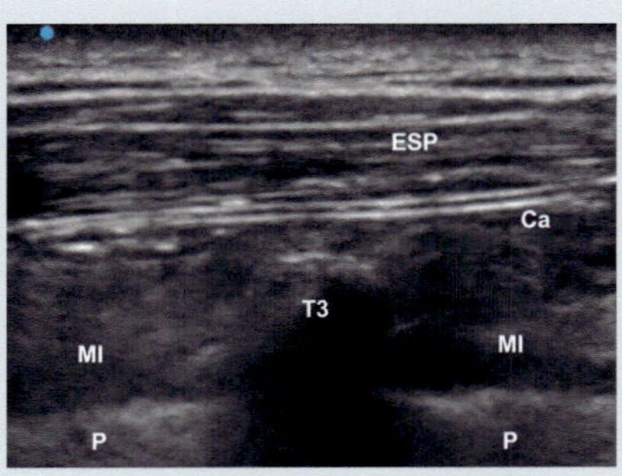

Figure 3.8 Catheter placement in deep plane of the erector spinae muscle. Ca: catheter; ESP: erector spinae plane; MI: intercostal muscles; P: pleura; T3: transverse process at T3 level.

medial (rib to target). Moving the probe medially from rib towards the target show a clear transition from the deeper triangular-shaped structure (costo-transverse union) to a slightly more superficial flat hyperechoic structure (tip of the transverse process). It may be easier to identify the target moving from lamina which is a flat and deeper bony structure 2-3 cm medial to the tip of the transverse process. As previously described it may be useful to reiterate the change in the sonoanatomy of the visualized structures during the transition from lamina to transverse process.

The lamina produced a pattern that resembled the head and neck of a horse, which we refer to as the "horse head sign", and the gap between adjoining lamina was the interlaminar space. The articular process appeared as one continuous hyperechoic wavy line with no intervening gaps. Finally, the transverse process appeared as a crescent-shaped hyperechoic reflection with its concavity facing anteriorly.

In both approaches, after a few minutes, the operator must test the dermatome level of the sensory block by means of an ice test and pinprick test. Following the administration of the initial bolus, it is also possible to perform a continuous blockade. US-guided ESP block lends itself well to insertion of an indwelling

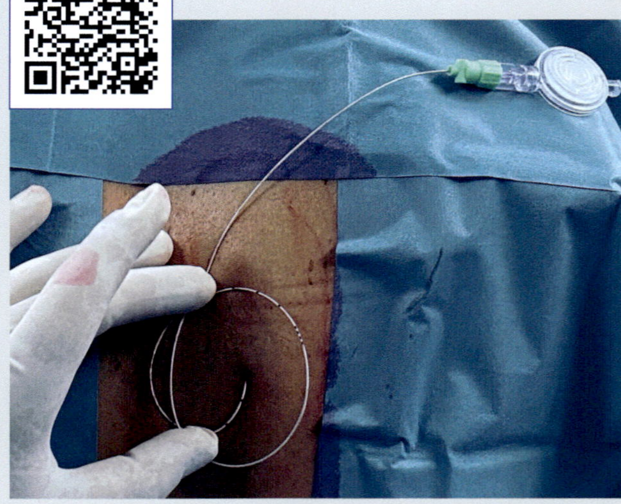

Figure 3.9 Continuous ESP block. In evidence catheter placement in order to prolong postoperative analgesia.

catheter which can be used to extend the duration of postoperative. We recommend to place the catheter after initial single shot bolus (usually 20 ml) to open up the space before threading the catheter. Generally, an echogenic peri-neural catheter or epidural catheter may be inserted and placed 4-5 cm beyond the tip of a regular 18 G Tuohy needle deep to the erector spinae plane in order to prolong the analgesia (**Figures 3.8**, **3.9**, **Video 3.3**). The defined interfascial plane and the thickness of erector muscle allow secure anchoring of the catheter. Different catheters for LA infusion have been successfully used in clinical practice (catheter over needle or catheter through needle). The preference of most of the authors is to use the later due to the fact that the catheter can be advanced and securely left into the erector spinae muscle. The catheter must be inserted under US-guidance and it may remain in place for 48-72 hours, as needed, paying particular attention to asepsis norms and the patient's haemocoagulative status before removal and subsequent resumption of any anticoagulant therapy (**Flow chart 3.1 online**).

Indications and dosage

ESP block has multiple indications thanks to the distribution of the erector spinae muscle from the neck to the lumbar region. The main advantage of this technique is that the injectate may reach the desired spinal level probably due to its spread to PVS.

The single-shot or continuous ESP block is an LRA technique that can be performed at various levels of the spine, finding a wide field of application in the management of various painful conditions of the thoracic and abdominal wall, as well as for analgesia of the lumbar and brachial plexus involving upper and lower limb surgeries (hip and shoulder analgesia).

This block can be used, in selected patients, as the main anesthetic technique appropriately combined with adequate sedoanalgesia, or as an analgesic strategy in the case of more complex operations involving general anesthesia. Recent evidence demonstrate that ESP block can be successfully used for management of acute postoperative pain in thoracic surgery. This technique has also shown promising results in breast surgery such as mastectomy, especially if combined with other fascial blocks such as PECS II or serratus anterior plane block when axillary lymph node dissection is involved. In literature, moreover, several case reports testify the analgesic efficacy of this technique in other types of operations, such as abdominal (laparoscopy or laparotomy), bariatric, gynecologic, urologic, vertebral, orthopaedic (postsurgical hip or shoulder pain), carotid surgeries. The efficacy in abdominal cavity procedure (gastric bypass) suggested the potential mechanism of visceral blockade in addition to the somatic blockade. As similar as other interfacial blocks (TAP block), the ESP block has been reported to be effective as rescue block after surgery in the thoracic-abdominal cavity, shoulder and lower extremities above the knee.

A fascinating field of application of the ESP block is its use in pain therapy, with particular reference to the management of post-traumatic chest pain (e.g. patients with multiple rib fractures) and neuropathic pain syndromes of various aetiologies (surgery, trauma, medical diseases such as herpes zoster, diabetes, neoplasms) which are often refractory to pharmacological therapies leading to the development of chronic pain. It is possible to perform the block unilaterally or bilaterally as needed, taking care not to exceed the maximum recommended doses of LA.

Usually, the level chosen for thoracic indications is between T2 and T5, and for abdominal-pelvic indications between T7 and T10 (**Table 3.1**).

The common dosages used in adults include 20 ml of LA long-acting (levobupivacaine or ropivacaine 0.25% at analgesic dosages; levobupivacaine 0.375-0.5% or ropivacaine 0.5-0.75% at anesthetic dosages) for single-shot block; in the case of continuous blockade, after the initial bolus, analgesia can be prolonged by a peri-neural catheter through continuous infusion of long-acting LA at low concentration (levobupivacaine 0.25% or ropivacaine 0.25%). Catheter placement can be unilateral or bilateral depending on the patient's needs. We recommend levobupivacaine or ropivacaine 0.2 for unilateral infusions, instead for bilateral infusions levobupivacaine or ropivacaine 0.125% at a rate that varies from 8 ml to 13 ml per catheter per hour.

The most common infusion methods are continuous infusion plus patient-controlled analgesia (PCA) or inter-

TABLE 3.1 INDICATIONS OF ESP BLOCK FOR DIFFERENT SURGERIES

Vertebral level	Surgery
T2-T3	Post-surgical shoulder pain Chronic shoulder pain syndrome
T4-T6	Open thoracotomy and VATS lobectomy (T5) Rescue after TE failiure after thoracic surgery (T5) Cardiac surgery-sternotomy (T5) Breast surgery with axillary lymph node dissection (T3) Rib fractures Metastatic ribs cancer (level of segments involved) Chronic postherpetic neuralgia (level of segments involved) Chronic post-thoracotomy pain (level of segments involved)
T7-T12	Nephrectomies (T8) Hysterectomies (T10) Laparoscopic ventral hernia repair with mesh (T7) Laparotomies (T7) Chronic postherpetic neuralgia (level of segments involved) Chronic abdominal pain syndrome (T7 to T10) Chronic pelvic pain syndrome (T10)
L4	Verterbral surgery Post-surgical hip replacement pain (L4)

mittent programmed boluses (IPB). A typical example will be levobupivacaine 0.25%: continuous infusion 5-8 ml/h plus PCA (5 ml lockout interval 60 minutes) or continuous infusion 5 ml/h plus IPB (10 ml/2 h). The most appropriate method of infusion has not been determined yet. However, IPB is lately gaining popularity due to the fact that pressure during injection appears to play an important role to improve analgesia during ESP continuous infusion. Regarding adjuvants, the most common one reported is dexamethasone or dexmedetomidine in the postoperative settings and methylprednisolone in the chronic pain setting.

Continuous ESP block has been used successfully for postoperative analgesia in different surgeries. Scimia et al. in 2017 described the application of continuous US-guided ESP block performed at T5 level for postoperative analgesia in a ASA III patient undergoing video-assisted thoracoscopic surgery (VATS) for lobectomy of the right upper lobe which received general anesthesia and one lung ventilation (**Figure 3.10**). After a single shot ESP block with a total of 0.5% ropivacaine 20 ml a catheter was inserted through a 18-Gauge Tuohy needle. Postoperatively PCA pump was connected to the catheter (0.20% ropivacaine at 8 ml/h, 5 ml bolus, lockout period of 60 minutes) in order to prolong postoperative analgesia. The patient reported a good quality opioid-free postoperative pain control (NRS <4) and the catheter was removed 72 hours after surgery. In recent years other case reports confirmed the effectiveness of US-guided ESP block for postoperative analgesia in thoracic surgery suggesting that this technique may represent a valid alternative to conventional regional techniques, such as thoracic epidural analgesia or PVB, especially when they could not be recommended.

Contraindications to the block

- Absolute contraindications: patient refusal, injection site infections, allergies to LA
- Relative contraindications: obesity (high BMI), vertebral fractures, severe scoliosis, coagulopathies and/or coagulation disorders

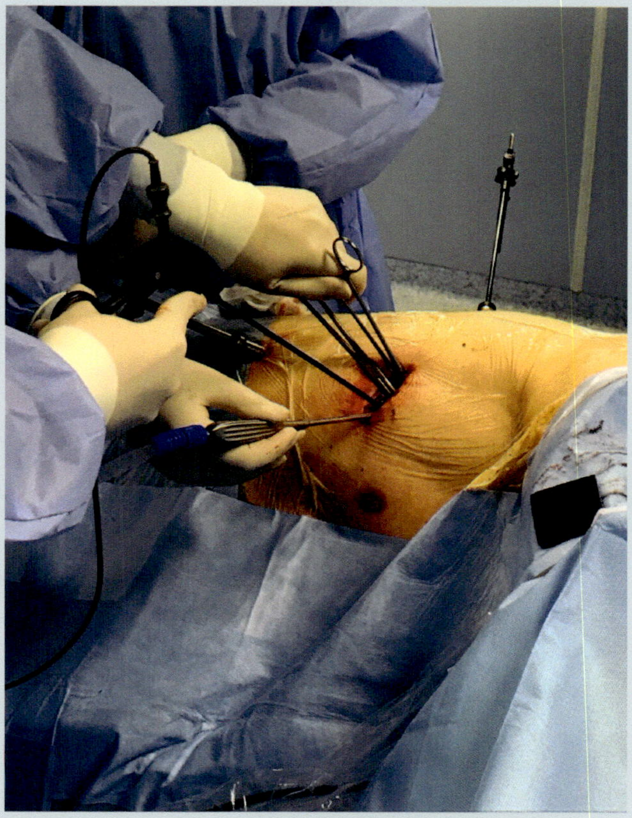

Figure 3.10 VATS lobectomy of the right upper lobe.

Complications and contraindications

US-guided ESP block is an easy and relatively safe technique in experienced hands.

Possible complications are the risk of local anesthetic systemic toxicity (LAST) and diffusion of the anesthetic solution into the peridural space. While LAST is to be considered especially in case of bilateral block because of the generous volumes used, the peridural diffusion of LA could be favored by a latero-medial direction of the needle tip or by a high injection pressure.

Although some authors consider ESP block to be a relatively safe LRA technique compared to PVB, as the transverse process is a useful sonoanatomical landmark to stop further needle advancement, misrecognition of target structures or poor visualization of needle tip progression may lead to the risk of accidental pleural puncture, resulting in iatrogenic pneumothorax. Regarding safety, only two reports of either complication or unexpected clinical effect have been published. One reported pneumothorax and the second reported transient motor block. However, the authors recommended careful administration of LA following safety maneuvers under monitoring to avoid or detect intravascular administration and local anesthetic toxicity events.

Absolute contraindications include lack of patient consent, infection at the injection site and known allergies to the LA used. Relative contraindications are high BMI, presence of vertebral fractures or high scoliosis. Although, for all intents and purposes, ESP block can be considered a more "peripheral" and superficial LRA technique than PVB, the presence of anatomical variants or morphological alterations of the tissues such as oedema and particularly represented subcutaneous panniculus adiposus could affect the correct visualization of the needle and nerve target, compromising the success of the block. ESP block cannot be considered a "deep" block like PVB, however, especially in "frail" patients or those at high anesthesiologic risk, the same restrictions as for central blocks should be observed in case of concomitant anticoagulant/antiaggregant therapy or thromboprophylaxis, in respect of patient safety.

Complications

- LAST from accidental intravascular injection or reabsorption of LA
- LA diffusion into the peridural space
- Accidental pleural puncture and pneumothorax (shallower target – reduced risk compared to PVB)

Chronic pain indication

Recent literature has highlighted the important role of ESP block in the treatment of chronic chest wall pain syndromes of different etiologies, sometimes refractory to common therapies. This technique has been successfully used in the management of chronic pain conditions of a post-traumatic or postsurgical nature (thoracotomy, mastectomy), or associated with medical pathologies (neoplasms, diabetic neuropathy, herpes zoster). The clinical efficacy of the block seems to be attributable to the partial diffusion of LA near the intervertebral foramina, proximal to the origin of the dorsal and ventral rami of the thoracic spinal nerves. Extension of application to chronic pain emerges in the case report. Because the target is away from the neuraxial compartment and thoracic cavity, ESP block is used increasingly in procedures previously considered for PVB. Furthermore, avoiding the neuraxial area and the superficial location of the target makes the ESP a more attractive alternative to patient on anticoagulants. Fusco et al. have recently described how, by virtue of this mechanism, ESP block may offer a valid alternative to PVB in the management of chronic neuropathic pain syndromes of the thoracic wall, guaranteeing long-lasting analgesia, with an excellent safety profile and an improvement in the patient's quality of life.

RECOMMENDED READING

- Forero M, Adhikary SD, Lopez H, Tsui C, Chin KJ. The erector spinae plane block: a novel analgesic technique in thoracic neuropathic pain. Reg Anesth Pain Med. 2016;41:621-7.
- Chin KJ, Malhas L, Perlas A. The Erector Spinae Plane Block Provides Visceral Abdominal Analgesia in Bariatric Surgery: A Report of 3 Cases. Reg Anesth Pain Med. 2017 May/Jun;42(3):372-6.
- Cornish PB. Erector spinae plane block: the "happily accidental" paravertebral block. Reg Anesth Pain Med. 2018;43(6):644–5.
- De Cassai A, Marchet A, Ori C. The combination of erector spinae plane block and PECS blocks could avoid general anesthesia for radical mastectomy in high risk patients. Minerva Anestesiol. 2018;84:1420–1.
- Ivanusic J, Konishi Y, Barrington MJ. A cadaveric study investigating the mechanism of action of erector spinae blockade. Reg Anesth Pain Med. 2018;43(6):567–71.
- Luftig J, Mantuani D, Herring AA, Dixon B, Clattenburg E, Nagdev A. Successful emergency pain control for posterior rib fractures with ultrasound-guided erector spinae plane block. Am J Emerg Med. 2018 Aug;36(8)1391-6.
- Nardiello MA, Herlitz M. Bilateral single shot erector spinae plane block for pectus excavatum and pectus carinatum surgery in 2 pediatric patients. Rev Esp Anestesiol Reanim. 2018 Nov;65(9):530-3.
- Schwartzmann A, Peng P, Maciel MA, Forero M. Mechanism of the erector spinae plane block: insights from a magnetic resonance imaging study. Can J Anaesth. 2018 Oct;65(10):1165-6.
- Ahiskalioglu A, Alici HA, et al. Ultrasound guided low thoracic erector spinae plane block for management of acute herpes zoster. J Clin Anesth. 2017 Dec 21;45:60-1.
- Fusco P, Di Carlo S, Scimia P, Luciani A, Petrucci E, Marinangeli F. Could the new ultrasound-guided erector spinae plane block be a valid alternative to paravertebral block in chronic chest pain syndromes? Minerva Anestesiol. 2017 Oct;83(10):1112-3.
- Fusco P, Petrucci E, Marinangeli F, Scimia P. Block failure or lack of efficacy? The "Double V" sign: a novel sonographic sign for a successful interfascial plane block. Minerva Anestesiol. 2019 Aug;85(8):917-918.
- Ranocchia S, Scimia P, Giordano C, Danzi V, Bignami E. Ultrasound-guided erector spinae plane block and dexmedetomidine cooperative sedation for non-intubated chest wall surgery. Minerva Anestesiol. 2019 Dec;85(12):1365-1366.
- Scimia P, Basso Ricci E, Droghetti A, Fusco P. The Ultrasound-Guided Continuous Erector Spinae Plane Block for Postoperative Analgesia in Video-Assisted Thoracoscopic Lobectomy. Reg Anesth Pain Med. 2017 Jul/Aug;42(4):537.
- Sepolvere G, Tognù A, D'Errico C, Tedesco M, Cristiano L, Scialdone VR, Borghi B. Bilateral erector spinae block combined with awake sedation for cancer breast surgery in a seriously ill patient. Minerva Anestesiol. 2021 Jan;87(1):117-118.
- Scimia P, Sepolvere G. Nuove prospettive anestesiologiche ed antalgiche nella moderna chirurgia della mammella. Explora Editor. 2021
- Peng P, Finlayson R, Lee SH, Bhatia A. Ultrasound for Interventional Pain Management. An Illustrated Procedural Guide. © Springer Nature Switzerland AG 2020.

CLINICAL CASE 1 – ULTRASOUND (US)-GUIDED ERECTOR SPINAE PLANE (ESP) BLOCK AND DEXMEDETOMIDINE (DEX) COOPERATIVE SEDATION FOR NON-INTUBATED CHEST WALL SURGERY

Clinical history and anamnesis We reported the use of US-guided ESP block as sole anesthetic technique and combined to DEX sedation in a 77-year-old man, ASA 3, which was scheduled for elective excision of right subscapular elastofibroma (**Figure 3.11**). The patient received antiplatelet therapy for previous myocardial ischemia treated with coronary stent implantation.

Materials and methods Written informed consents to surgery and anesthesia were obtained. After sedoanalgesia with fentanyl 50 µg and midazolam 2 mg, a unilateral single shot US-guided ESP block was performed at T8 level.

Technique description A high-frequency linear US-probe (12 MHz) was placed in a longitudinal plane 3 cm from the midline and trapezius, rhomboid major, and erector spinae muscles with their fasciae were identified. In asepsis a 22 G 90 mm echogenic needle (SonoPlex stim Pajunk®) was inserted in caudad-to-cephalad direction to reach the block target between deep layer of the erector spinae muscle and the tip of transverse process. The correct position of the needle tip was confirmed by hydrolocation and a total of 20 ml of 0.5% levobupivacaine was injected assessing dermatomical extension of the sensory block by pinprick and cold tests after 20 minutes. During surgery patient received intravenously sedation (Ramsay 3) with DEX in a loading dose of 1 mcg/kg over 15 minutes followed by an infusion of 0.2-0.4 µg/kg/h maintaining spontaneous breathing and hemodynamic stability (**Figure 3.12**). Supplemental oxygen (4 l/min) was administered by Venturi mask and end-tidal CO_2 was monitored. Postoperatively pain score was assessed by Numerical Rating Scale (NRS) both at rest and movement and also during cough. Scheduled postoperative analgesics were acetaminophen 1 g and ketorolac 30 mg every eight hours, providing a dose of Tramadol 100 mg if NRS was >5. The patient reported a good postoperative pain control (NRS <4) without needing opioids and he was discharged from the hospital 48 hours after the surgery.

Conclusions Our experience seems to confirm that the use of US-guided ESP block associated to DEX cooperative sedation may represent a valid technique for non-intubated chest wall surgery. We believe that this approach could provide a reliable strategy for implementing enhanced recovery after surgery pathways.

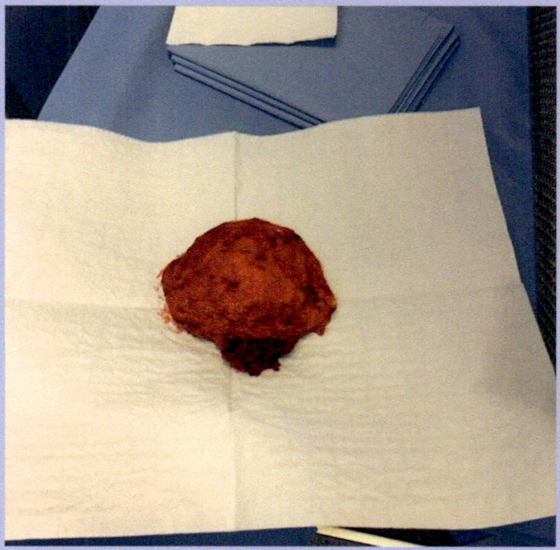

Figure 3.11 Elastofibroma dorsi is a benign soft-tissue tumor of the chest wall which typically presents as an ill-defined mass adjacent to the inferior pole of the scapula.

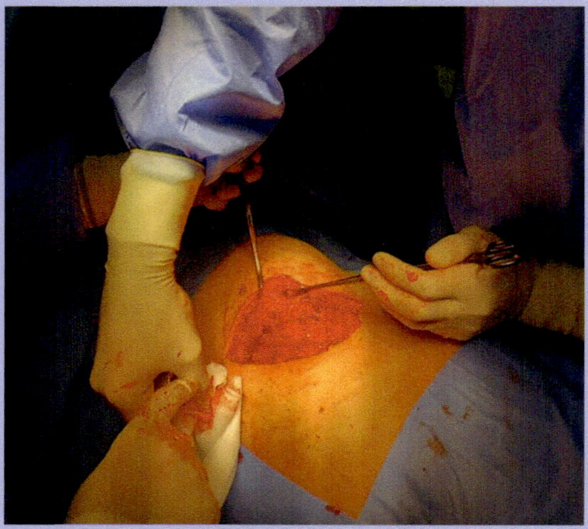

Figure 3.12 Surgical excision of elastofibroma dorsi. Patient underwent cooperative sedation with DEX (Ramsay 3) maintaining spontaneous breathing during surgery.

CLINICAL CASE 2 – BILATERAL ULTRASOUND (US)-GUIDED ERECTOR SPINAE PLANE (ESP) BLOCK COMBINED WITH AWAKE SEDATION FOR BREAST CANCER SURGERY IN A SERIOUSLY ILL PATIENT

Clinical history and anamnesis We reported the use of US-guided ESP block as a single anesthetic technique combined with mild sedation for breast cancer surgery. A 64-year-old woman, ASA 3, affected by hypertensive cardiopathy, atrial fibrillation in anticoagulation therapy and chronic obstructive pulmonary disease, was scheduled for bilateral modified radical mastectomy without axillary lymph-node dissection.

Materials and methods Written informed consents to surgery and anesthesia were obtained. US-guided ESP block was bilaterally performed at T4 level (**Figure 3.13**).

Technique description With the patient in sitting position a linear US-probe was placed at T4 level 3 cm laterally from the midline in order to identify the ESP. In asepsis a 21 G 100 mm echogenic needle (SonoPlex stim Pajunk®) was positioned between deep layer of the erector spinae muscle and the tip of transverse process. After hydrolocation by normal saline, a total of 20 ml of 0.5% levobupivacaine plus dexamethasone 4 mg was injected. Oxygen by facemask was administered at a flow rate of 5 l/min and Propofol TCI started at the rate of 1 ng/ml to obtain a Ramsay sedation scale level of 3. The patient was comfortable maintaining spontaneous breathing and hemodynamic stability throughout the procedure (**Figure 3.14**). Only 1 g of acetaminophen every eight hours was systematically administered and no supplemental opioids were required. Postoperative nausea and vomiting and other complications were absent.

Conclusions Our experience suggests that the US-guided ESP block could have a good anesthetic potency for breast cancer surgery and be a valid alternative to conventional techniques, especially in seriously ill patients.

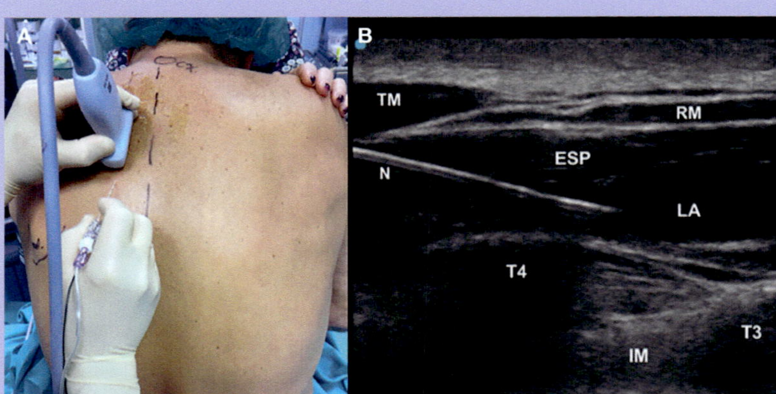

Figure 3.13 A Probe and patient position: a linear US-probe was longitudinally placed at T4 level 3 cm laterally from the midline bilaterally. **B** US-guided ESP block. Note spread of LA within the interfascical plane between erector spine muscle and the tip of transverse processes. ESP: erector spinae plane; IM: intercostal muscle; LA: local anesthetic; N: needle; RM: rhomboideus muscle; T: transverse process; TM: trapezius muscle.

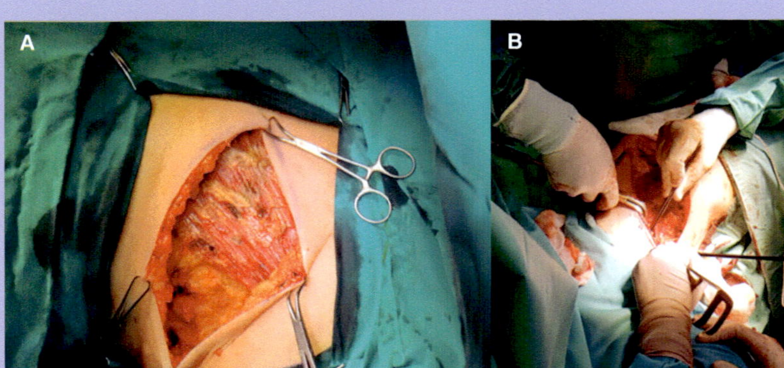

Figure 3.14 A Patient underwent left mastectomy in mild sedation maintaining spontaneous breathing. **B** Right mastectomy.

CHAPTER
4

Deep and superficial serratus plane block and intercostal nerve block

Vito Torrano, Gianluca Russo, Antonio Giorgi, Paolo Scimia, Giuseppe Sepolvere, Pierfrancesco Fusco

DEEP AND SUPERFICIAL SERRATUS PLANE BLOCK

Recent literature has shown the importance of a rational choice of analgesic strategies in order to improve surgical outcome while reducing postoperative comorbidities. With regard to pain management in breast cancer surgery, one of the most studied techniques is the paravertebral block (PVB which, especially when used in combination with general anesthesia, is able to provide optimal pain control. Systemic analgesia, namely the intravenous administration of opioids, provides good pain control at rest (static analgesia), but is not equally effective on pain symptoms during movement (dynamic analgesia); moreover, it is associated with dose-dependent side effects like postoperative nausea and vomiting (PONV). As a consequence opioids may not ensure adequate quality in terms of functional recovery after surgery. These clinical observations clearly suggest the need of alternative analgesic techniques which may allow to spare usage of opiates and reduce their related side effects.

Ultrasound-guided serratus plane block (US-SAP block), is a locoregional anesthesia technique (LRA) recently described by Blanco et al. This technique was introduced in an attempt to ensure adequate pain control in anterolateral thoracic wall surgery and, simultaneously, to provide a less invasive alternative method that was equally effective, safer and easier to perform compared to paravertebral block.

A recent international consensus made by representatives from both the American Society of Regional Anesthesia and Pain Medicine (ASRA) and European Society of Regional Anaesthesia and Pain Therapy (ESRA), has defined nomenclature in abdominal wall, paraspinal, and chest wall regional anesthetic techniques:

- a superficial approach called "Superficial serratus anterior plane (SAP) block": Injection in the plane superficial to the serratus anterior muscles;
- a deeper approach, called "Deep serratus anterior plane block (SAP)": Injection in the plane between the posterior surface of the serratus anterior muscle and the periosteum of the rib.

The results obtained demonstrate, through Nuclear Magnetic Resonance (NR) reconstructions, the real effectiveness of the block in terms of dermatomeric distribution after injection of a LA and gadolinium, whether the mixture is injected over the serratus or under the muscle itself, thus showing a better diffusion of the anesthetic solution both in the anteroposterior direction and along the hemithorax in case of superficial injection. Instead, more recent evidence seems to prove the analgesic non-inferiority of a deep injection compared to superficial serratus plane injection. However, few studies have demonstrated at present the analgesic efficacy of the superficial approach compared to the deep approach.

ANATOMY AND SONOANATOMY

The anatomy of the anterolateral chest wall essentially consists of 5 muscles (**Figure 4.1**):

1. The Musculus latissimus dorsi (LTD) forms the posterior wall of the axillary cavity. The muscle is divided into four parts:

- Vertebral, between the lumbodorsal fascia, which fits on all the lumbar vertebrae and on the midsacral crest, and the last 6 thoracic vertebrae;
- Scapular (inconstant), originating from the inferior angle of the side edge of the scapula;

- Iliac, originating from the back lip of the iliac crest;
- Costal, originating from the last four ribs.
- IT is innervated by the thoracodorsal nerve (TDN), collateral branch of the posterior secondary trunk of the brachial plexus (C6-C8). The skin that covers the muscle is innervated by the dorsal and ventral branches of roots T4 to T12 and by the dorsal branches of roots L1 to L3.

2. The pectoralis major Muscle (PM) is located in the upper half of the anterior surface of the thoracic wall. It has a clavicular insertion originating from the medial wall of the anterior surface of the clavicle and a sternocostal insertion originating from the anterior surface of the handlebar and from the body of the sternum, from the anterior face of the first six ribs and from the aponeurosis of the external oblique muscle of the abdomen. The muscle, through a tendon, fits on the inner lip of the intratubercular sulcus of the humerus.
   The pectoralis major (PM) is the most superficial muscle of the thoracic wall, lying in front of the smaller pectoralis minor, innervated at the ribs and at the anterior dentate part by the medial pectoral nerve (C8 and T1) and by the lateral pectoral nerves (C5, C6, C7), while the clavicular part is innervated by C5 and C6. The skin that covers the PM is innervated by nerve roots T2 to T6.
3. The teres major (TM) is a large rounded muscle that originates from an oval-shaped area on the dorsal surface of the scapula. Together with the LTD, it forms the back of the axilla. It is inserted along the medial lip of the intratubercular sulcus of the humerus. The tendon is covered with a bursa throughout its extension, which separates it from the tendon of the latissimus dorsi muscle.
   The teres major (TM) is innervated by the inferior subscapular nerves (C6 and C7), which originates from the posterior cord of the brachial plexus.

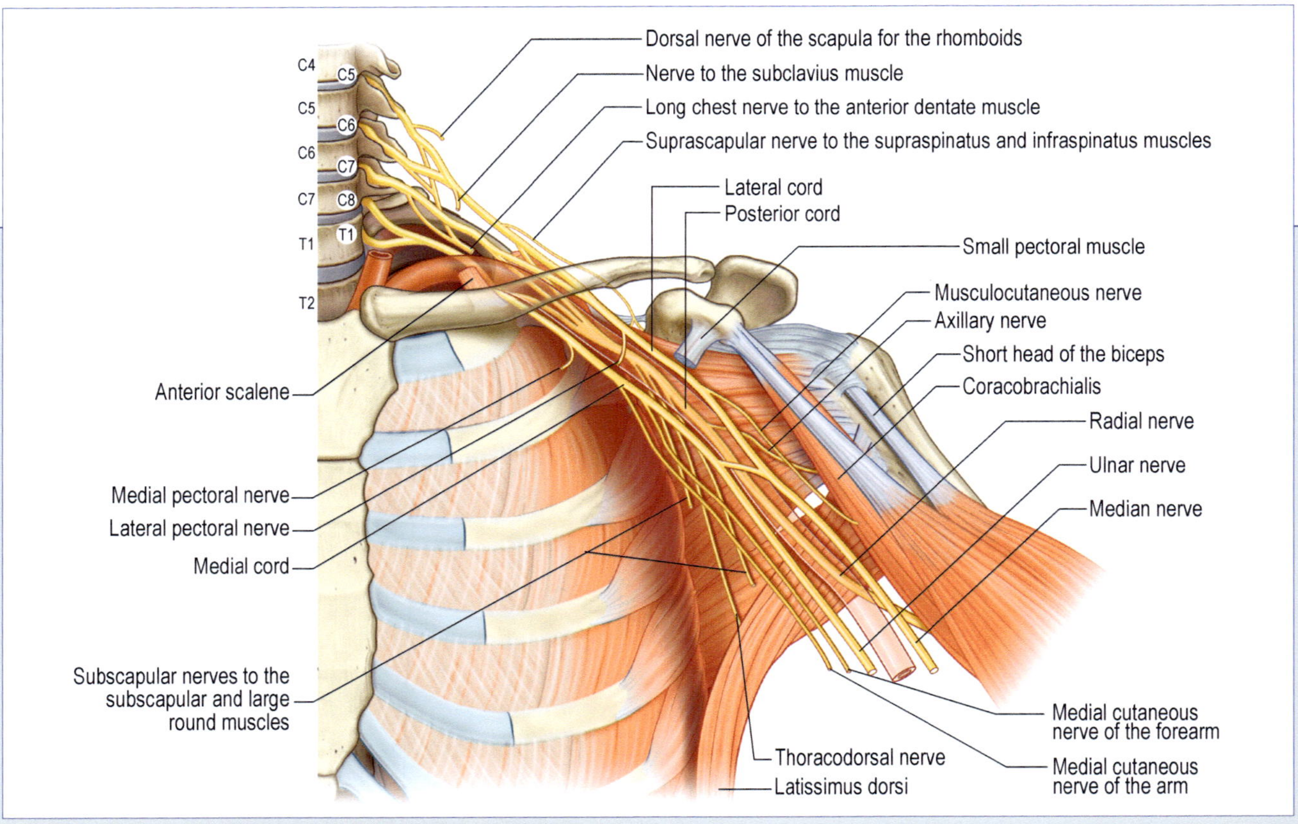

Figure 4.1 Brachial plexus, its branches and innervation muscles.

4. The pectoralis minor muscle (Pm) is a muscle located deeper than the PM and mainly performs the function of inspiratory muscle. It starts with three insertions from the outer face and posterior edge of the III, IV and V ribs. The bundle of muscles then head upwards and converge to the apex and medial edge of the coracoid process of the scapula. It is innervated by the medial pectoral nerve, which perforates and, at the level of the axilla, communicates with the lateral pectoral nerve, ensuring a double innervation. The nerve roots involved are C6, C7 and C8.
5. The Serratus anterior muscle (Sm) located on the side wall of the thorax fits into the vertebral edge of the scapula and originates on front of the first 10 ribs; it is innervated by the long chest nerve . The long thoracic nerve (LTN) is a purely motor nerve that innervates the Sm and originates from the ventral roots of C5, C6, and C7. The Sm is usually divided, due to its extension, into 3 parts, depending on where it originates on ribs and where it fits exactly on the scapula:
   - originates from the 1st to the 10th rib and fits on the upper part of the scapula;
   - originates from the 2nd to the 4th rib and fits onto the intermediate part;
   - originates from the 5th to the 9th (and sometimes 10th) rib and fits on the inferior part.

In addition to the 5 muscles described above, it is important to remember that the intercostal region consists of 3 muscle planes. From the surface to the depth, the muscle planes are:

- the external intercostal muscle;
- the internal or intermediate intercostal muscle;
- an inner muscle layer composed of the subcostal, internal intercostal, and transverse thoracic muscles.

As regards the neuroanatomy of the anterolateral thoracic wall, the main nerve structures to be kept in mind consist of the pectoral (lateral and medial) nerves, the intercostal nerves (lateral and anterior branches), the long thoracic (LTN) and thoracodorsal (TDN) nerves. Although, for educational purposes, the neuroanatomy of the anterolateral thoracic wall can be schematized as follows, it is fundamental to remember that the innervation of the thoracic mammary and axillary region receives an important contribution from branches of the cervical and brachial plexus .

The (lateral and medial) pectoral nerves are important nerves that branch off from the brachial plexus, which innervate pectoral muscles (**Figure 4.2**). The lat-

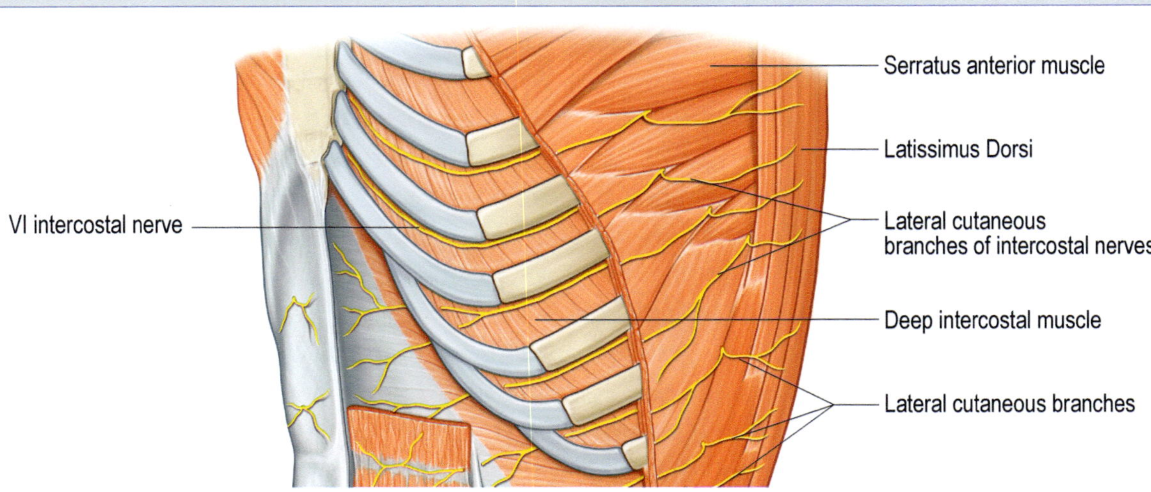

Figure 4.2 Cutaneous branches of the last intercostal nerves and of the lumbar nerves (from Gray's Anatomy – Foundations, R.L. Drake A.W. Vogl A.W.M. Mitchell – Edra 2015).

eral pectoral nerve most commonly arises from C5, C6 and C7, and the medial pectoral nerve from C8 and T1. The lateral pectoral nerve runs between the major and minor pectoral muscles on a fascial plane in the proximity of the pectoral branch of the thoracoacromial artery and innervates the Pm. The medial pectoral nerve runs below the Pm. Various Authors agree that the medial pectoral nerve crosses the Pm in 62% of patients, while it lies on its lateral margin in the remaining cases.

A second series of nerves involved consist of the anterior divisions of thoracic intercostal nerves T2 to T6. They are located posteriorly, between the pleura and the posterior intercostal membrane. Intercostal nerves divide into lateral and anterior branches (see **Figure 4.2**):

- Lateral branches: the nerves pierce the external intercostal muscles and the Sm at the mid-axillary line and then divide into anterior and posterior terminal branches. The cutaneous lateral branch of the second intercostal nerve does not divide into anterior and posterior branches and is called intercostobrachial nerve.
- Anterior branches: the nerves cross in front of the internal mammary artery and pierce the internal intercostal muscles.

Most of the skin sensitivity of the breast comes from intercostal nerves. At the exit of the intervertebral foramina, the spinal nerves of the thorax divide into dorsal and ventral branches. Dorsal branches innervate the skin and muscles of the medial spine.

Ventral branches pass through the paravertebral space to subsequently become intercostal nerves, which run in the intercostal space, just below the lower edge of the upper rib, and are accompanied by the vein and the intercostal artery. The intercostal nerves run in the plane between the innermost layer and the internal intercostal muscle. Close to the midpoint between the spine and the sternum, the skin branch unravels from each intercostal nerve and pierces the internal intercostal, external intercostal and Sm muscles. The lateral cutaneous branches then divide into anterior and posterior divisions that provide cutaneous innervation to the lateral portion of the breast. The continuation of each intercostal nerve ends as an anterior cutaneous branch (ACB), which pierces the fascial extension of the external intercostal muscle close to the lateral edge of the sternum, providing cutaneous innervation to the medial chest and sternum. The third series of nerves are the long thoracic nerve (LTN) and the thoracodorsal nerve (TDN). The LTN, also known as anterior dentate nerve, originates from C5 to C7 and then enters the axilla behind the rest of the brachial plexus, resting on the anterior dentate muscle. It innervates this muscle and, when it is damaged by trauma or radical mastectomy, it causes the deformity of the winged scapula (scapula alata). During surgery, the dentate muscle is dissected along with the pectoral muscles to create a pocket necessary for the positioning of the expanders.

The LTN is a branch of the posterior cord, composed of the three posterior divisions of the trunks of the brachial plexus. It innervates the back wall of the armpit. It runs in depth, and is important for breast reconstruction.

The TDN, or middle subscapular nerve, originates from C6-C8, and is therefore a branch of the posterior cord of the brachial plexus. This nerve runs in the axillary cavity, accompanied by the thoracodorsal artery, and provides innervation to the LTD muscle. This nerve has a deep course and plays an important role in reconstructive breast surgery of the latissimus dorsi flap.

The sonoanatomy of the lateral thoracic wall, with sagittal scan at the level of the fifth rib on the mid axillary line (approach described by Blanco et al.), shows three muscle structures starting from the skin and subcutaneous tissue, separated by hyperechoic bands: from the outside towards the inside, the ultrasound image (**Figure 4.3**) will show:

a) the following muscles:
- (superficial and posterior) latissimus dorsi;
- (upper and most proximal) teres major (TM);
- Serratus anterior muscle;

b) the underlying ribs, visible through the typical hyperechoic rounded image and the corresponding posterior shadow cone.

The nerves of the thoracic wall cannot be displayed within the SM bands, although their identification is not necessary for the execution of the block.

DESCRIPTION OF THE TECHNIQUE

The purpose of the block is to position the needle tip between LTD and Sm, and inject the anesthetic solution into this interfascial plane to block the thoracic nerves running through these muscles. The injection of LA into the SAP provides unilateral analgesia of the skin, muscles and bones of the anterolateral thoracic wall. The block has been described and introduced with an ultrasound-guided technique that allows for an accurate injection of the LA into the target neurovascular plane, which also provides ultrasound confirmation of the correct "opening" of the plane. The block should be performed after inducing general anesthesia or, in any case, after adequate sedoanalgesia in case of awake surgery, and always before the procedure. The use of the SAP block in a multimodal context may certainly be beneficial both in terms of perioperative pain control and to avoid opioid analgesics and reduce their related side effects.

The following material is required for this block:

- ultrasound system equipped with a high-frequency linear probe (6-12 MHz);
- probe cover, not necessarily sterile, for single-shot block;
- standard LRA tray;
- antiseptic agent for skin disinfection and gloves, not necessarily sterile, for single-shot;
- 50-100 mm, 20-21 G TAP block (Sonotap®) needle;
- 20-40 ml of LA;
- 10 ml syringe containing saline and a 3-way stopcock (for hydrolocalization).

The presence of a nurse is recommended for the LA injection and to help with preinfusion aspiration, thus providing a further safety measure. The block can be performed either on an awake patient, after adequate sedoanalgesia, or, more commonly, with the patient under general anesthesia.

The positioning of the needle tip and the injection of the LA into the SAP are guided by ultrasonography, using the technique described by Blanco; this will confirm the "opening" of the target interfascial plane. The ultrasound probe must be protected by the special protective sheath and covered with ultrasound gel. With the patient in the supine position, with an arm along the flank or abducted at 90° (**Figure 4.4**), after careful disinfection of the skin, a high-frequency linear probe (6-18 MHz) is placed at the level of the deltoid-pectoral sulcus with a sagittal scan plane.

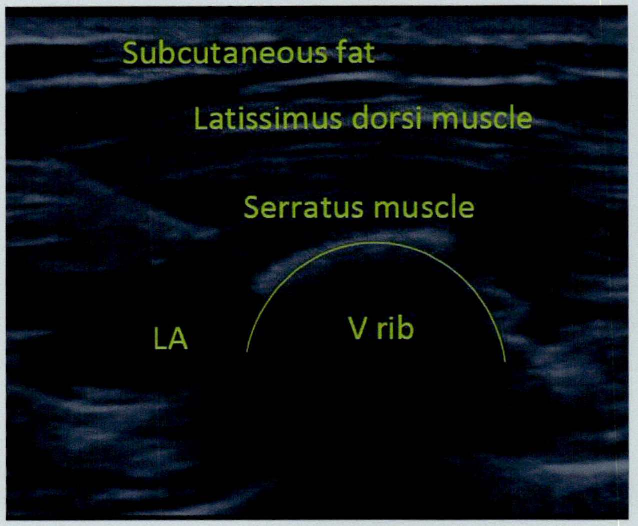

Figure 4.3 Sonoanatomy SAP block. Ultrasonography performed at the level of the fifth rib on the mid-axillary line with sagittal scan.

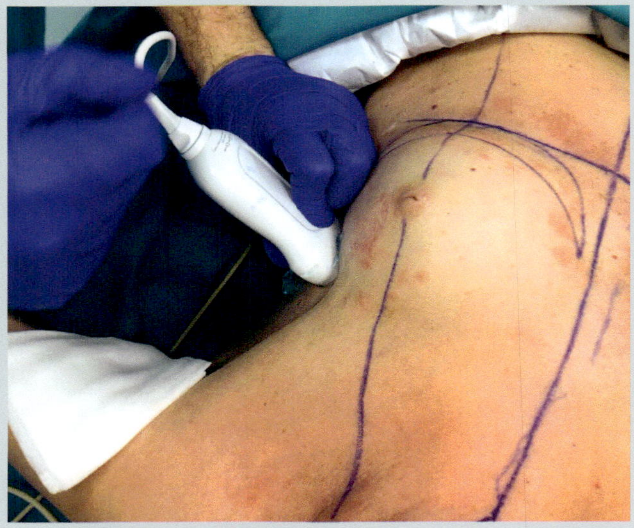

Figure 4.4 SAP block. Patient position.

Subsequently, after slightly medializing the probe, the probe is moved in the inferior and lateral areas counting down the ribs until the fifth rib is identified at the level of the mid-axillary line. At this level, the superficial and posterior latissimus dorsi, the upper teres major and the deep and lower anterior dentate muscles can be easily viewed above the fifth rib. As a further sonoanatomical landmark, we recommend using the toracodorsal artery, as it helps identifying the surface plane at the dentate muscle that separates it from the LTD muscle. Alternatively, the surgeon may start from the lower costal arch and go up with the scan plane counting up the ribs above until the fifth rib is identified on the mid-axillary line. The needle is introduced with an in-plane technique with a cranio-caudal and anteroposterior direction, until it reaches the fifth rib on the mid-axillary line (**Figures 4.5**, **4.6**, **4.7**). Under continuous ultrasound guidance, the local anesthetic (LA) mixture is injected at the level of the target fascial plane; this allows to evaluate its spreading and to monitor the needle and its tip throughout the procedure. As previously described by Blanco, an injection may be made at the superficial plane or in depth with respect to the Sm. In the first case, the correct execution of the block will be highlighted by the "opening" of the fascial plane between the Sm and the LTD, and by the spreading of the LA inside it (**Figure 4.8**). If using deep injection, the success of the technique will be shown by a homogeneous and linear spreading of the LA above the costal plane and simultaneously by the "lowering" of the external inter-

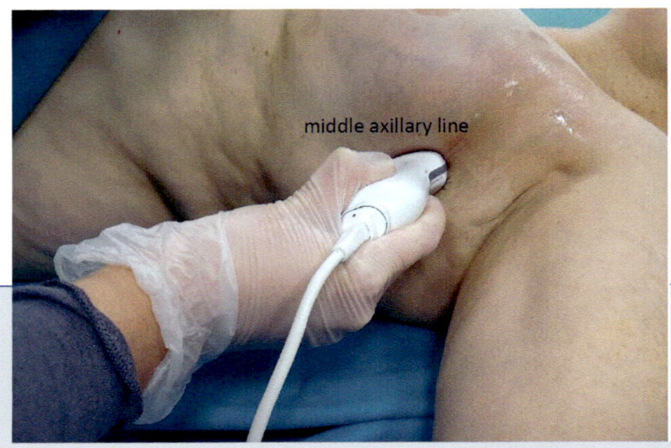

Figure 4.6 SAP block. Puncture in the cranio-caudal and antero-posterior direction.

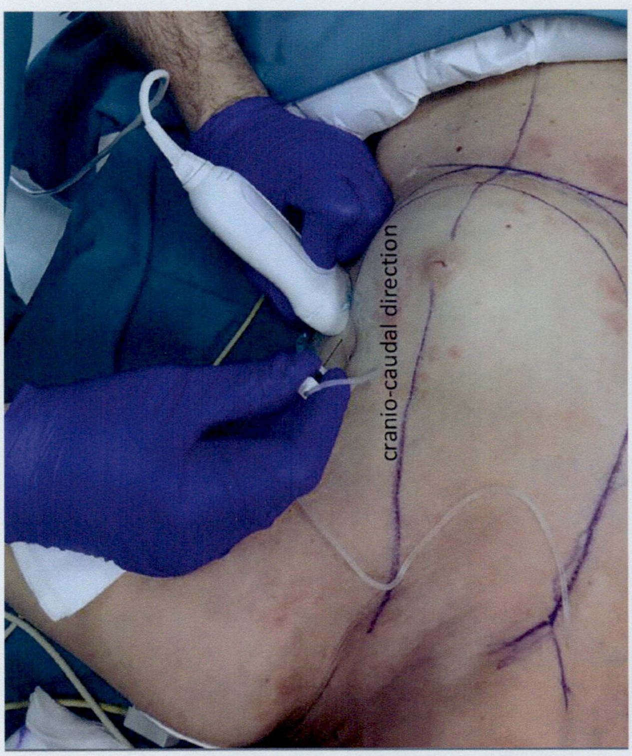

Figure 4.5 SAP block. Positioning of the probe and probe-needle alignment.

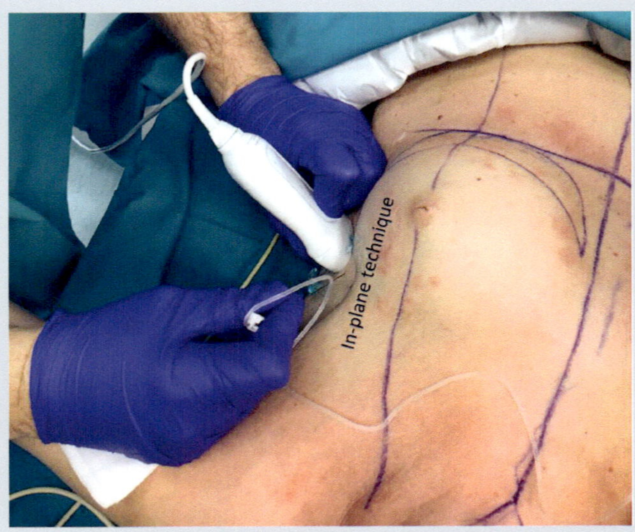

Figure 4.7 SAP block. In-plane ultrasound-guided technique and probe-needle (SonoPlex stim Pajunk®) alignment.

costal muscle downwards by the anesthetic solution (**Figure 4.9**, **Video 4.1**). For a correct injection in the deep plane of the Sm, the Authors suggest to position the tip of the needle at the lateral edge of the fifth rib. In the original study by Blanco et al., the injection of the anesthetic mixture below the Sm showed a lower efficacy and dermatomeric extension (T2-T6 versus T2-T9 in the superficial approach), in addition to being less easy to perform because of being deeper and closer to the pleura. However, we point out that the Deep SAP block may be particularly useful in cases where the plane between Sm and LTD muscles is not properly outlined due to the presence of scar tissue; for example, after radical mastectomy and axillary lymph node dissection. In such circumstances, the injection at the surface plane of the Sm may be difficult to perform, resulting in an incorrect spreading of the LA.

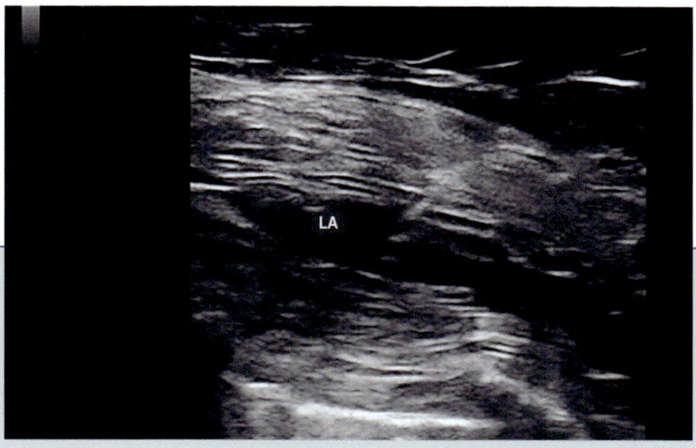

Figure 4.8 Superficial SAP block. Dissection of the plane between SM and LTD after injection of a LA. SM: serratus anterior muscle; LTD: Latissums dorsi.

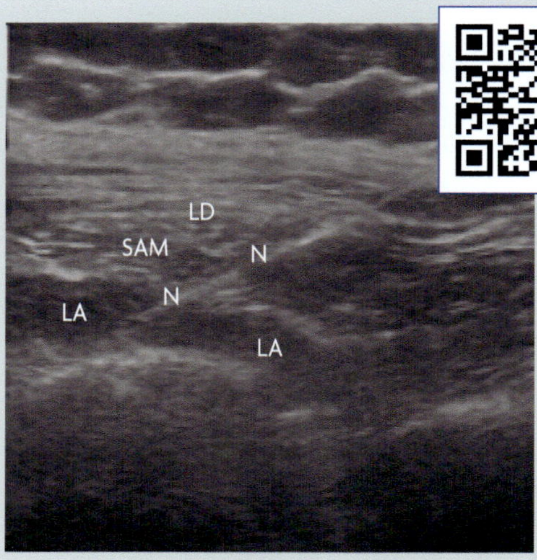

Figure 4.9 Spread of local anesthetic confirmed by ultrasound guidance. LA: local anesthetic; LD: Latissimus dorsi; N: needle; SAM: serratus anterior muscle.

The efficacy and safety of this blockade has not been validated at the present time by a large number of clinical studies. Moreover, it is important to remember that, although the SAP block provides adequate analgesia in the hemithorax by blocking the lateral branches of the thoracic intercostal nerves, this technique does not block the anterior branches of the same nerves for an analgesic coverage of the medial region of the breast.

Although there are only a few studies on this topic in literature, continuous SAP block may also be used. Data on the actual feasibility and efficacy of the technique are currently limited.

A case report showed the efficacy of the continuous SAP block in the control of post-thoracotomy pain by injecting a continuous infusion of bupivacaine 0.1% and fentanyl 1 mcg/ml at a rate of 7 ml/h.

A further contribution was made by the Torrano et al. group, who used a continuous catheter positioned in a patient undergoing radical mastectomy and reconstruction surgery with temporary expanders.

At the end of the procedure, an ultrasound-visible-catheter over the needle (E-Cath®) was inserted into the anatomical space created by the local anesthetic spread in the posterior plane of the serratus anterior muscle, giving a continuous infusion of levobupivacaine 0.125% 10 ml/h (**Figure 4.10**).

Sterility must be ensured for the continuous positioning of catheters, in order not only to avoid iatrogenic complications, but, above all, not to nullify the analgesia obtained. The in-plane approach of the needle to the ultrasound probe is recommended. The echogenic needle is (SonoPlex stim Pajunk®) available to obtain a better visibility of the needle through the muscle planes of the chest wall.

Once the "opening" of the target fascial plane has been achieved, the catheter can be inserted, thus displaying the tip and facilitating progression within the plane.

The use of adhesive fasteners and polyester patches is recommended, as well as only clear antimicrobial dressings with chlorhexidine gel. An initial bolus of 10-20 ml of anesthetic solution can be injected from the catheter.

Continuous infusion of the LA may be obtained either by a programmed PCA pump with 0.2% ropivacaine or other anesthetic solutions such as levobupivacaine 0.375%, 0.125%, 0.25%. Fascial blocks may be a viable alternative to peridural infusion in cases where neuraxial anesthesia and deep peripheral blocks are not recommended for patient therapy (anticoagulants and antiaggregating agents) or in certain clinical conditions (coagulopathies) (**Flow chart 4.1 online**).

LOCAL ANESTHETIC INDICATIONS AND DOSAGES

The ultrasound-guided SAP block may be a viable alternative in the cases where epidural analgesia and PVB are contraindicated, unfeasible or rejected by the patient. At present, analgesic/anesthetic efficacy has been documented in:

- breast cancer surgery (mastectomy, mastectomy with axillary lymph node dissection, quadrantectomy, quadrantectomy with axillary lymph node dissection);
- breast reconstruction surgery (with positioning of expander or prostheses);
- anesthetic breast surgery;
- analgesia in S-ICD implantation;
- analgesia in rib fractures (and thoracic drainage in polytrauma patients (**Figure 4.11**).

The SAPB clinically provide anterolateral and posterior analgesia (Rose, P. et al).

The mechanism of analgesic efficacy of the SAP block in posterior rib fractures is not clear. Johnston, D.F. et al have found in a cadaveric study that the mechanism is likely due to rib trauma, because the disrupted tissue planes appear to facilitate spread of injectate through the muscle planes to the intercostal nerves, allowing for posterior coverage. Local anesthetics could extend deep to iliocostalis and longissimus thoracis muscles based on the cadaveric finding of further posterior extent of SP spread in the fractured specimens.

- Analgesia in patients with chest trauma hospitalized in ICU, favoring early weaning from mechanical ventilation;
- Thoracic surgery (video-assisted thoracic surgery-VATS lobectomy, alternative to epidural analgesia in post-thoracic pain control);
- Orthopedic surgery (anesthetic coverage of the thoracic component in shoulder surgery, LTD muscle reconstruction).

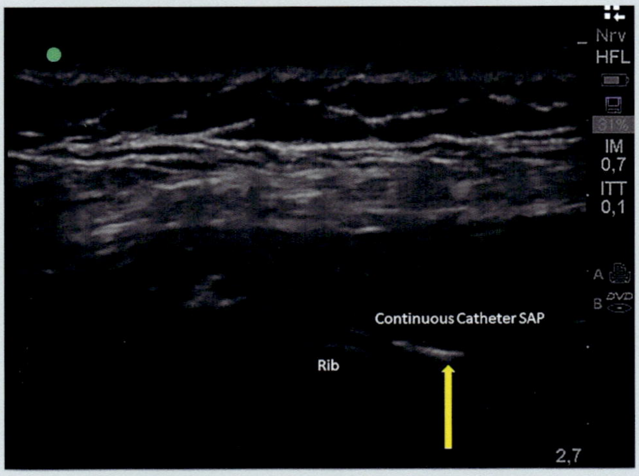

Figure 4.10 Continuous catheter positioned in the deep serratus plane block.

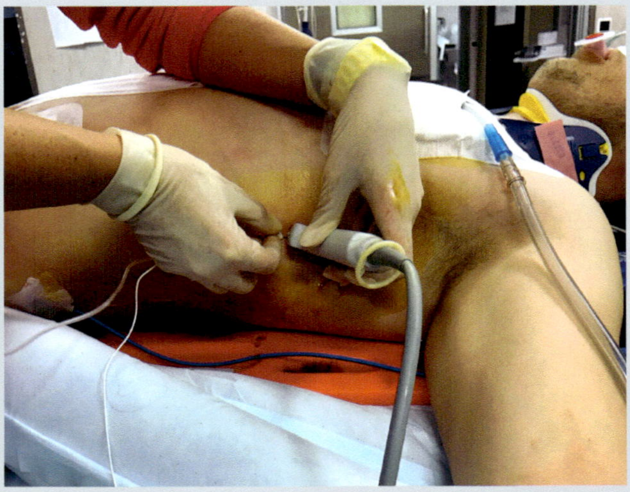

Figure 4.11 Deep serratus plane block in Thoracic Trauma.

With regard to execution timing, the SAP block should be carried out before surgical incision to exploit the analgesic/intraoperative anesthetic effect, to have intact muscle landmarks, and not to have situations of conflict with the surgical site and wound dressings. The effectiveness of the blockade is related to the spread of the LA rather than its concentration, and it is volume-dependent. This concept is fundamental, since the SAP block, being a compartment block, requires generous volumes of LA to ensure the blockade of the lateral branches of the intercostal nerves and to ensure adequate coverage of the lower thoracic dermatomes. A dosage of 0.4 ml/kg may be used for the calculation of the volume to be used (**Table 4.1**). Saying this, providing the block before surgery, and so before tissues disruption, may allow the provider to exploit the fascial sheets integrity in order to guarantee a wider spread of LA through the target plane.

COMPLICATIONS AND CONTRAINDICATIONS

The SAP block, if carried out by experienced operators and with an ultrasound-guided technique, is a relatively simple technique and could prove to be very safe for superficial target structures and for the distance from "noble" structures, such as the vessels and the pleura.

Complications have not been described at the moment; however, as with the TAP block, the need for generous volumes of local anesthetic, especially if performed bilaterally, may result in high plasma concentrations of LA, increasing the risk of LAST.

There are currently no contraindications or documented complications in the literature for patients under anti-aggregation and anticoagulation therapy or with coagulopathies.

Cases where the block is NOT recommended

Contraindications:

- Patient's refusal
- Allergy to the LA
- Infection at the injection site

Complications

- Vascular puncture (if performed by inexperienced operators)
- Pneumothorax (if performed by inexperienced operators)
- Increased risk of LAST (linked to high volumes of LA used or to failure to comply with maximum recommended dosages)

PEDIATRIC APPLICATION

The SAP block is also indicated in the pediatric area, in the surface surgery of the lateral thoracic wall, which involves the lateral branches of the thoracic intercostal nerves T2-T6, with variable extension up to T9. In recent years, the introduction of ultrasound guidance in LRA has significantly increased the application of peripheral nerve blocks, and especially of fascial plane blocks, in the pediatric population as well. Some case reports in literature have documented the efficacy of the SAP block in pediatric patients undergoing minimally-invasive thoracic surgery (VATS) or thoracotomy for aortic coarctation repair. However, the block must be performed by experienced operators with pediatric anesthesia skills.

Strict compliance with the maximum allowable dosages is also recommended, as the SAP block, being a

TABLE 4.1 DOSAGES AND VOLUMES OF LOCAL ANESTHETIC TO BE USED IN THE SAP BLOCK

	Local anesthetic volume	Concentration and local anesthetic recommended
Adult	20-40 ml	Ropivacaine 0.25% or 0.375%, Levobupivacaine 0.25% or 0.375%
Child	0.25-0.75 mg/kg	Ropivacaine (Evidence B1)

volume-dependent block, may require generous LA volumes, resulting in an increased risk of LAST. Recent ASRA/ESRA recommendations suggest that the dose of bupivacaine or ropivacaine of 0.25-0.75 mg/kg (Evidence B1) should be observed in fascial plane blocks.

INDICATIONS IN CHRONIC PAIN

In the light of the proven analgesic efficacy of the SAP block, several pieces of evidence suggested potential applications of the technique in the management of chronic pain syndromes of the thoracic wall.
In literature, several studies have documented the successful use of the SAP block in the management of postmastectomy or post-thoracotomy chronic pain syndromes refractory to drug therapy, with a considerable improvement in the quality of life of treated patients.

SERRATUS ANTERIOR PLANE BLOCK IN CARDIAC SURGERY

Thanks to the growth of minimally invasive cardiac surgery and specifically with the use of nonsternotomy incisions such as mini-thoracotomy, the use of ultrasound nerve blocks for postoperative pain management has increased. Thoracotomy is a surgical incision between the intercostal space that produces direct trauma to cartilage tissue, ribs, muscles or peripheral nerves inducing more intense postoperative pain than the one resulting from median sternotomy. On this basis, optimal analgesia became an integral part of enhanced recovery after surgery (ERAS) protocols designed to reduce postoperative complications, hospitalization time and improve patients' outcome.
Pain management after cardiac surgery is very important to enhance the deep breathing, coughing and early ambulation which are critical for respiratory care, early recovery and prognosis. Pain is most severe during the first 24 hours and decreases on subsequent days, because it is a self-limiting phenomenon. In the early postoperative period, within the first 24 hours, the most painful areas are those directly related to thoracotomy like the chest, mediastinal and pleural drain-placement sites (**Figure 4.12 A**) and can often compromise a patient's respiratory dynamics, increasing the risk of respiratory complications, especially in severe chronic obstructive pulmonary disease (COPD) patients, and late extubation. Both aortic or mitral valve replacement and coronary artery bypass grafting can be treated by mini-thoracotomy surgery where the sternum is not opened. For this reason, exacerbation of postoperative pain is also influenced by the extent of traumatization of the intercostal nerves when the intercostal space is opened. This maneuver increases the risk of damage to the nerve inflicted by the rib in cases of fracture or by compression exerted by dilator during surgery (**Figure 4.12 B**) Moreover, the presence of postoperative drainages intensifies the parietal pleura innervated by the intercostal and phrenic nerves.

Cardiac surgery pain management

The opioid administration represents the mainstay for cardiac-surgery pain management even if it is associated with several adverse effects, including sedation, nausea, vomiting, ileus and respiratory depression. A particularly dangerous sequel of severe pain after cardiac surgery procedures are dysfunctions of the respiratory system. Pain is the cause of reflex muscular tension and impairs the patient's activity or even immobilizes them. It leads to a shortness of breath and to a reduction in tidal volume, vital capacity, functional residual capacity and pulmonary compliance. The fear of pain also impairs the exptectoration of secretions accumulating in the bronchial tree, which may result in atelectasis, pulmonary infections and hypoxemia of arterial blood, myocardial ischemia or infarction, cerebrovascular accidents, thromboembolism, delayed wound healing. There is growing and emerging scientific evidence for the analgesic/anesthetic fascial plane blocks efficacy in cardiac surgery with a reduced side effect profile in an opioid-free/opioid-sparing anesthetic protocols. A successful introduction of ERAS protocols is possible, but a multidisciplinary approach is imperative for success. In particular, an adequate analgesia after thoracotomy incision is important because pain is a key component in the alteration of lung function that leads to increased morbidity and prolonged hospital stay.

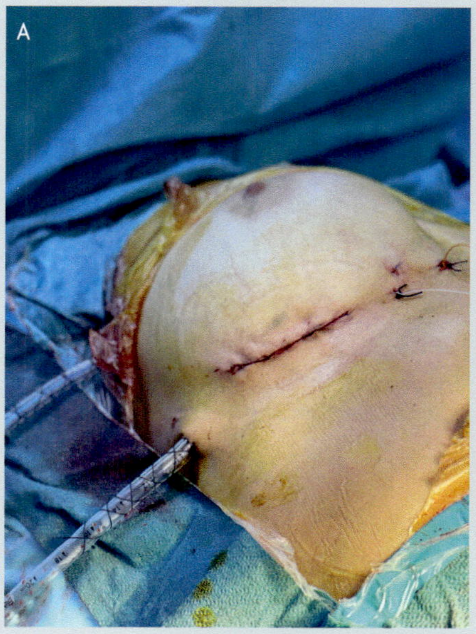

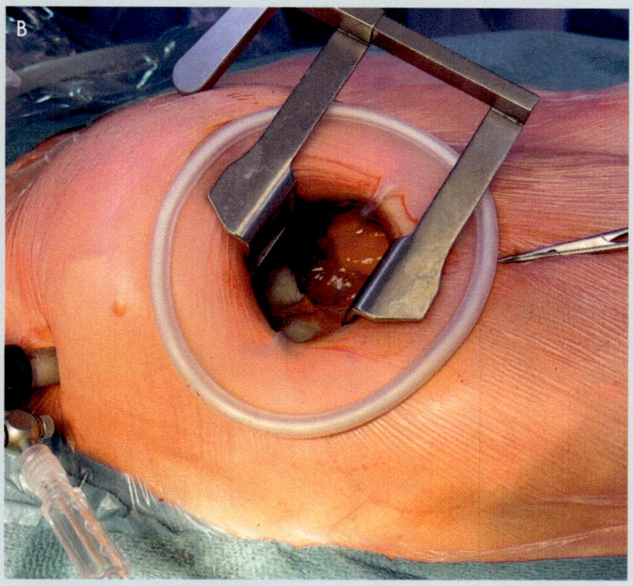

Figure 4.12 A The most painful areas are those directly related to thoracotomy like the chest, mediastinal and pleural drain-placement sites. **B** Postoperative pain deriving from thoracotomy is also influenced by the extent of traumatization of the intercostal nerve when the intercostal space is opened.

Serratus plane block: indications, dosages and technique description

The surgery of anterolateral chest wall is often accompanied by severe postoperative pain, leading to postoperative infection, atelectasis and prolonged hospitalization. Paravertebral block and thoracic epidural analgesia have indisputably comparable postoperative analgesic profiles following thoracotomy. However, the use of neuraxial blocks in cardiac surgery is controversial due to the risk of bleeding or spinal hematoma in the setting of anticoagulation therapy. Recently, the ultrasound-guided serratus anterior plane block (SAPB) has improved the safety and the success rate of cardiac surgery operations with a similar analgesic efficacy of neuraxial blocks profile. SAPB is performed using ultrasound at the level of the midaxillary line and the fifth rib, and the local anesthetic is injected either superficially or deeply into the serratus anterior muscle, blocking the third to sixth intercostal nerves, the long thoracic and thoracodorsal nerves. The trial by Toscano et al. stated that SAPB has a promising role for analgesia after cardiac surgery. In a small, randomized controlled trial comparing the analgesic efficacy of SAPB versus thoracic epidural for pain after thoracotomy, Khalil et al. demonstrated no significant differences in the visual analog pain scores or rescue morphine requirement. In a recent randomized trial, Hanley et al. reported the noninferiority of the SAPB as compared to paravertebral blockade for pain after thoracotomy. SAPB in cardiothoracic surgery is performed both as a single shot and continuous local anesthetic infusion technique. The single shot is usually used in emergency conditions to abolish the pain deriving from rib fractures or from the chest tube insertion for pneumothorax or pleural effusion management (**Figure 4.13 A**, **B**, **Video 4.2**)

The continuous technique is performed for intra and postoperative analgesia management in patients undergoing mini-thoracotomy approach such as video-assisted thoracic surgery (VATS), mitral valve replacement (MVR) or coronary artery bypass grafting (CABG), at least 30 ml of local anesthetic is required

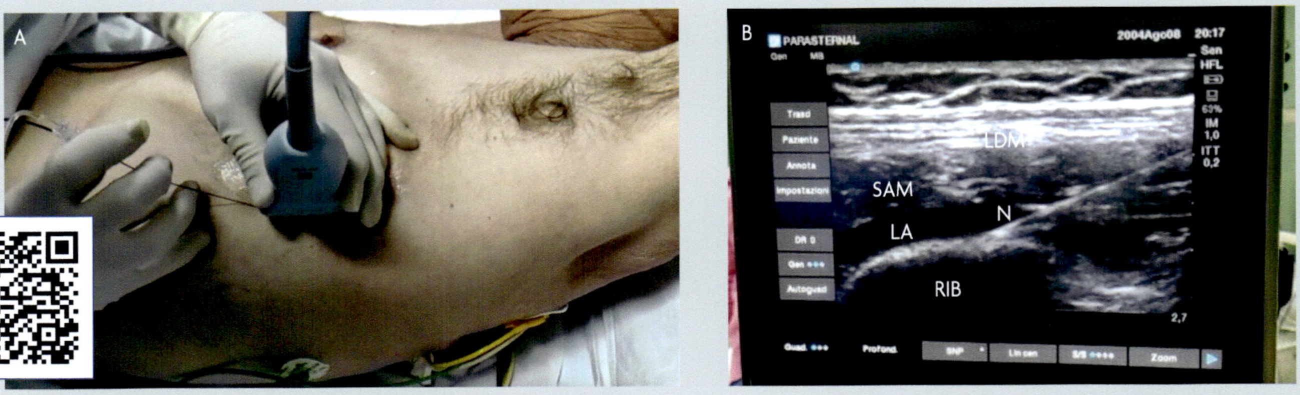

Figure 4.13 A Patient, needle (SonoPlex stim Pajunk®) and probe position. **B** Deep serratus anterior plane block; LA: local anesthetic; LDM: latissimus dorsi muscle; N: needle; RIB: rib; SAM: serratus anterior muscle.

to perform the SAPB. The continuous postoperative analgesia is realized by an infusion of local anesthetic at 7-10 ml/h for at least 24 hours.

The single-shot or continuous serratus anterior plane block (C-SAPB) is performed with the patient in a supine position. A high frequencies linear probe is placed on the midaxillary line and a 100 mm 20 g SonoPlex stim Pajunk® needle is used to perform the single-shot procedure while a needle Tuohy is used to realize the continuous technique. Via an in-plane approach in a caudal to cephalad direction, local anesthetic is injected into the interfascial plane between the latissimus dorsi (LDM) and serratus anterior muscle (SAM) realizing the superficial serratus anterior plane block (S-SAPB) or into the interfascial plane between SAM and external intercostal muscles (EIM) performing the deep serratus anterior plane block (D-SAPB) or BRILMA (The block of the lateral branches of the intercostal nerves in the middle axillary line) When used, in order to better fix and avoid its displacement, it is useful to place the catheter at level of fifth intercostal space in a caudal to cranial direction between the SAM and the EIM and ribs realizing the continuous deep serratus anterior plane block (CD-SAPB) (**Figures 4.14 A**, **B**, **C**). SAPB provides analgesia to the hemithorax from the 2nd (T2) to the 9th (T9) thoracic dermatomes making the technique similar to the Erector spinae block (ESP). Both the procedures could be used to manage the thoracotomy pain even if some substantial considerations are required. It is advisable to perform monolateral ESP before general anesthesia with the patient in lateral decubitus to minimize dangerous hemodynamic instability (hypertension, hypotension, arrhythmia, lipothymia, bradycardia) that may occur with cardiac critically ill patients in a sitting position. On this basis, in order to drastically reduce the hemodynamic complications, it seems useful to perform CD-SAPB with the patient in a supine position after general anesthesia induction. Furthermore the SAPB and Pecs II blocks are simple single-shot effective alternatives to ICNB with a prolonged analgesic duration following thoracotomy and can potentially enhance pain-free recovery after cardiac surgery.

Conclusions

The ultrasound-guided serraturs anterior plane block in cardiac surgery represents an integral part of ERAS protocols reducing the length of stay, respiratory complications and opioid adverse effects. Its main advantage is represented by performing it with the patient in supine position avoiding dangerous hemodynamic instability such as hypertension, hypotension, arrhythmia, lipothymia, bradycardia that may occur with cardiac critically ill patients in a sitting position. Moreover, SAPB has a high success rate, fewer compli-

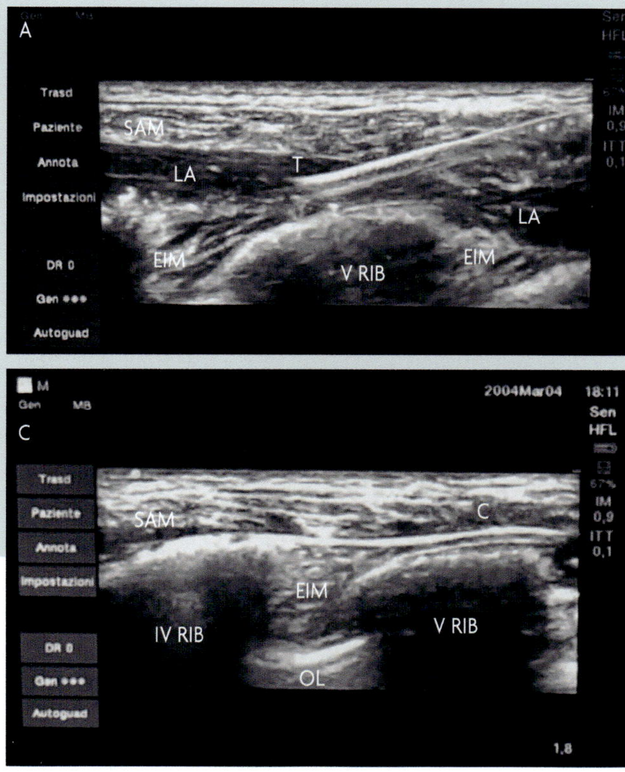

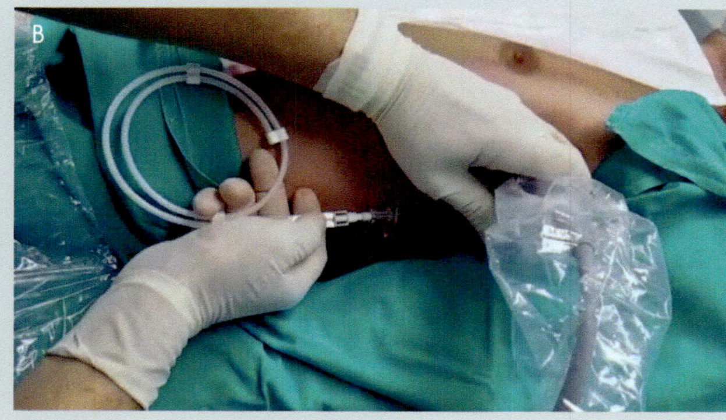

Figure 4.14 Continuous deep serratus anterior plane block. **A** Needle (E-Cath® insertion and local anesthetic injection. **B** Catheter insertion. **C** Catheter placement. C: catheter; EIM: external intercostal muscle; LA: local anesthetic; PL: pleura; RIB: rib; SAM: serratus anterior muscle; T: Tuohy needle.

cations and simpler effective postoperative analgesia compared with thoracic epidural analgesia and thoracic paravertebral block.

SERRATUS PLANE BLOCK IN THORACIC SURGERY AND TRAUMA

Serratus plane block (SAPB) is an ultrasound (US) guided interfascial plane block described for the first time in 2013 by Blanco. The use of Serratus plane block is increasing especially for the anesthesia and analgesia in thoracic surgery, breast surgery and in thoracic trauma. The SAPB is an alternative that has become popular due to its efficacy, relative easy, and limited side-effects profile compared with the anesthetic techniques most used in the past in surgery and thoracic trauma, such as: paravertebral block and thoracic epidural anesthesia. Pain control in Thoracic surgery and thoracic trauma, plays a fundamental role in improving patient outcome. Uncontrolled chest pain is responsible for the alteration in the respiratory dynamics of the rib cage, with an increase in the incidence of atelectasis, pneumonia and respiratory distress with prolonged ICU stay and therefore in mortality and morbidity.

In recent years the literature has concentrated on and validated the use of the SAPB in multiple ribs fracture. Actually intravenous opioids are a mainstay of treatment in multiple ribs fracture, but have side effects, including respiratory depression, depressed cough reflex, and delirium in the elderly. Several trials have been carried out and have highlighted the superiority of this locoregional anesthesia technique over conventional pharmacological therapies. Furthermore the total opioid consumption significantly lower in patient group that receive an analgesia by serratus plane block. To date, the major interest in SAPB is aimed at pain control and the prevention of the development of chronic pain after Video-assisted thoracic surgery (VATS). A gold standard for regional analgesia for VATS procedures has not yet surfaced, the studies published so far are very heterogeneous. Paravertebral block (PVB) and catheter techniques might have a positive effect on pain scores, but this technique is more difficult to perform and has more side effects than SAPB. For this reason, to date, an implementation of the use of this technique and the creation of a standard of pain management in thoracic surgery is fundamental in the perspective of a future based on ERAS protocols.

However a recent study by Rodney A Gabriel et al, show that the SAPB provided inferior analgesia compared with paravertebral blocks.
There is still a long way to go to create a standard in chest pain treatment, however, it can be said that the SAPB will play a fundamental role in this context.
In conclusion the SAPB can play an important role in management of pain after thoracic surgery by reducing both pain scores and 24-h postoperative opioids consumption. In addition, there is less incidence of PONV (Post Operativ Nausea and Vomiting) . Furthermore US guided SAPB is an opioid sparing effective interfascial plane block which is safe and should be considered early in all patients who sustain multiple ribs fracture.

The prospect Working Group of the European Society of Regional Anesthesia and Pain Therapy recently performed a systematic review of the scientific literature which highlighted how the use of SAPB single shot represents the ideal choice for the management of perioperative pain in VATS (grade A).
The use of continuous SAPB is also increasing more and more, because it is believed to provide pain relief for a longer duration, facilitate early mobilization, physiotherapy and initial discharge from the ICU. Although to date the grade of evidence is still low (grade D), due to the continuous benefits of the SAPB, research in this regard is making great strides. Is it the beginning of a new era (**Figure 4.15**)?!

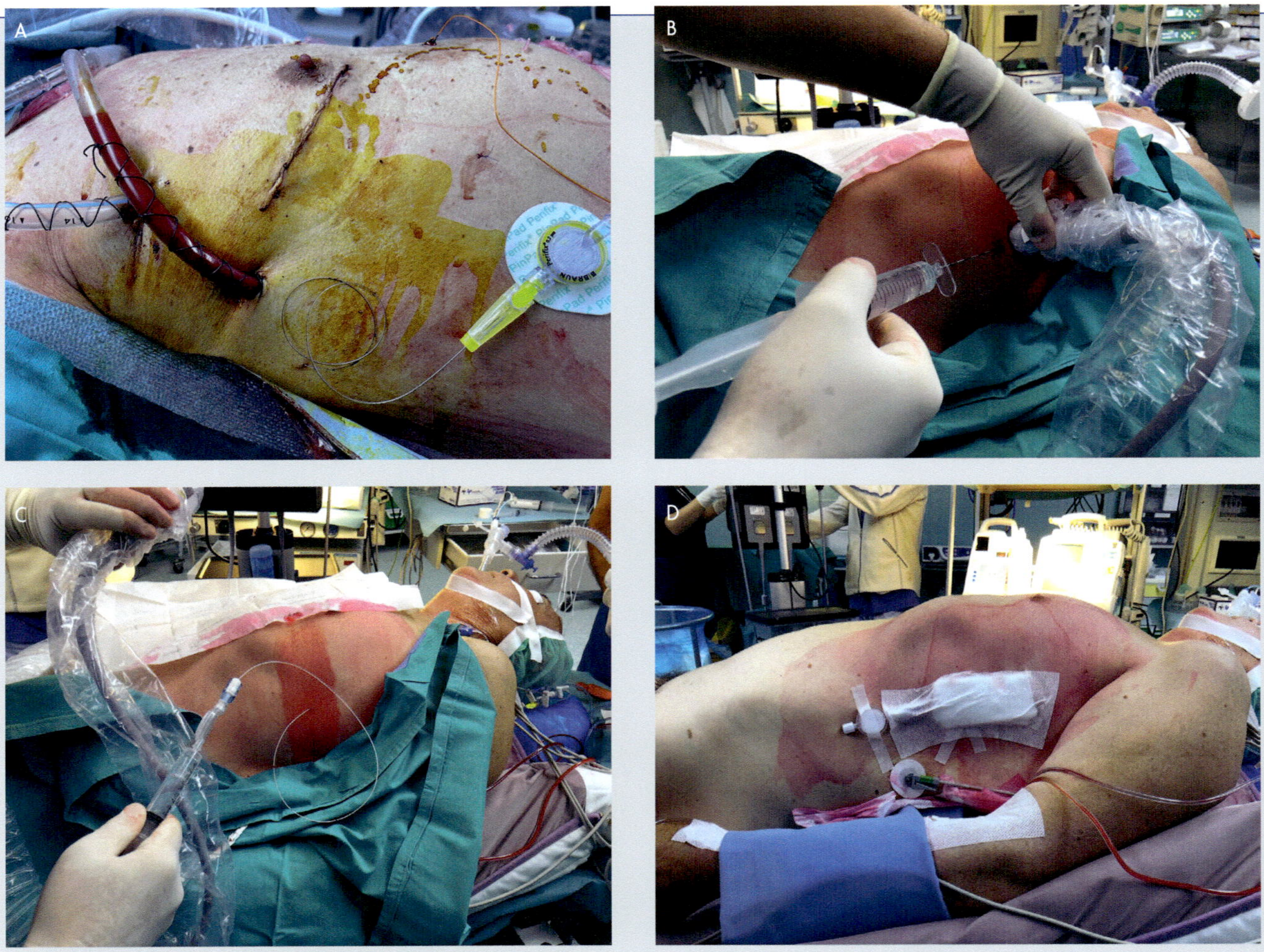

Figure 4.15 Continuous deep serratus plane block in thoracic surgery.

INTERCOSTAL NERVE BLOCK

Intercostal nerve block is a technique that provides segmental anesthesia-analgesia of the chest wall at selected levels. This block is indicated for postoperative anesthesia and analgesia in thoracic (thoracotomy, thoracostomy) and upper abdominal wall surgery (gastrostomy, and cholecystectomy). It has a documented beneficial effect on respiratory function, as well as in the treatment of acute and chronic pain conditions of various etiologies (post-traumatic pain, neuralgia, causalgia), which are unresponsive to conventional therapies.

The mechanism of action at the basis of the effectiveness of the technique is attributable to the blocking of the lateral cutaneous rami of the intercostal nerves which run, within the selected intercostal space, along the inferior margin of the overlying rib (**Figure 4.16**).

Anatomy and sonoanatomy

The thoracic spinal nerves are 12 pairs and emerge from the spinal cord with two roots: the dorsal sensory root and the ventral motor root.

The roots of the thoracic spinal nerves, after emergence from their respective intervertebral foramina, divide mainly into dorsal and ventral primary rami, as well as issuing meningeal rami that innervate the spinal canal and the meninges, white and grey communicating rami that anastomose with the adjacent ganglia of the sympathetic trunk to supply the viscera and vessels, and sympathetic fibres for the spinal cord.

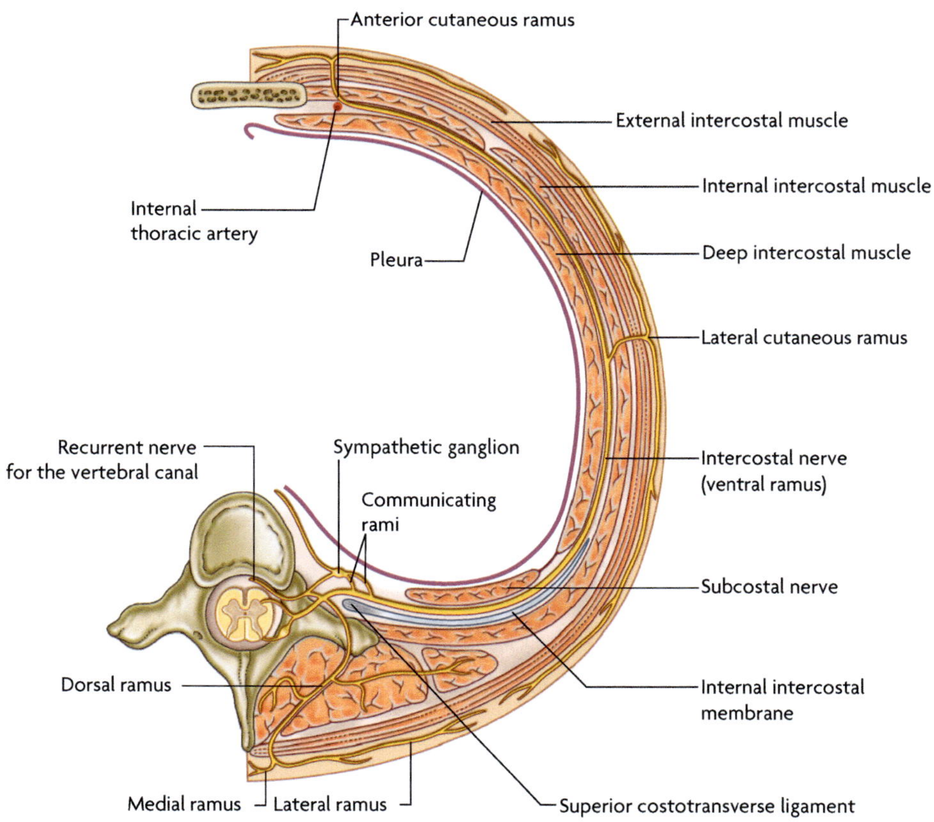

Figure 4.16 Course of a typical intercostal nerve.

The dorsal ramus of the thoracic spinal nerves provides the innervation of the skin and muscles of the para-vertebral region; the ventral ramus continues laterally as the intercostal nerve.

The intercostal nerves have a segmental distribution and are responsible for the innervation of the skin and muscles of the thoracic and abdominal wall. These nerves, after the emergence from the PVS, perforate the internal intercostal membrane approximately 3 cm lateral to the intervertebral foramen, and run between the external and internal intercostal muscles, to subsequently enter the subcostal groove, where they run in the vascular-nervous bundle, inferior to the intercostal artery and vein (**Figure 4.17**).

It should be remembered, because of this anatomical arrangement, that special care must be taken during invasive procedures carried out at this level, due to the close proximity of the nerves to the blood vessels, which could lead to accidental intravascular injection, with the possibility of reaching toxic concentrations of LA in the systemic circulation.

The 11 upper nerves are pure intercostal, in that they travel at least partially in the intercostal spaces. The twelfth, however, runs along the lower margin of the twelfth rib and is called the subcostal nerve. Initially, the intercostal nerves run between the parietal pleura and the internal intercostal membrane. Near the costal angle, these nerves make the rest of their journey in the space between the internal intercostal muscles and innermost intercostal (intercostalis intimi) muscles, running caudally to the intercostal vessels. At the mid-axillary line, the intercostal nerves then give rise to the lateral cutaneous rami, which cross the internal and external intercostal muscles to provide innervation of the muscles and skin of the lateral thoracic, abdominal, and axillary region. The last nerve endings of the intercostal nerves are represented by the anterior cutaneous rami, responsible for the innervation of the skin and muscles of the anterior region of the trunk, including the skin of the suprasternal region and the rectus abdominis.

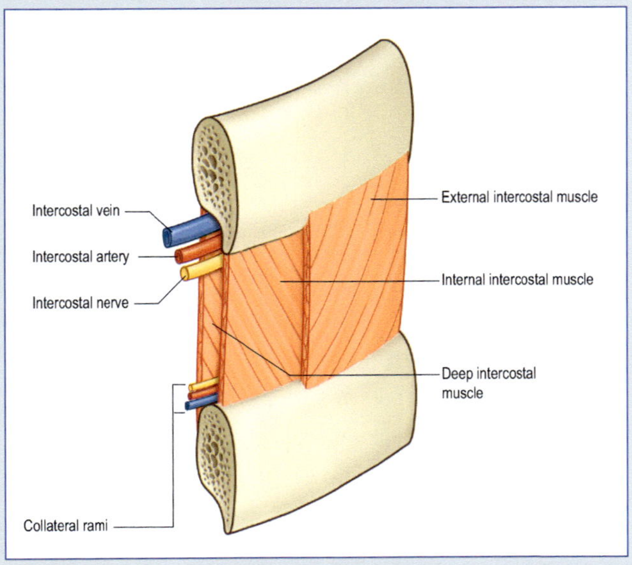

Figure 4.17 Dissection of part of an intercostal space. Note the position of the intercostal vessels and nerves relative to the intercostal muscles.

Description of the technique (anatomical and ultrasound findings)

Intercostal nerve blocking can be performed with the patient in a sitting, lateral decubitus, or prone position. Although this technique is relatively easy to perform due to the presence of palpable bone landmarks and does not cause excessive discomfort to the patient, the contact of the needle with the periosteum may cause some discomfort.

For this reason, the authors suggest that adequate sedation-analgesia should always be ensured before performing the block, especially when the technique is performed with the patient awake, using a combination of benzodiazepines and opioids (midazolam 0.02 mg/kg^{-1} + fentanyl 1-2 mcg/kg^{-1} or sufentanyl 0.1-0.15 mcg/kg^{-1}). Blockade can be performed using the blind technique or with the aid of ultrasound guidance. The anatomical landmarks for estimating the position of the ribs are the 12th rib (the last rib of the costal arch that can be palpated caudally) and the 7th rib (the lowest rib covered by the angle of the scapula). After identification of the landmarks by palpation, the lower margin of the selected rib can be marked on the skin with an "X" at the costal angle about 6-8 cm from the midline, which will indicate the needle insertion site.

After thorough disinfection of the skin with an antiseptic solution, a subcutaneous infiltration at the planned injection site is performed with 1-2 ml of diluted LA. Stabilising the skin with the fingers of the non-dominant hand, to avoid unwanted movement, a 22 G 50 mm needle will be inserted at an angle of approximately 20° to the skin plane, "in-plane", advancing approximately 3 mm below the lower margin of the selected rib, to position the tip in the space containing the vascular-nervous bundle.
After a negative aspiration test for blood or air, a volume of 3-5 ml of LA will be injected, repeating the procedure at the other desired levels. For the ultrasound-guided technique, a high-frequency (12-15 MHz) linear probe will be used, as the target structures are very superficial. The transducer is positioned perpendicular to the course of two adjacent ribs, so that the intercostal space, intercostal muscles, and pleura are identified.
The target of the block is the intercostal nerve, which runs deep in relation to the internal intercostal muscle, caudal to the inferior margin of the selected rib, usually at a distance of less than 5 mm from the pleura. The Authors consider the ideal injection site to be the costal angle (approximately 7 cm from the interspinous line), since at this level the rib reaches its maximum thickness, the costal groove is wider and deeper, the internal intercostal muscle is easier to identify, and the lateral skin ramus has not yet detached from the intercostal nerve.
It is also advisable to measure the distance between the skin and the pleura before performing the block, so that the needle does not cross the safety zone. A further suggestion is to use the Echo Colour Doppler function before performing the block, to avoid accidental intravascular injection due to the close proximity between the intercostal nevi and the accompanying vessels.
The probe will be positioned in the sagittal plane to obtain a transverse scan of two adjacent ribs. A 22 G 50 mm needle is inserted "in-plane" with respect to the ultrasound beam, until its tip passes the internal intercostal muscle to reach the target intercostal nerve of the block which runs, accompanied by the intercostal vessels, at the inferior margin of the selected rib (**Figure 4.18**).
At this point, after performing a negative aspiration test for blood and air and a hydro localisation by injection of 2-3 ml of saline solution to confirm the correct positioning of the needle tip, a volume of 3-5 ml of LA will be injected in fractionated boluses for each segment to be blocked, taking care to verify its diffusion by ultrasound. After performing the multi-level block, the authors suggest always scanning the pleura to document the absence of pneumothorax. The ultrasound presence of pleural sliding, B lines or comet-tail artefacts, the M-mode seashore sign, and the absence of a lung point allow the presence of pneumothorax to be excluded, with a sensitivity and negative predictive value of 100%.
A few minutes after the end of the procedure, the operator should test the dermatome level of the sensory block by ice test and pinprick test. It is also possible, after the initial bolus, to continue the continuous infusion of LA by means of a peri-neural catheter positioned in the chosen intercostal space, in order to prolong the analgesic effect obtained (**Flow chart 4.2 online**).

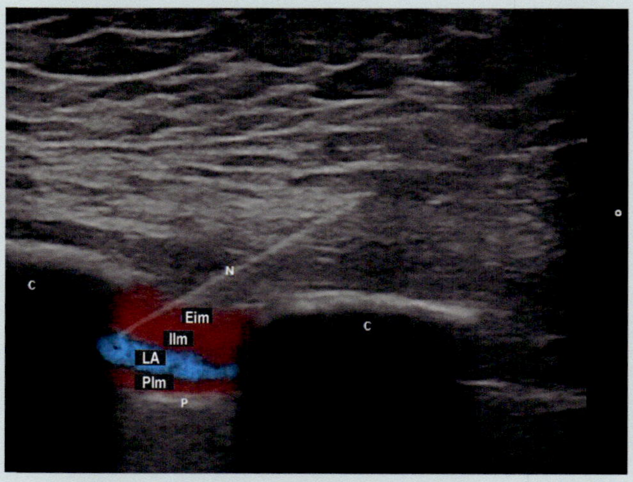

Figure 4.18 US-guided block of the intercostal nerve. Highlighted the tip of the needle that passes the Ilm to reach the target intercostal nerve and the spread of the LA. Eim: external intercostal muscle; Ilm: internal intercostal muscle; LA: local anesthetic; P: pleura; Plm: posterior intercostal muscle.

Deep and superficial SAP block and IC nerve block

Indications and dosages

Intercostal nerve block can provide ipsilateral metameric anesthesia/analgesia of the thoracic wall at selected segments. This technique is an excellent anesthetic option for superficial chest wall surgery and chest drain placement. This block is also indicated for postoperative pain control in thoracic, breast, or upper abdominal wall surgery. The intercostal nerve block may play a role in other painful conditions, with both diagnostic and therapeutic applications.

This technique may be used in the differential diagnosis of some cases of chest pain of uncertain etiology to discern a somatic or autonomic origin of the pain symptoms.

For therapeutic purposes, intercostal blockade may be useful for analgesia in patients with single or multiple rib fractures or thoracic contusions, to relieve pain from muscle spasms or chest wall injuries by promoting the cough mechanism and deep breathing, or in the acute phase of shingles in combination with a somatic PVB. With regard to the dosages for performing the blockade, a total volume of 3-5 ml of levobupivaine 0.5% or ropivacaine 0.5% per segment is sufficient. In the case of continuous blockade, after the initial bolus, a continuous infusion of low-concentration long-acting LA (levobupivacaine 0.2% or ropivacaine 0.2%, at an infusion rate of 4-8 ml/h, lock out 20 min, and the possibility of 2 ml rescue boluses) is recommended.

Intercostal nerve block is the procedure in which the highest blood levels of LA per mg injected are reached, due to the marked speed of absorption of the same with the risk of overdose; it is therefore advisable to calculate the maximum individual dosage allowed and not exceed it, to avoid the possible onset of LAST.

Contraindications to the block

- Absolute contraindications: patient refusal, injection site infections, allergy to LA
- Relative contraindications: patients who are too thin, severe chronic obstructive pulmonary disease (COPD), coagulopathies and/or coagulation disorders

Complications and contraindications

Although intercostal nerve block has a good safety profile, especially if performed by experienced operators and with the aid of ultrasound guidance, it is not without risk of possible complications, the most feared of which are pneumothorax, infection, intravascular injection and LAST. Rarer complications are represented by the risk of visceral or peritoneal puncture, by the possible diffusion of the anesthetic solution in the PVS, and by spinal anesthesia due to the contact of the needle with a dural sheath that can extend up to 8 cm from the median line, with consequent spread of the anesthetic in the subarachnoid space and onset of cardio-respiratory instability linked to the sympathetic block. Contraindications are absolute (patient refusal, infections and skin diseases at the injection site, known allergy to LA) and relative (patients who are too thin, chronic obstructive disease with poor pulmonary reserve, anticoagulant/antiplatelet therapy).

Intercostal nerve block provides ipsilateral chest wall analgesia, but an unresolvable limitation is that the spread of LA after a single injection is limited to the target thoracic segment of the block. Although intercostal blocks are an excellent choice for analgesic purposes, sometimes it is necessary to combine them with other anesthetic techniques to achieve complete surgical anesthesia. Compared to PVB, longitudinal cranio-caudal spread of anesthetic between adjacent levels is much less likely, although it can be achieved by large volume injection and/or near the midline of the thoracic spine, factors which may favor spread from the solution to the PVS. This limitation of intercostal nerve block justifies the need for multiple injections to extend the effect to adjacent dermatomes.

In addition, multiple injections can be painful and time-consuming, while increasing the risk of complications such as pneumothorax. With this in mind, the authors believe that more recently introduced alternative techniques, such as the ultrasound-guided serratus plane block (US-SAP block), may be more suitable for surgical anesthesia and analgesia of the lateral thoracic wall because, with a single injection, it allows to obtain multi-dermatome analgesia, with variable extension from T2 to T9, thanks to the block of the lateral skin rami of the intercostal nerves.

Complications

- Pneumothorax
- Injection site infections
- Accidental intravascular injection with LAST
- Visceral or peritoneal puncture
- Diffusion of anesthetic solution into the PVS
- Diffusion of LA into subarachnoid space with spinal anesthesia/sympathetic blockade

Pediatric applications

Intercostal nerve block is a simple technique that can also be used in pediatric medicine, provided that the indications and maximum doses of the above-mentioned drugs are observed. The main indications are postoperative analgesia in thoracic or upper abdominal wall surgery, as well as pain control in pediatric trauma patients with single or multiple rib fractures or chest wall contusions.

Indication for chronic pain

The intercostal nerve block may also be used to treat chronic pain conditions that are refractory to pharmacological therapy involving the intercostal region (neuralgia and causalgia), of post-traumatic origin (single or multiple rib fractures), or associated with a medical pathology (neoplasms, diabetic neuropathy, herpes zoster) (**Figure 4.19**).

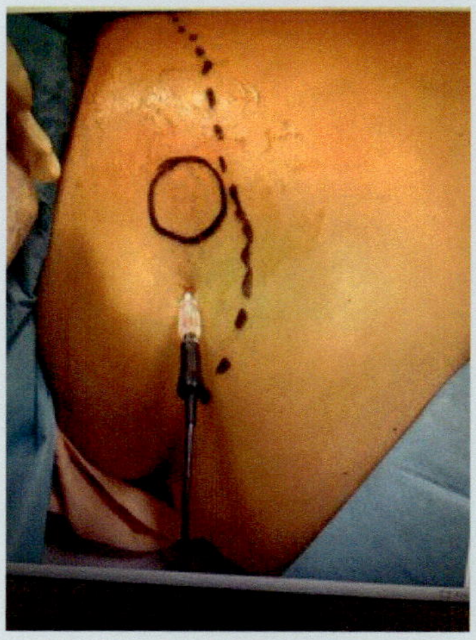

Figure 4.19 Radiofrequency of the intercostal nerve.

RECOMMENDED READING

- Fusco P, Scimia P, Di Carlo S, Testa A, Luciani A, Petrucci E, Marinangeli F. Ultrasound-Guided Serratus Plane Block and Fast-Track Tracheal Extubation in the Operating Room for Thoracic Trauma Patients: A case report. A A Case Rep. 2017 Dec 1;9(11):305-307.
- Patel SJ, Augoustides JGT. Serratus Anterior Plane Block-A Promising Technique for Regional Anesthesia in Minimally Invasive Cardiac Surgery. J Cardiothorac Vasc Anesth. 2020 Nov;34(11):2983-2985. doi: 10.1053/j.jvca.2020.07.011. Epub 2020 Jul 11. PMID: 32739085.
- Sepolvere G, Tedesco M, Fusco P, et al. Ultrasound-guided thoracic wall nerve blocks for effective pain control in cardiac surgery. Minerva Anestesiol. 2020 Jun;86(6):681-683. doi: 10.23736/S0375-9393.20.14368-2. Epub 2020 Feb 17. PMID: 32068984.
- Sepolvere G, Tedesco M, Fusco P, Scimia P, Cristiano L. Fascial plane blocks in cardiac surgery: a future to discover. Minerva Anestesiol. 2021 Mar;87(3):382-383. doi: 10.23736/S0375-9393.20.15271-4. Epub 2020 Dec 17. PMID: 33331755.
- Capuano P, toscano a, rinaldi M, Brazzi l. Ultrasound- guided thoracic wall nerve blocks in cardiac surgery: has the best yet to come? Minerva anestesiol 2021;87:381–2.
- Smith LM, Barrington MJ; St Vincent's Hospital, Melbourne. Ultrasound-guided blocks for cardiovascular surgery: which block for which patient? Curr Opin Anaesthesiol. 2020 Feb;33(1):64-70. doi: 10.1097/ACO.0000000000000818. PMID: 31833864.
- Coppolino F, Sansone P, Passavanti MB, Pace MC, Sepolvere G, Aurilio C. the role of an Ultrasound-guided Block of the Deep Plane of the Serratus Muscle in a Modified ERAS Protocol for cardiac surgery. the open anesthesia Journal. 2020;14:49–51.
- Blanco R, Parras T, McDonnell JT, Prats-galino A, Serratus plane block: a novel ultrasound-guided thoracic wall nerve block. anaesthesia 2013;68:1107–13.
- Zubrzycki M, Liebold A, Skrabal C, Reinelt H, Ziegler M, Perdas E, Zubrzycka M. Assessment and pathophysiology of pain in cardiac surgery. J Pain Res. 2018 Aug 24;11:1599-1611. doi: 10.2147/JPR.S162067. PMID: 30197534; PMCID: PMC6112778.
- Liu X, Song T, Xu HY, Chen X, Yin P, Zhang J. The serratus anterior plane block for analgesia after thoracic surgery: A meta-analysis of randomized controlled trails. Medicine (Baltimore). 2020 May 22;99(21):e20286. doi: 10.1097/MD.0000000000020286. PMID: 32481308; PMCID: PMC7249988.
- Marshall K, McLaughlin K. Pain Management in Thoracic Surgery. Thorac Surg Clin. 2020 Aug;30(3):339-346. doi: 10.1016/j.thorsurg.2020.03.001. Epub 2020 Apr 29. PMID: 32593366.
- Southgate SJ, Herbst MK. Ultrasound Guided Serratus Anterior Blocks. 2021 Jul 31. In: StatPearls [Internet]. Treasure Island (FL): StatPearls Publishing; 2021 Jan–. PMID: 30860711.
- Feray S, Lubach J, Joshi GP, Bonnet F, Van de Velde M; PROSPECT Working Group *of the European Society of Regional Anaesthesia and Pain Therapy. PROSPECT guidelines for video-assisted thoracoscopic surgery: a systematic review and procedure-specific postoperative pain management recommendations. Anaesthesia. 2021 Nov 5. doi: 10.1111/anae.15609. Epub ahead of print. PMID: 34739134.

CLINICAL CASE 1 – A CASE REPORT ON ULTRASOUND-GUIDED SERRATUS PLANE BLOCK AND FAST-TRACK TRACHEAL EXTUBATION IN THE OPERATING ROOM FOR THORACIC TRAUMA PATIENTS: IS IT POSSIBLE?

Clinical history and anamnesis We report the use of a continuous ultrasound-guided serratus plane block (US-SPB) in a 28-year-old man with thoracic trauma after a fall and displaced fractures of the anterior arches of eighth, ninth, and tenth ribs, a left basal pneumothorax with maximum thickness of 5 mm, and an ipsilateral pleural effusion. The abdomen computerized tomographic images showed a splenic laceration with serum-effusion in the perisplenic and perihepatic area.

Technique description Under aseptic conditions we performed a US-SPB followed by the insertion of a catheter for continuous infusion of local anesthetic. A high-frequency linear probe (12.5 MHz) was positioned at the level of the fifth rib along the midaxillary line (**Figure 4.20**). Two separate injections were performed under ultrasound guidance because we did not have an optimal visualization of the target plane due to the thoracic trauma. A 22-Gauge 50 mm needle was introduced in-plane with a cranial-to-caudal direction. The plane between serratus anterior and fifth rib was identified. Once the tip of the needle was directed on the top of the rib underneath the serratus anterior muscle, 3 to 4 ml of saline solution was injected to open this plane. Afterward, a total of 30 ml of 0.375% levobupivacaine was injected, and a catheter (E-Cath®) was inserted over the needle, deep to the serratus anterior muscle. The correct spread of local anesthetic was confirmed by ultrasound guidance (**Figure 4.21**).

The patient spent the first night after surgery in the intensive care unit quietly and spontaneously breathing. No patient discomfort, infections, side effects of local anesthetics, nor other complications were observed.

Materials and methods Written informed consent was obtained. Electrocardiogram, heart rate, arterial blood pressure, and Spo2 were monitored. An IV induction of general anesthesia was performed with 100 μg of fentanyl, 200 mg of propofol, and 0.6 mg/kg of rocuronium, and the patient was intubated and ventilated mechanically. Sevoflurane and remifentanil maintained anesthesia. The surgeon performed an exploratory laparotomy and a splenectomy. Before emergence, we performed a continuous US-SPB.

Conclusions The US-SPB provided complete anesthesia of hemithorax, facilitated a fast-track extubation in a patient with traumatic rib fractures, and perhaps avoided reintubation.

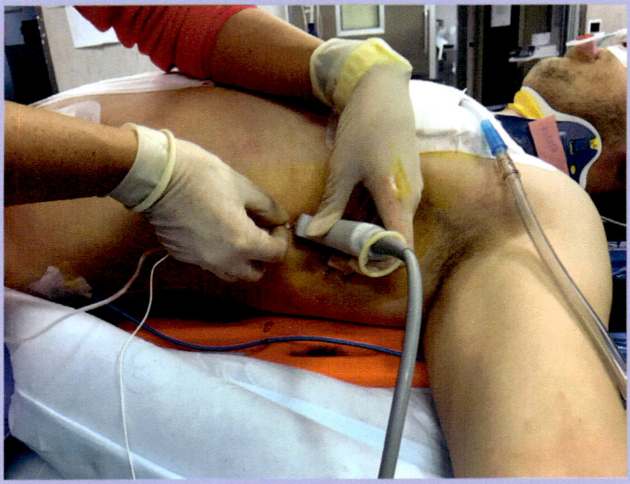

Figure 4.20 Patient on the operating table, after the surgery, during the execution of the serratus plane block at the fifth rib level. We can observe the chest tube on the II intercostal space.

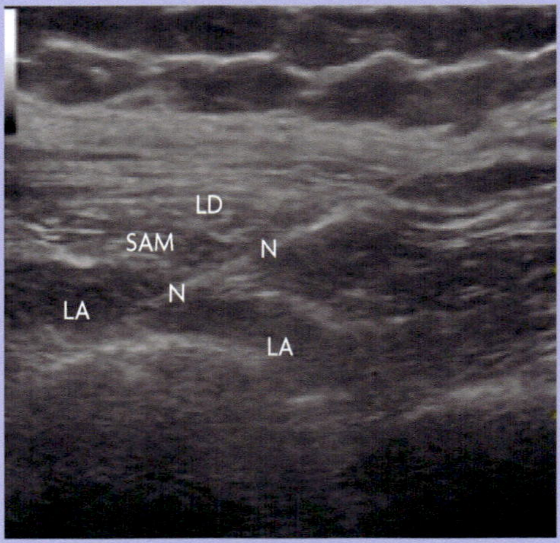

Figure 4.21 Spread of local anesthetic confirmed by ultrasound guidance. LA: local anesthetic; LD: Latissimus dorsi; N: needle; SAM: Serratus anterior muscle.

CLINICAL CASE 2 – SERRATUS ANTERIOR PLANE BLOCK IN MINI-THORACOTOMY AND PNEUMOTHORAX PAIN MANAGEMENT

Clinical history and anamnesis We report a case of a young patient affected by severe mitral valve insufficiency scheduled to undergo mini-thoracotomy mitral valve replacement. The patient reported two acute pulmonary edema before cardiac surgery and referred allergic reaction to nonsteroidal anti-inflammatory drugs (NSAIDs). On the fifth postoperative day the patient presented a spontaneous right pneumothorax and subcutaneous emphysema for which a chest tube was inserted.

Technique description At the end of surgery, under aseptic conditions, using a linear probe and a needle Tuohy in-plane approach, a continuous deep serratus anterior plane block was performed to manage postoperative pain deriving from mini-thoracotomy. 30 ml of 0.375% levobupivacaine was injected and a catheter over the needle (E-Cath®) was inserted into the anatomical space created by the local anesthetic spread. An infusion of 0.125% levobupivacaine started at 5-7 ml/h for the next 24 hours (**Figure 4.22**) Patient reported a good postoperative analgesia (numerical rating scale <3) and NSAIDs or opioids were administered. On the fifth postoperative day, with the patient in left lateral position, 30 ml of mepivacaine 2% was used to perform a single shot DSPB in order to manage pain deriving from the chest tube insertion due to right spontaneous pneumothorax (**Figure 4.23**). No pain was reported and spontaneous breathing was maintained during the procedure.

Materials and methods Written informed consent to the procedures was obtained. The patient received total intravenous and controlled infusion anesthesia (TIVA-TCI) by a target infusion of propofol and remifentanil 3 mcg/ml for the whole surgery period. A light sedation with midazolam 5 mg was used to manage the chest tube insertion in spontaneous breathing. Vital and respiratory parameters (Hr, Invasive blood pressure, SaO_2%) were monitored.

Conclusions Serratus anterior plane block represents a safe and effective regional technique both to manage postoperative pain deriving from thoracotomy incision and emergency conditions such as chest tube insertion or ribs fractures. It's a part of ERAS protocols reducing pulmonary complications, length of stay and avoiding the opioid adverse effects.

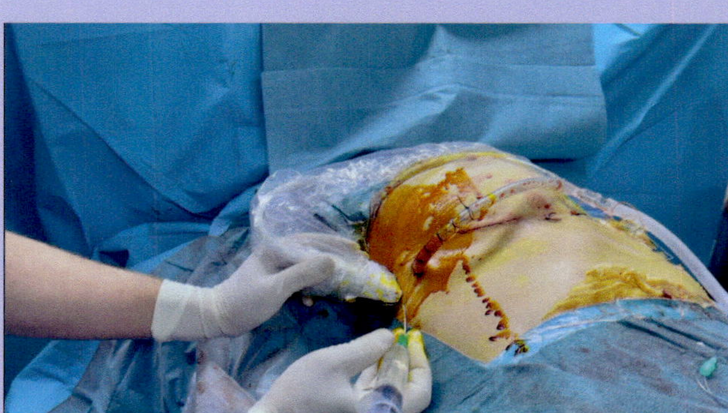

Figure 4.22 Continuous deep serratus plane block.

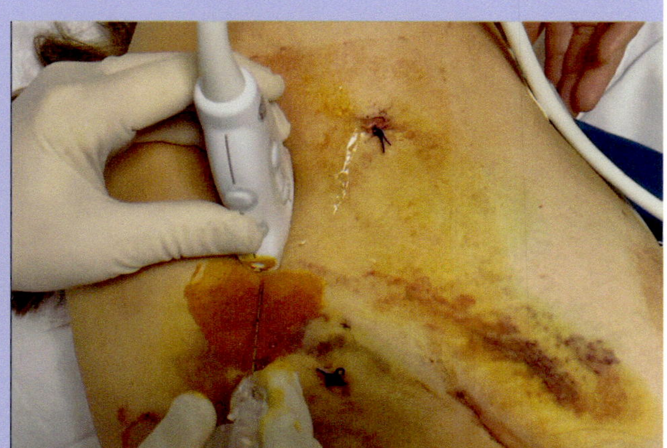

Figure 4.23 Single-shot deep serratus plane block.

Interpectoral plane block (IPP) and Pectoserratus plane block (PSP) (PECS 1 and PECS 2 blocks)

Pierfrancesco Fusco, Stefano Di Carlo, Emiliano Petrucci, Giuseppe Sepolvere, Rafa Blanco

Breast cancers are one of the most frequent oncological pathologies in women, representing 31% of all the cases of neoplasia in the female population on an annual basis.

Breast surgery, frequently extended to the axillary region, is currently one of the most common procedures performed in hospitals. These surgical interventions cause the onset of an acute postoperative pain of moderate to severe intensity which, if not properly treated, like other surgical procedures, can increase perioperative morbidity and hospitalization times/costs, as well as cause the development of a chronic pain (postmastectomy pain syndrome) in 25-60% of the cases, with the significant impairment of the quality of life.

To date, the control of the post-operative pain in breast and axillary surgery is frequently unsatisfactory. Generally, the treatment of postoperative pain in breast surgery is based on a multimodal approach that involves the use of analgesic drugs via systemic administration, with opioids representing the most important ones.

However, these drugs are characterized by the onset of related and dose-dependent side effects such as respiratory depression, nausea, vomiting, itching, sedation, delayed canalization, hypotension, and urinary retention, in addition to immunosuppressive and pro-metastatic effects. In oncological patients, the acute postoperative pain can cause a change in the immunological response, while the association of an opioid treatment, with further depression of the immune system, can cause neoplastic proliferation and tumor/metastatic relapses, in addition to infections. However, scientific evidence shows how breast surgery, female sex, young age, general anesthesia, volatile anesthetics, and the use of systemic opioids are risk factors for the onset of postoperative nausea and vomiting (PONV).

The related literature highlights the importance of adopting locoregional anesthesia/analgesia (LRA) techniques to achieve better antalgic control and avoid the use of opioids, particularly in patients with risk factors for PONV. Nowadays, the concept of "preventive analgesia" is widely acknowledged: in other words, the execution of LRA techniques before surgery can allow to achieve an excellent control of the acute postoperative pain and a rapid recovery of the normal physiological functions, thus preventing at the same time central sensitization phenomena underlying the development of a persistent postoperative pain.

Currently, thoracic epidural analgesia and paravertebral block are the main LRA techniques for postoperative analgesia in breast surgery. However, although these techniques allow to achieve excellent pain control, they are not always easy to perform, and frequently are even contraindicated, due to the possible onset of systemic side effects or procedural complications.

The recent introduction of new ultrasound-guided blocks of the chest wall, described by Raphael Blanco, can open new horizons in the management of postoperative pain in breast surgery. The new generation of superficial and thus less invasive interfascial nerve blocks include the PECS 1 block, the PECS 2 block, and the Serratus plane block. They offer an effective and safe alternative in the conventional regional techniques for postoperative anesthesia and postoperative analgesia in chest wall surgery.

The recent first international consensus led by representatives of both ASRA and ESRA on the nomenclature and anatomical descriptions of abdominal wall blocks, chest wall and paraspinal blocks established that the PECS I and II blocks will change their name and therefore the Interpectoral plan block (IPP) has been proposed to replace the PECS I and the Pectoserratus plan (PSP) block for the PECS II.

For this reason in this chapter we will use the interpectoral plane block (IPP) instead of PECS 1 and the Pectoserratus plane block (PSP) instead of PECS 2 Block.

The recent literature, albeit insufficient, suggests that these techniques, when as part of a multimodal therapeutic scheme, allow to achieve an excellent postoperative pain control and to reduce the consumption of analgesics, with a lower risk of complications. However, it is important to remember the correct execution and the clinical efficacy of these blocks are intricately linked to the expertise of the operator, which should include the knowledge of anatomy and the sonoanatomy of the target structures.

ANATOMY AND SONOANATOMY

The breast is a modified sweat gland that is covered by the skin and that lies on the fascia of the pectoralis major muscle. The breast and this fascia are separated from each other by an adipose layer, which continues with the one interposed between the glandular elements. The main muscles of the chest wall include the pectoralis major and minor muscles, the anterior serratus muscle, and the latissimus dorsi muscle (**Figure 5.1**).

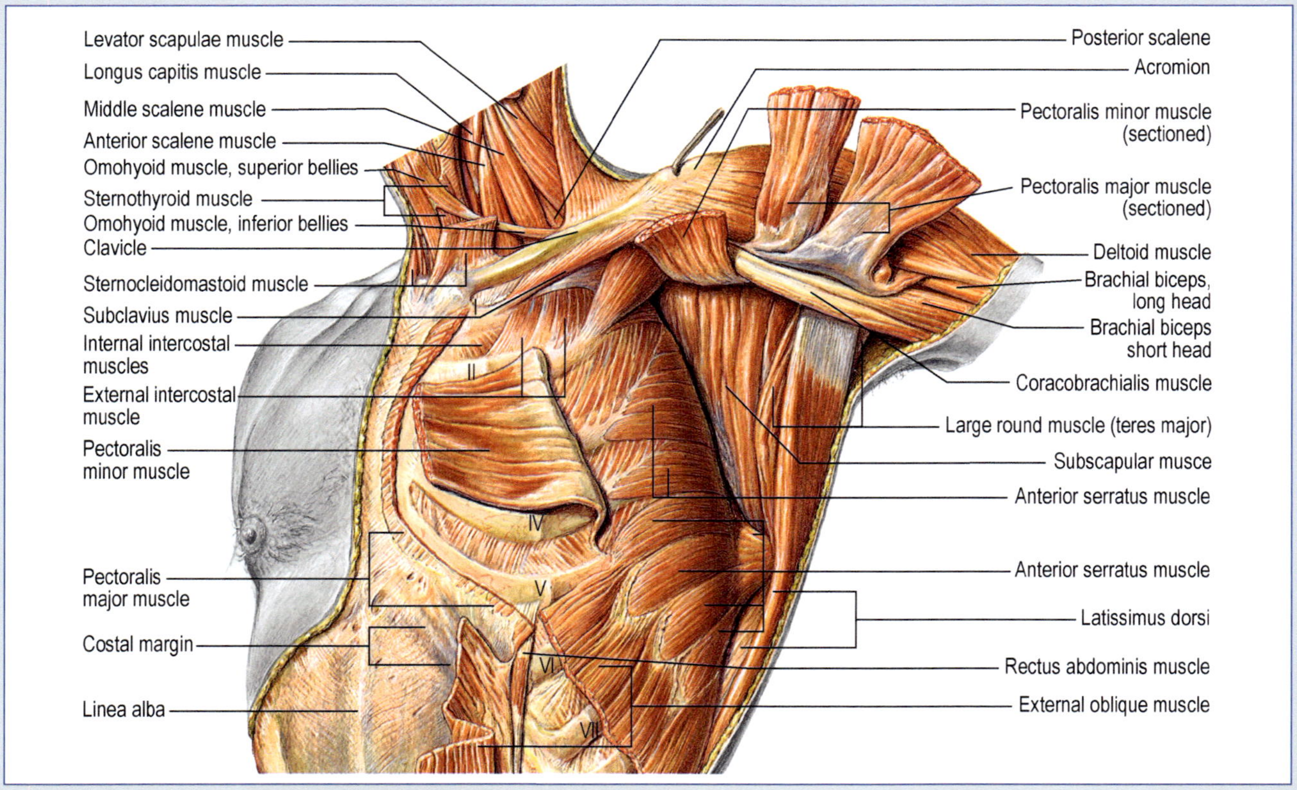

Figure 5.1 Muscles of the chest wall.

The innervation of the mammary and axillary region receives an important contribution by the branches of the cervical and brachial plexus and is basically composed of three main groups of nervous structures: pectoral nerves, intercostal nerves, the long thoracic nerve, and the thoracodorsal nerve.

The pectoral nerves are major nerve branches that derive from the brachial plexus (**Figure 5.2**).

The lateral pectoral nerve (LPN) is the largest among the two nerves and usually originates from C5-C7 and runs along the fascial plane between the pectoralis major and pectoralis minor muscles. It is constantly adjacent to the pectoral branch of the thoracoacromial artery and gets to innervate the pectoralis major muscle (PMm).

The medial pectoral nerve (MPN) originates from C8-T1 and innervates the pectoralis minor muscle (Pmm) (**Figure 5.3**).

Some authors believe that in 62% of the cases MPN passes through Pmm and reaches the inferior third of this muscle, after crossing the two layers of the clavipectoral fascia. In the remaining 38% of the cases, MPN completes its journey up to the lateral margin of Pmm. Although pectoral nerves are described as pure motor nerves, many experts hypothesize that they also carry proprioceptive and nociceptive fibers, as other nerve motors (**Figures 5.4**, **5.5**).

The thoracic intercostal nerves T2-T6 are localized between the pleura and the posterior intercostal membrane and run within a plane laying between the intercostal muscles up to the sternum. These nerves give rise to lateral and anterior branches, respectively responsible for the sensory innervation of the lateral and medial region of the breast (**Figure 5.6**). The lateral branches of the intercostal nerves cross the external intercostal muscle and the serratus anterior muscle

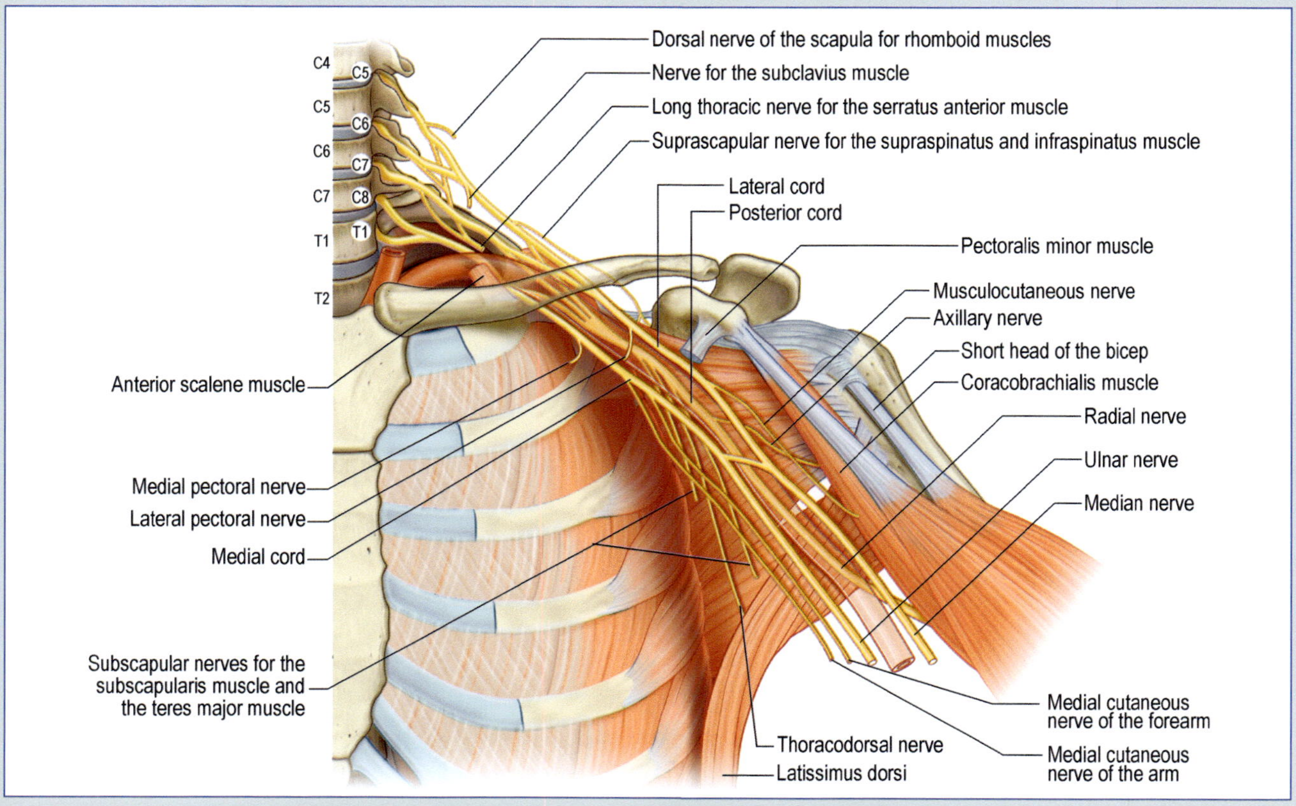

Figure 5.2 Brachial plexus, with its branches and the innervated muscles.

along the mid-axillary line, to get to the anterior and posterior terminal branches (**Figure 5.7**).

The lateral cutaneous branch of the second intercostal nerve does not split in anterior and posterior branches and is called intercostobrachial nerve.

The anterior branches of the intercostal nerves meet in front of the internal mammary artery, crossing the internal intercostal muscle, the intercostal membranes and PMm, until they get to innervate the medial region of the breast.

The large intercostal brachial nerves or brachial cutaneous nerves, which cross the axillary space, provide sensitivity to the surface of the upper branch and to the skin of the chest wall along the posterior margin of the armpit. The severing of these nerves, which occasionally takes place during axillary dissection, can cause skin anesthesia in these areas. The long thoracic nerve (or external respiratory nerve of Bell) arises from C5-C7, enters the axillary cavity posteriorly to the brachial plexus, and gets to innervate the serratus anterior muscle. The lesion of this nerve during axillary dissection can lead to a deformity called "winged scapula". The serratus muscle is frequently dissected during surgery, together with the pectoral muscles, to achieve a "pocket" which is necessary for positioning breast tissue expanders (**Figures 5.8**, **5.9**, **5.10**).

The thoracodorsal nerve (or mid-subscapularis) arises from C6-C8 and is, therefore, a branch of the posterior cord of the brachial plexus (**Figure 5.2**).

This nerve makes its journey in the axillary cavity, where it follows the thoracodorsal artery and heads towards the space below the axillary vein, until it gets to the medial surface of the latissimus dorsi muscle to innervate the latter.

This nerve has a deep course and plays an important role in the reconstructive surgery of the latissimus dorsi flaps. The thoracodorsal nerve is preserved during the removal of the axillary lymph nodes, unless its sacrifice is not necessary for the complete removal of the lymph nodes.

To complete the anatomical overview of the mammary and axillary region, it is fundamental to know the structures involved in this type of nerve blocks: the clavipectoral fascia and the Gerdy's ligament.

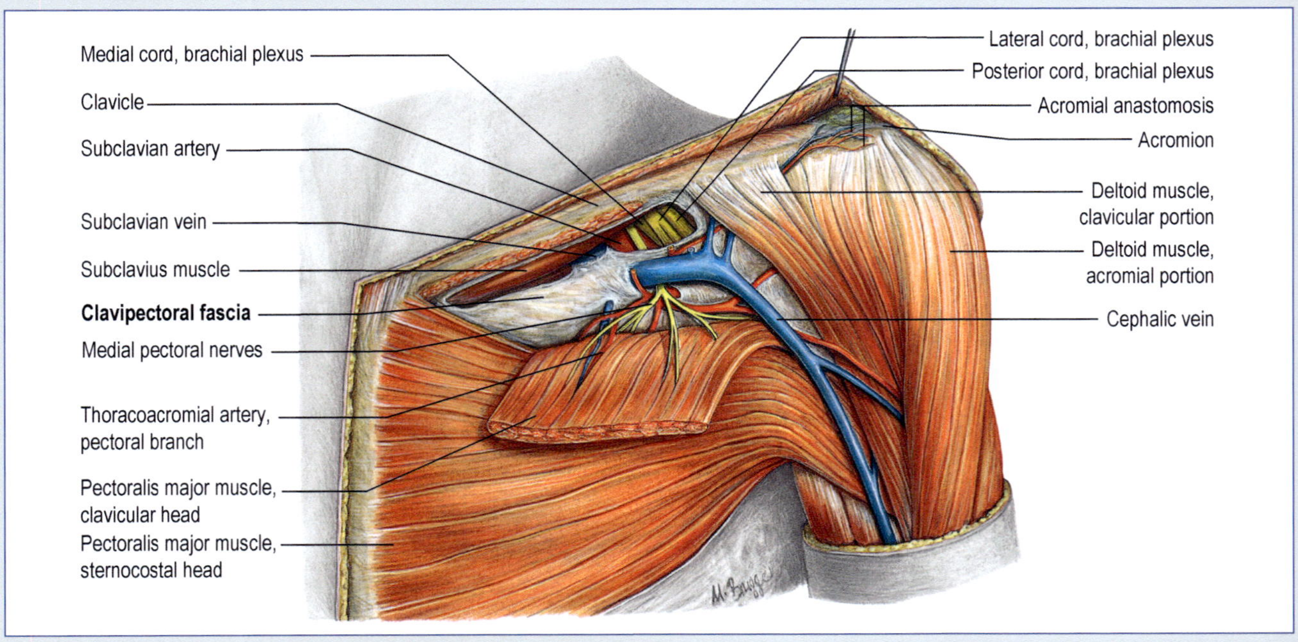

Figure 5.3 Pectoral nerves and muscles.

The fascia the covers the superficial region of PMm is the so-called clavipectoral fascia (**Figure 5.3**), while the resistant fascia located on the lateral margin of this muscle is the Gerdy's ligament (or suspensory ligament of the axilla), in other words, a connective tissue that helps maintain the concave shape of the armpit.

The mammary gland in women is richly vascularized by the branches of the axillary arteries and the internal mammary arteries.

To correctly identify the sonoanatomy in the target regions of the block and to guarantee an adequate spread of AL, the proper orientation of the probe and its subsequent sequences are fundamental. There are various approaches, but here only the in-plane approach in a proximal and medial to a distal and lateral direction, at the level of T2-T3 dermatomes, will be described. If the probe is positioned at the infraclavicular level near the deltopectoral groove, with an oblique orientation and a marker with cranial direction, it is possible to identify pectoralis minor muscle from the surface towards the lower part of the pectoralis major muscle, with the underlying axillary artery and vein (**Figure 5.11**).

Subsequently, the operator moves the probe obliquely in the cranial-caudal direction towards the armpit and the anterior axillary line, to reach the lateral margin of the pectoralis minor muscle and the continuation of the clavipectoral fascia with the Gerdy's ligament. At this level, after counting the succession of ribs, the ribs III and IV ribs are met, above which it is possible to view via ultrasound, as for the TAP block, three muscular bellies that include, moving towards the deep layers, the pectoralis major muscle, the pectoralis minor muscle and the serratus muscle immediately above the ribs themselves (**Figure 5.12**).

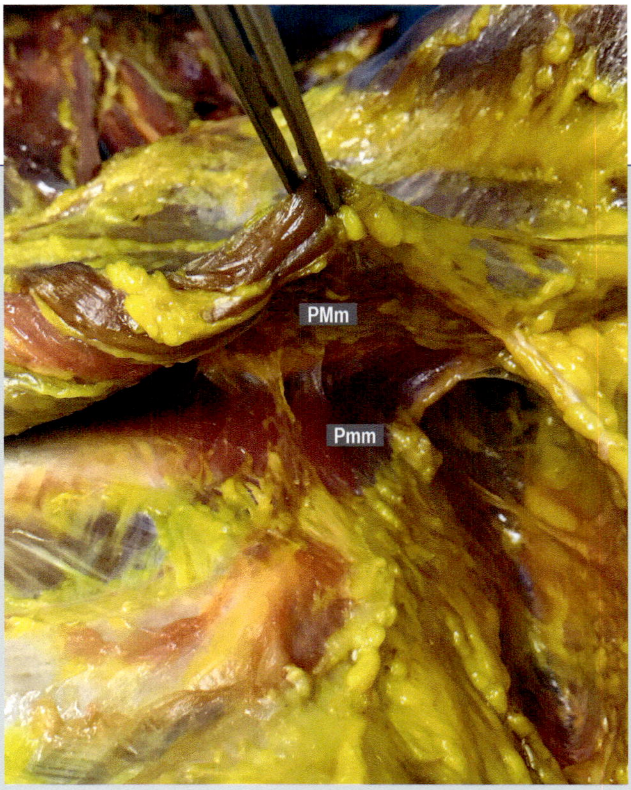

Figure 5.4 Anatomical preparation of pectoral muscles and clavipectoral fascia. PMm: pectoralis major muscle, Pmm: pectoralis minor muscle.

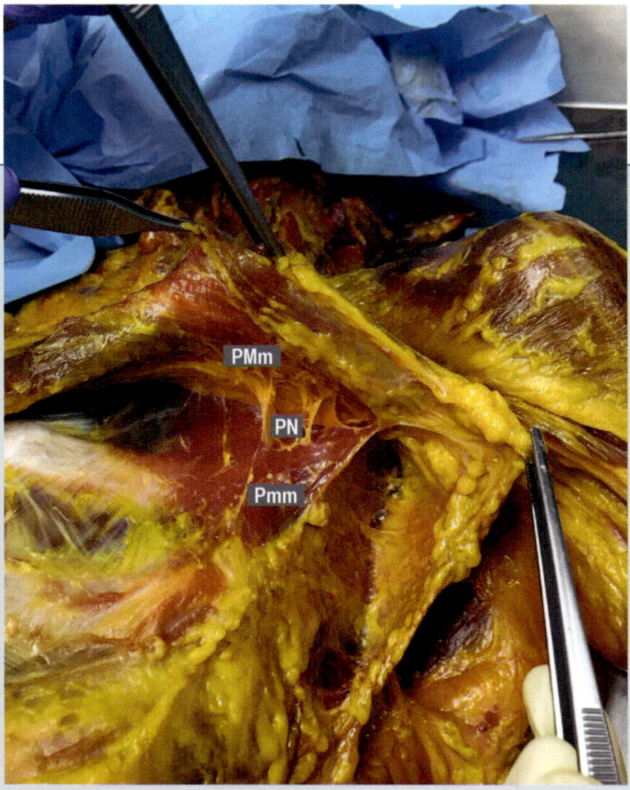

Figure 5.5 The pectoral muscles are in evidence. PMm: pectoralis major muscle; Pmm: pectoralis minor muscle; PN: pectoral nerve (courtesy of Dr. Behr and Prof. Stecco).

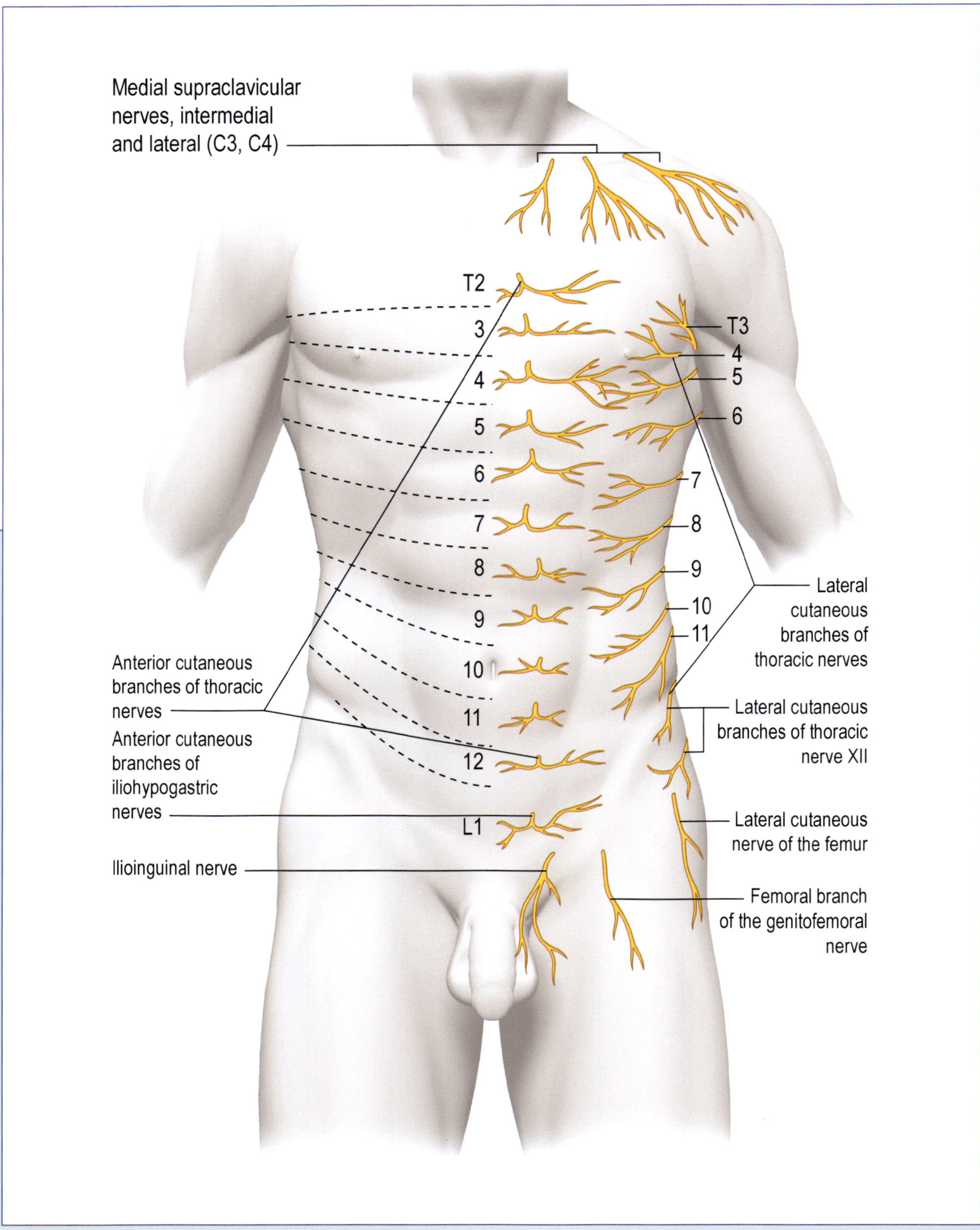

Figure 5.6 Anterior and lateral cutaneous branches of thoracic intercostal nerves.

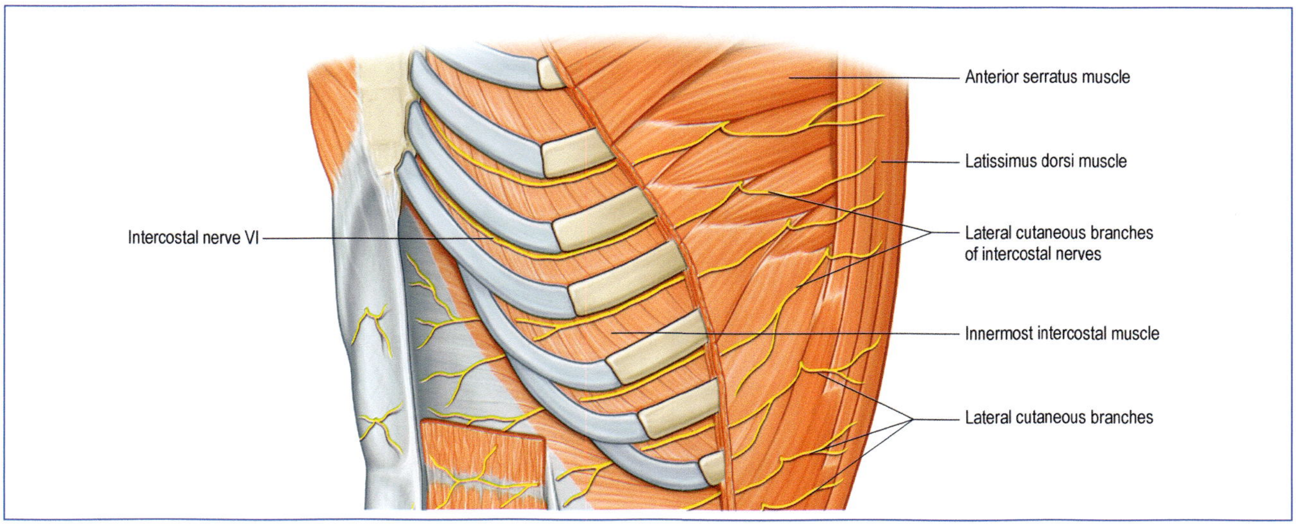

Figure 5.7 Lateral cutaneous branches of intercostal nerves.

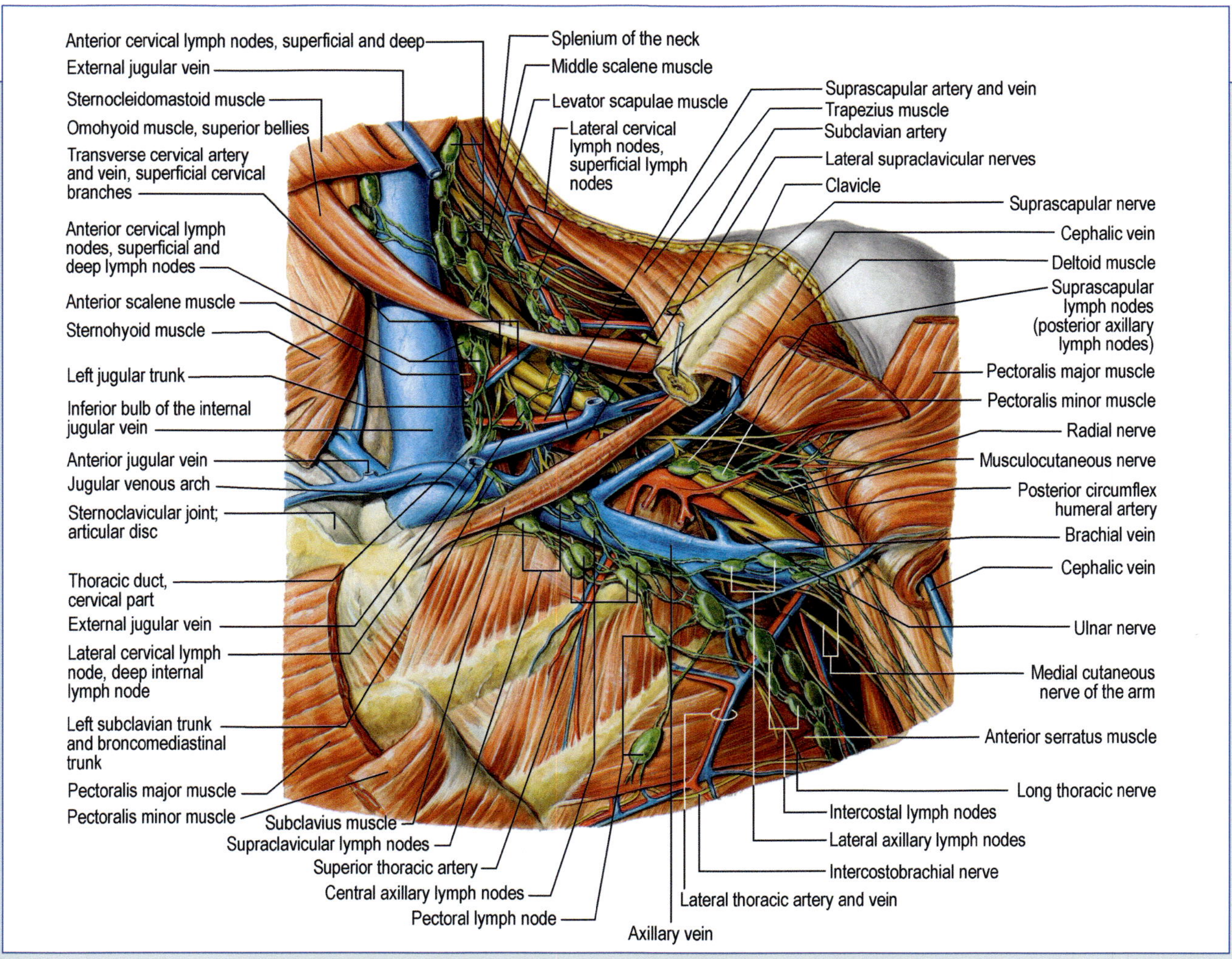

Figure 5.8 Brachial plexus, innervation of the chest wall, and mammary region.

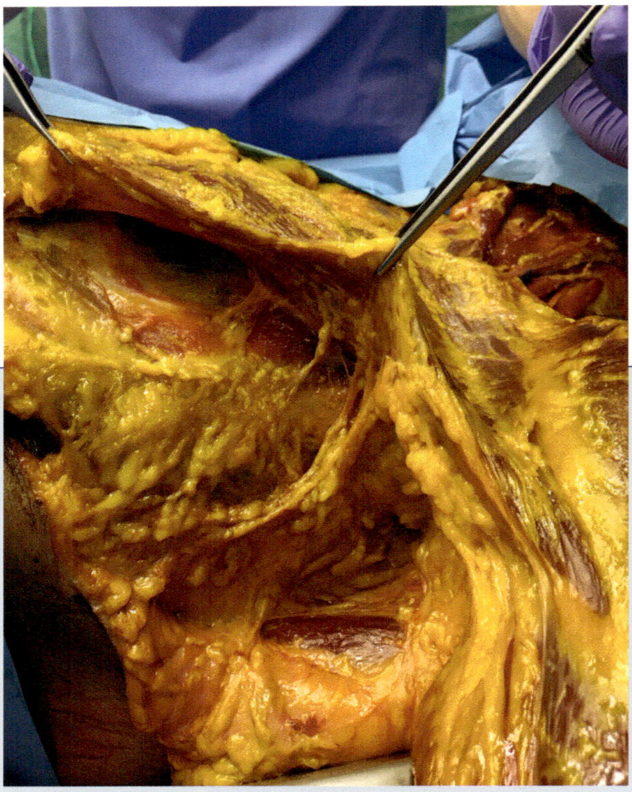

Figure 5.9 Anatomical preparation of chest and axillary cavity. The pectoralis major muscle, the pectoralis minor muscle, and the axilla are in evidence.

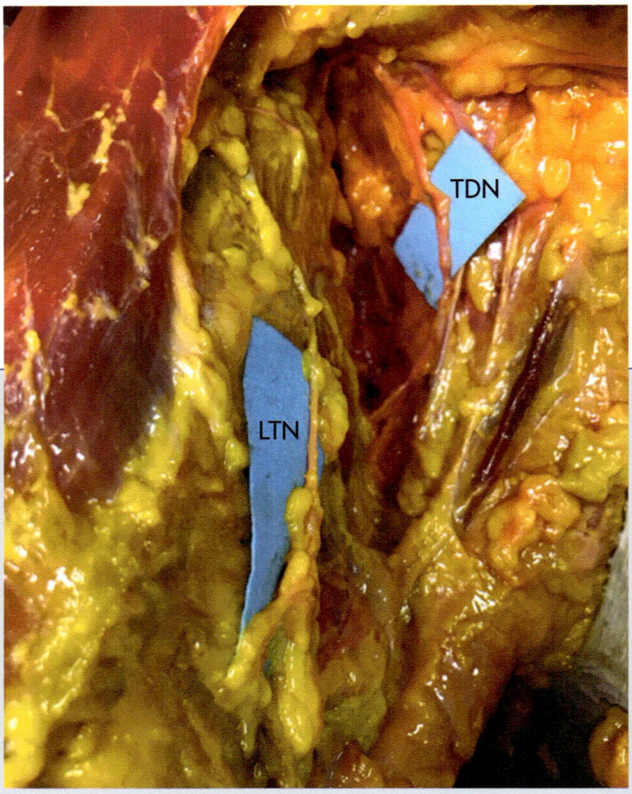

Figure 5.10 Anatomical preparation of the chest and upper limb: detail of the long thoracic nerve and the thoracodorsal nerve. LTN: long thoracic nerve; Pmm: pectoralis minor muscle; TDN: thoracodorsal nerve (courtesy of Dr. Behr and Prof. Stecco).

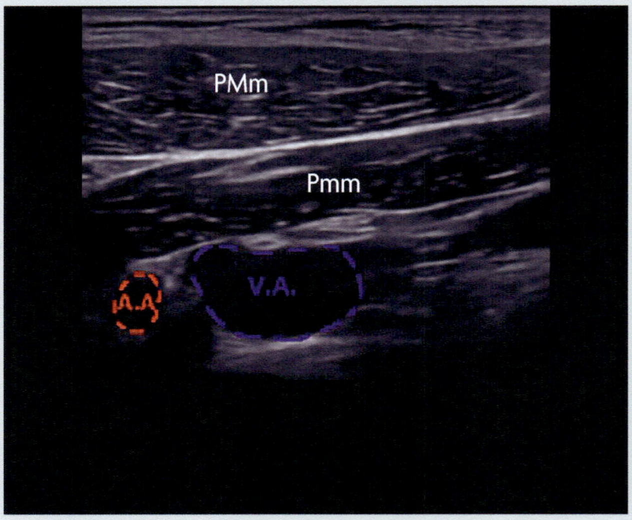

Figure 5.11 Ultrasound scan of the infraclavicular region: the vessels (axillary artery and axillary vein) with the overlying pectoralis minor muscle (Pmm) and pectoralis major muscle (PMm) are in evidence.

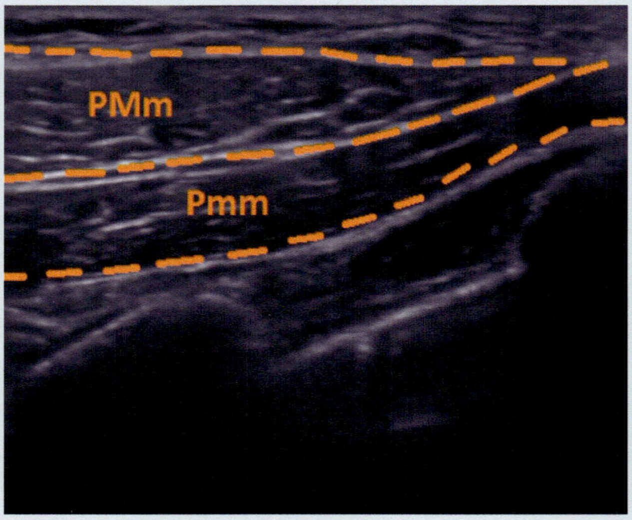

Figure 5.12 Ultrasound scan along the direction of the anterior axillary line. The pectoralis major muscle (PMm) and the pectoralis minor muscle (Pmm) are clearly visible. The pectoralis major muscle ends, as can be seen in the upper right corner of the figure, to make way for the Gerdy's ligament.

TARGET OF THE BLOCK

IPP Block: the goal of the block is to position the needle tip in the interfascial plane between PMm and Pmm, and to inject 10 ml of LA near the pectoral branch of the thoracoacromial artery with the opening of the plane itself.

It allows to obtain the block of the pectoral nerves LPN and MPN that innervate Pmm and PMm (**Figures 5.13**, **5.14**)

PSP Block: the object of this block, in addition to performing **IPP** as previously described, requires to position the needle tip below the lateral margin of Pmm and above the anterior serratus muscle, at the level of the rib IV, as well as the subsequent 20 ml injection of AL in the interfascial place between the two muscle layers. This technique allows to block the lateral branches of the intercostal nerves from T2 to T6, the long thoracic nerve, and the thoracodorsal nerve (**Figure 5.15**).

DESCRIPTION OF THE TECHNIQUES

To perform the block, it is necessary to use the following materials:

1. ultrasound system equipped with a high frequency linear probe (6-12 MHz);
2. sterile probe cover and sterile gel (in obese patients a convex probe might be needed);
3. standard cart for nerve blocks;

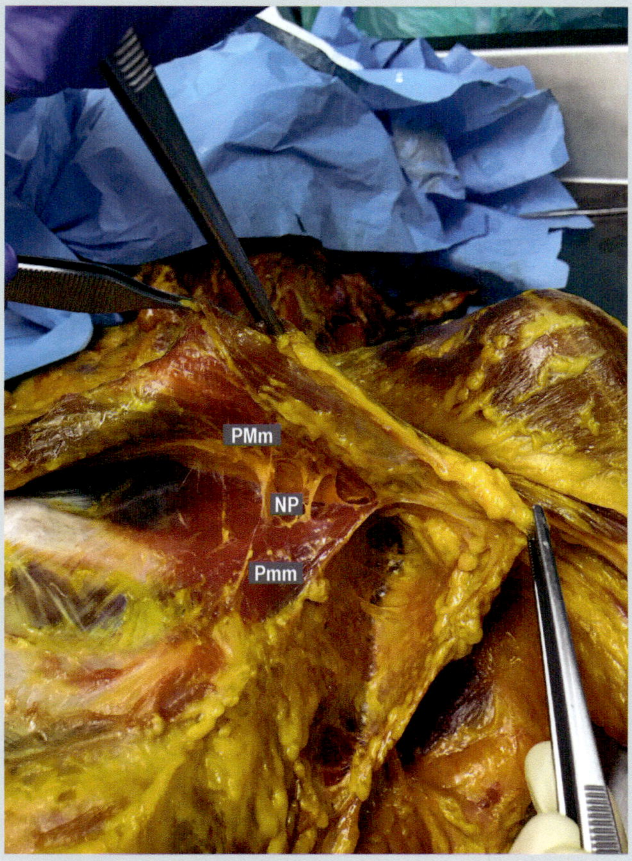

Figure 5.14 Anatomical preparation with the pectoralis major muscle duly lifted and visualization of the fascial compartment between the pectoralis major muscle, the pectoralis minor muscle, and the pectoral nerves. PMm: pectoralis major muscle; Pmm: pectoralis minor muscle; PN: pectoral nerve (courtesy of Dr. Behr and Prof. Stecco).

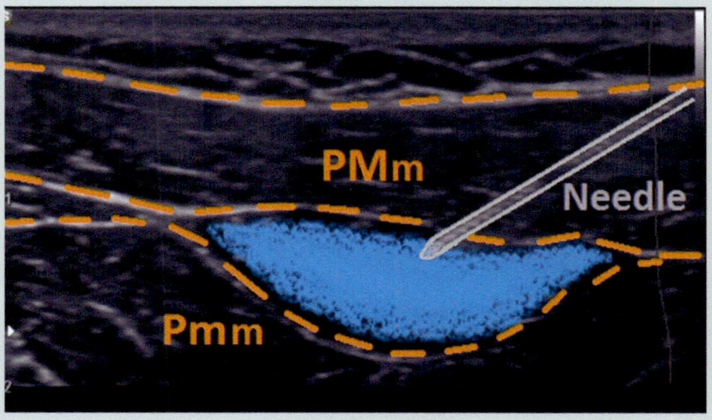

Figure 5.13 IPP, injection of the local anesthetic (in blue) between the pectoralis major muscle (PMm) and the pectoralis minor muscle (Pmm).

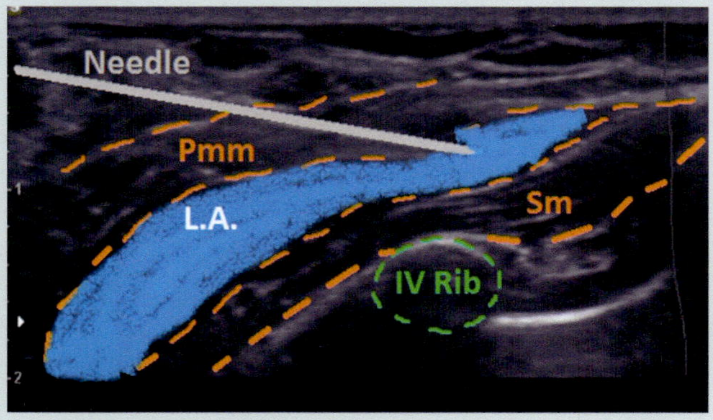

Figure 5.15 PSP block, injection of the local anesthetic (in blue) between the pectoralis minor muscle (Pmm) and the serratus muscle (Sm) at the level of the rib IV. The echogenic needle (SonoPlex stim Pajunk®) in white.

4. 10% chlorhexidine or povidone-iodine solutions for skin disinfection;
5. sterile gloves;
6. 50-100 mm needle (SonoPlex stim Pajunk®), 20-21 G;
7. a 20 ml syringe containing a local anesthetic, a 10 ml syringe containing a physiological solution, and a three-way stopcock.

It is important to stress the importance of an adequate monitoring of the patient's vital parameters, in addition to the checking of the availability of drugs for cardiopulmonary resuscitation and 20% lipid emulsion (Intralipid®). The block can be performed both with the patient awake, after adequate analgosedaction, and with the patient under general anesthesia. If the block is performed before induction, the puncture site on the skin can be infiltrated with 2% lidocaine.

The authors suggest the use of a three-way stopcock, connecting the main channel to the syringe that contains the physiological solution and the second channel to the syringe that contains the local anesthetic.

Technique for IPP Block

The purpose of **IPP** is to block the LPN and MPN that innervate the PMm and Pmm muscles.

The operator should place the monitor of the ultrasound machine in front of themself, on the same side of the block execution, preferably positioning themself at the patient's head, and should choose the most comfortable position to maneuver probe and needle, with the patient in a supine position and the homolateral arm to the breast to be treated abducted by 90° (**Figure 5.16**). Accurate asepsis of the skin in the affected anatomical region is recommended using an antiseptic containing chlorhexidine. Furthermore, it is necessary to protect the ultrasound probe with a sterile sheath and an ultrasound gel. At this point, a high-frequency linear probe (6-18 MHz) is placed, on a parasagittal plane, cadually to the lateral third of the clavicle, in the deltopectoral groove, positioning the probe in the same way as the infraclavicular block, so as to identify PMm and Pmm and, under them, the axillary vessels (**Figures 5.17**, **5.18**).

It is important to remember that the pectoral branch of the thoracoacromial artery runs between two pectoral muscles, while LPN is constantly adjacent to it. Therefore, it is always recommended to make an assessment with Eco-color-Doppler and an aspiration test before the injection of anesthetics, to prevent accidental intravascular injection. This vessel is an important landmark for AL injection. By rotating the probe in a position parallel to the clavicle, the 50-80 mm needle (SonoPlex stim Pajunk®) is inserted with an in-plane approach in relation to the probe itself and the PECS 1 block is performed, as previously described, by injecting 10 ml of long-acting AL, with 0.25% (analgesic dosage) or 0.5% (anesthetic dosage) levobupivacaine (**Figures 5.19**, **5.20**, **5.21**, **Video 5.1**). For a correct execution of all the fascial blocks of Fusco et al. described the double V sign due to the spread of the LA within the fascial plane (**Figure 5.21**).

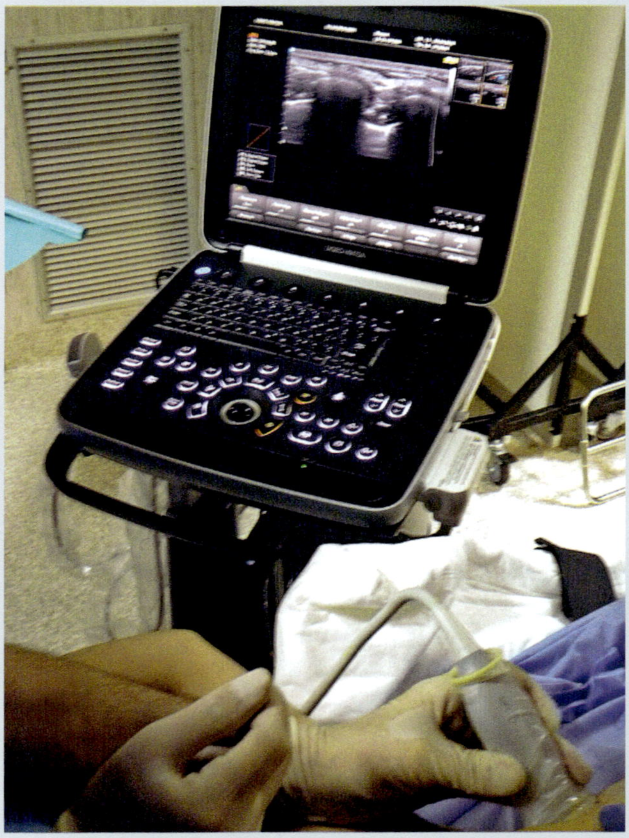

Figure 5.16 Correct positioning of the ultrasound machine and the probe to perform the IPP block for the left side of the thorax.

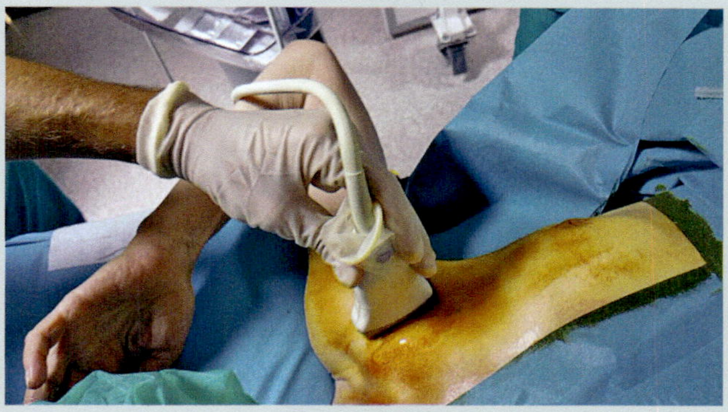

Figure 5.17 Alignment of the ultrasound probe to perform the IPP block, caudally to the third lateral of the clavicle in the deltopectoral groove.

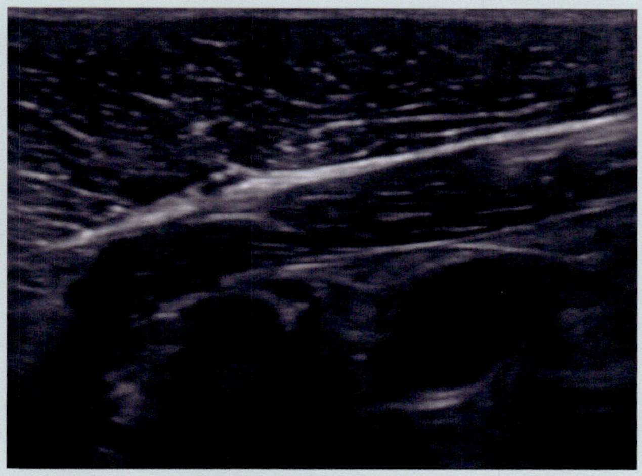

Figure 5.18 Ultrasound visualization after positioning the probe in the deltopectoral groove: the axillary vessels (vein and artery), the pectoralis major muscle, and the pectoralis minor muscle are in evidence.

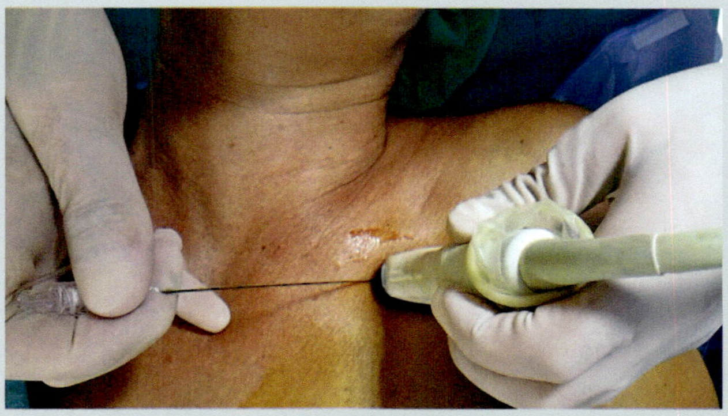

Figure 5.19 "In-plane" introduction of the needle (SonoPlex stim Pajunk®) after rotating the probe by 90° (to get to be parallel to the clavicle).

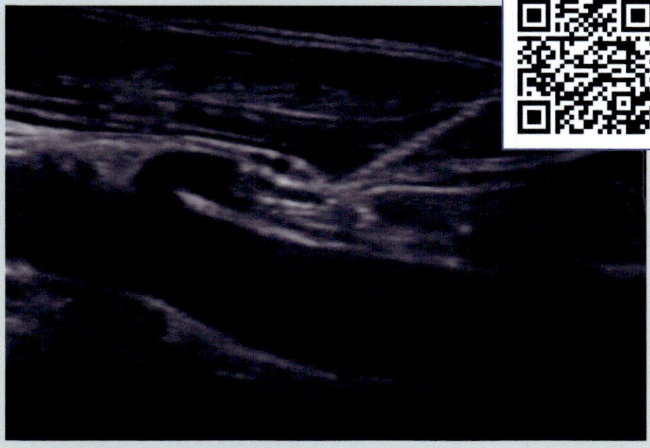

Figure 5.20 Once getting to the fascia between the pectoralis major muscle and the pectoralis minor muscle, the operator observes a resistance against the movement of the needle (SonoPlex stim Pajunk®) and, subsequently, also a loss of resistance that indicates that the needle has passed.

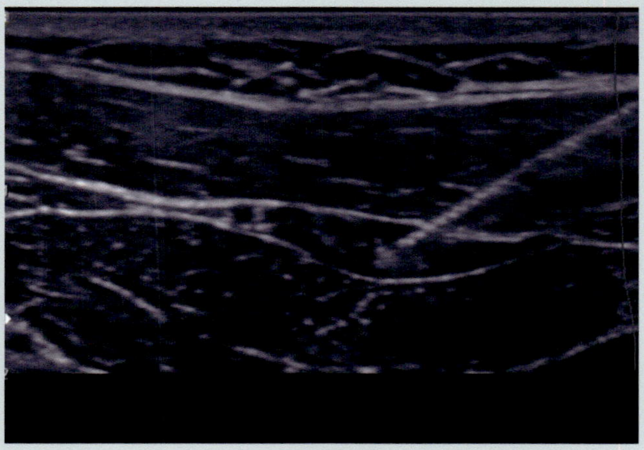

Figure 5.21 The tip of the needle (SonoPlex stim Pajunk®) inside the fascial plane and the injection of LA, together with the double V sign due to the spread of the LA within the fascial plane between the pectoralis major muscle and the pectoralis minor muscle.

Blanco suggests that the interfacial plane between the pectoral muscles can also be used for positioning a perineural catheter to prolong postoperative analgesia. There is a variant of the **IPP** execution technique in relation to this approach, which will be described in the next paragraph.

Technique for PSP Block

This technique allows to block the lateral branches of the intercostal nerves from T2 to T6, the long thoracic nerve, and the thoracodorsal nerve. The patient can assume two positions: supine position with the head rotated contralaterally to the block site and arm abducted by 90° or in a lateral position with the side to be blocked upwards and the arm abducted by 90° (**Figure 5.27 A**, **B**)
After obtaining accurate asepsis of the skin in the surrounding anatomical region and protecting the ultrasound probe with a sterile sheath, a high-frequency linear probe (6-18 MHz) is positioned on the chest wall, near the deltopectoral groove, as previously described. Subsequently, it is possible to visualize the second rib under the axillary vessels with a gradual lateral displacement of the probe itself (**Figures 5.22**, **5.23**, **5.24**).
Hence, a further movement of the probe in distal and medio-lateral direction towards the axillary cavity and the anterior axillary line will allow to reach the lateral margin of Pmm, under which the ribs III and IV can be identified (**Figures 5.25**, **5.26**). Near rib III, the sonoanatomical image highlights the fasclal plane formed by the PMm, Pmm and the anterior serratus muscle. At this level, Pmm lies over the serratus muscle, while the clavipectoral fascia continues with the axillary cavity as Gerdy's ligament. This point marks the entrance to the axillary cavity (**Figures 5.27**, **5.28**).

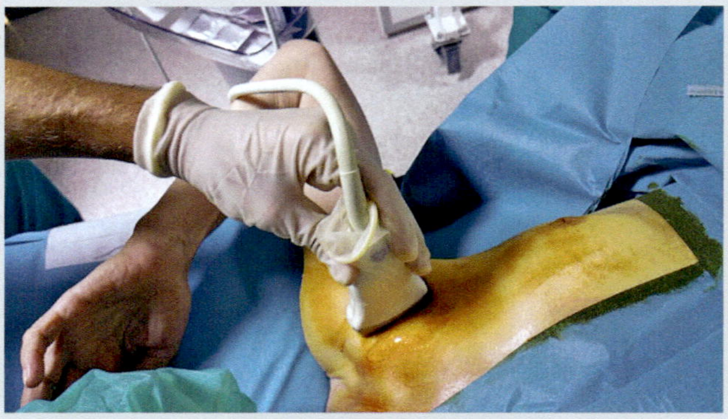

Figure 5.22 Initial positioning of the probe in the deltopectoral groove.

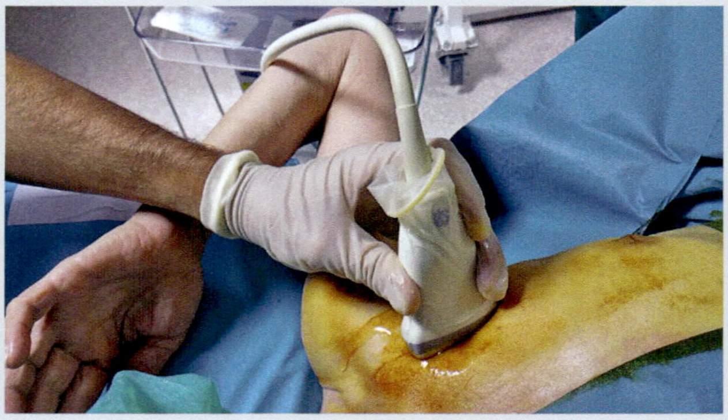

Figure 5.23 Slight lateral movement of the probe to visualize the ribs.

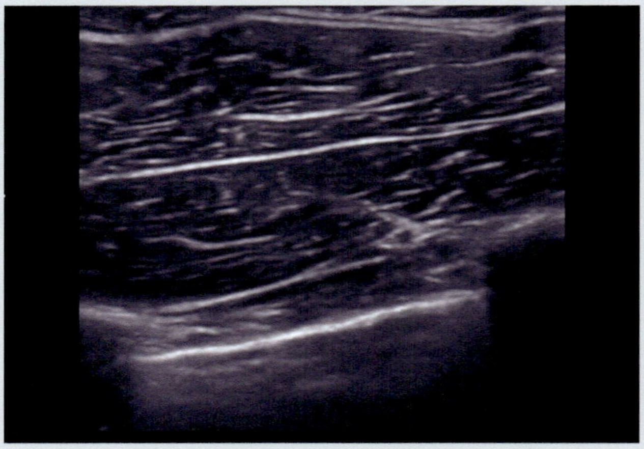

Figure 5.24 Ultrasound visualization after laterally moving the probe from the deltopectoral groove. Ribs II and III are easily identifiable.

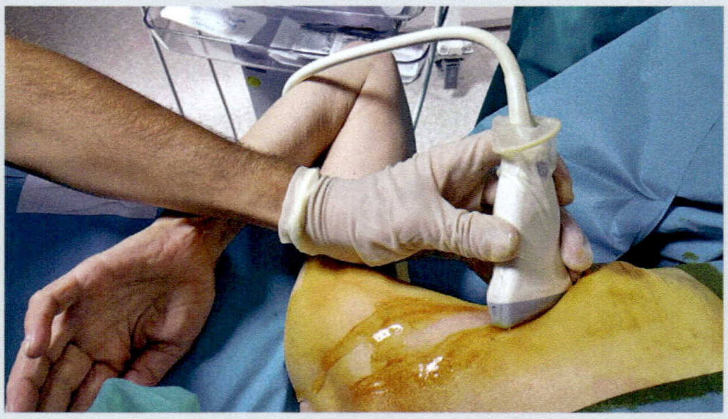

Figure 5.25 Positioning of the probe after the further distal and lateral movement.

After obtaining an optimal sonoanatomy image and positioning the target area of the block at the center of the screen of the ultrasound machine, the subcutaneous tissue is infiltrated in the entry point of the needle with some ml of 2% lidocaine (if the patient is awake and conscious); the needle (SonoPlex stim Pajunk®) is inserted with the in-plane technique on an oblique plane, with proximal/medial-distal/lateral orientation, and subsequently moved towards the interfascial plane (**Figure 5.29**).

To optimize the needle-probe alignment, it is recommended to insert the needle on a sagittal plane, at 1-2 cm from the probe itself, further increasing this distance in obese patients, where the target plane can turn out to be deeper due to a thick adipose panniculus.

If visualizing accurately the needle (SonoPlex stim Pajunk®) turns out to be difficult, it might be useful to move it with in-out micro-movements (jiggling) to generate a visible tissue movement near the tip, and to use an hydrolocation technique with a three-way stopcock, which requires the injection of a 1-2 ml physiological solution that will let the visualization of a small anechoic "pocket" near the tip itself. Only after checking the correct positioning of the needle tip, in the interfascial plane between Pmm and the ante-

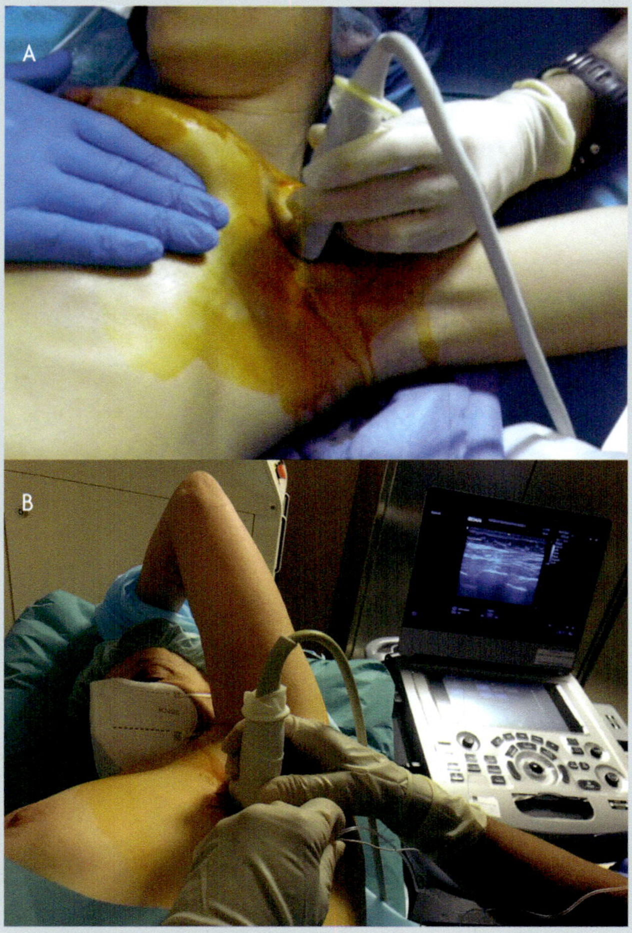

Figure 5.27 A Supine position of the patient and the correct positioning of the probe after performing the PSP block. **B** Lateral position of the patient and the correct positioning of the probe before the block is executed.

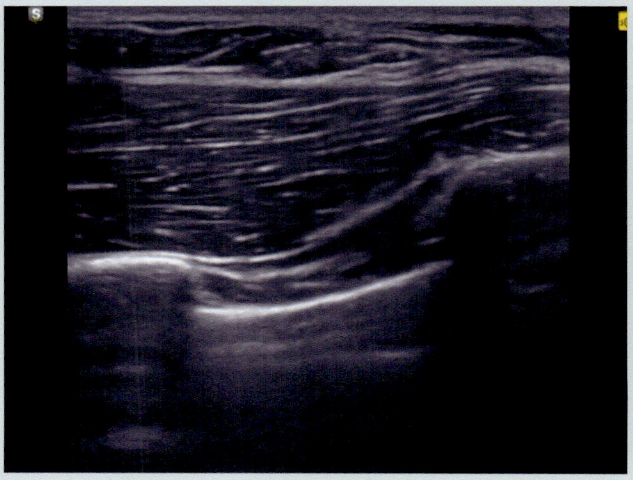

Figure 5.26 III and IV rib at the level of the anterior axillary line.

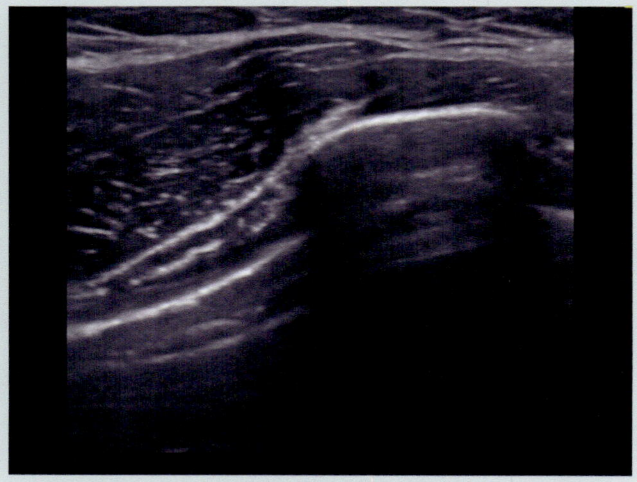

Figure 5.28 Ultrasound image of the IV rib (target block).

rior serratus muscle, above the IV rib, prior to due aspiration and resistance test, is it possible to inject the physiological solution through the three-way stopcock and to have ultrasound confirmation with the opening of the target interfascial plane.
Subsequently, 20 ml of 0.25% (analgesic dosage) or 0.5% (anesthetic dosage) levobupivacaine will be injected at this level, trying to move the needle within the plane to facilitate the opening and making sure that the anesthetic has distributed in the latero-medial direction at the end of the injection. For a correct execution of all the fascial blocks, Fusco et al. described the double V sign due to the spread of the LA within the fascial plane (**Figure 5.30 A**, **B**, **Video 5.2**). A variant to the described technique has been suggested, especially indicated in complex cases, which involves positioning the tip of the needle on the 4th rib and subsequent injection of anesthetic on the same plane.
At this point, if necessary, the operator can complete the block by removing the needle and positioning the tip on the interfascial plane between PMm and Pmm and, as previously described, can proceed with the block by injecting 10 ml of 0.25% (analgesic dosage) or 0, 5% (anesthetic dosage) levobupivacaine. Although PSP Block allows to block the lateral branches of the intercostal nerves T2-T6, the long thoracic nerve, and the thoracodorsal nerve it does not allow to anesthetize the anterior parasternal branches which provide sensory innervation to the medial breast side. Therefore, the authors think it is useful to integrate **PSP Block** with parasternal block in breast surgery, which involves the incision of the internal and central quadrants (see Chapter 6) (see **Flow chart 5.1 online**).

INDICATIONS AND DOSAGES

The recent literature is showing an increasing interest in new ultrasound-guided blocks of the chest wall. IPP and **PSP** blocks, described by Blanco and characterized by a lower invasiveness and a lower risk of

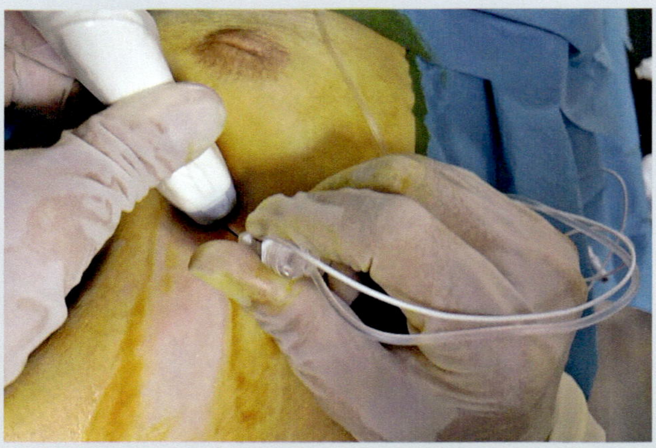

Figure 5.29 In-plane needle insertion for the PSP Block.

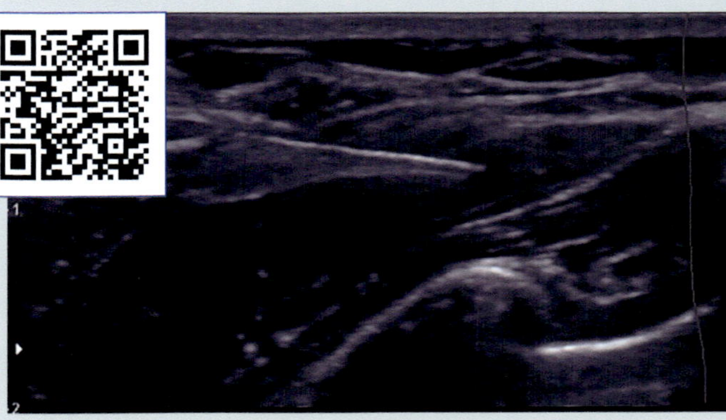

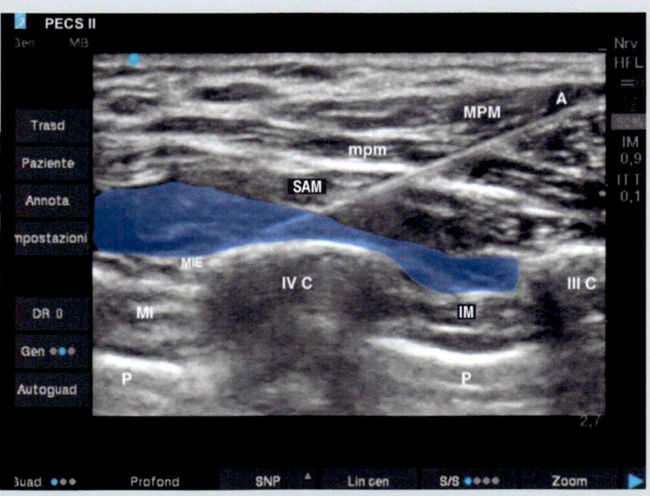

Figure 5.30 A The tip of the needle, at the level of the fourth rib, inside the fascial plane with diffusion of the local anesthetic and opening of the fascial plane (double V sign) between Pmm and the anterior serratus muscle. **B** The tip of the needle, on the fourth rib, with diffusion of the local anesthetic above the rib plane. IM: intercostal muscle; MPM: pectoral major muscle; mpm: pectoral minor muscle; P: pleura; SAM: serratus anterior muscle.

complications, are innovative interfacial nerve blocks that currently offer a valid alternative to epidural analgesia and paravertebral block for postoperative anesthesia and analgesia in breast surgery. The block of the pectoral nerves is a superficial, simple, and reproducible block, whose description is inspired by the infraclavicular block and by the transversus abdominis plane (TAP) block. IPP Block has as target LPN and MPN, which run along the interfacial plane between PMm and Pmm. For this reason, it is indicated in minor surgeries which involve PMm and Pmm such as the positioning of breast tissue expanders or subpectoral prostheses in breast reconstruction. Other possible indications include traumatic thoracic injuries, iatrogenic dissections of the pectoral muscle, positioning of internal automatic cardiac pacemakers/defibrillators (ICD), port-a-caths, and chest drainages. Furthermore, Blanco suggests how the interfascial plane between the pectoral muscles can be also used for the positioning of perineural catheters, so as to guarantee a prolonged postoperative analgesia if the pain intensity and duration are such to neutralize the effect of a single AL administration. Wallaert et al. have described how the administration of levobupivacaine via a catheter positioned on the plane between the fasciae of PMm and Pmm in patients undergoing breast surgery allows to achieve an excellent postoperative analgesia in the absence of side effects and complications.

In addition to blocking the pectoral nerves, PSP Block also has the purpose of blocking the lateral branches of the intercostal nerves T2-T6, which exit at the level of the axillary line and get to innervate the lateral side of the mammary gland and the corresponding cutaneous dermatomes, the intercostobrachial nerve, the long thoracic nerve, and the thoracodorsal nerve. PSP Block is also indicated in breast surgeries extended to the axilla such as mastectomies, large tumorectomies, dissections of sentinel lymph nodes, or surgeries that involve the intercostal innervations T2-T4 with extension up to T6. The studies performed through RMN with contrast medium have confirmed the efficacy of this technique, highlighting the uptake of the contrast solution at the level of the axilla passing over the serratus muscle, an anatomical area in which run the long thoracic nerve, the thoracodorsal nerve, and the lateral branches of the intercostal nerves, in the point where they emerge from the midaxillary line. In recent years, experiences regarding the use of PSP blocks in breast surgery have multiplied and have shown an excellent analgesic technique, thus allowing to reduce the consumption of opioids and the incidence of the related complications.

The association of adjuvants, in particular ketamine, with local anesthetics seems to guarantee a better analgesia without a higher incidence of complications. Further experiences have also been made in the minimally invasive cardiac surgery, where the application of IPP and PSP blocks has allowed to achieve a good analgesic control. These are experiences limited to case reports which will have to be validated by clinical trials to confirm the results obtained.

The onset time of the analgesic block is 20 minutes on average, whereas the duration of the analgesia can last up to 8 hours in the postoperative period, with a variability connected to the pharmacokinetics of the anesthetics used. According to the experts, the paravertebral block turns out to be the gold standard for postoperative analgesia in breast surgery. However, as the paravertebral space communicates with the epidural space, is close to the pleural space, and contains the arteries that vascularize the spinal cord, this technique can be associated to severe complications such as pneumothorax, epidural block, total spinal anesthesia, or intravascular injection. Furthermore, as the paravertebral block does not allow to achieve the block of MPN, LPN, the long thoracic nerve, and the thoracodorsal nerve, the component of the postoperative pain deriving from the brachial plexus does not turn out to be covered adequately, making this technique ineffective in breast surgery extended to the axillary cavity. The recent introduction of the new ultrasound-guided blocks of the chest wall allows to overcome these limits. Although the literature shows no statistically significant prospective randomized studies that highlights the analgesic superiority (or at least the analgesic non-inferiority) of the PSP Block compared to TPVB, this technique is currently a good candidate, above all in prospect, as valid alternative to the conventional regional techniques for postoperative anesthesia and analgesia in breast surgery. PSP Block is an easy to perform superficial technique that, in expert hands, offers the advantage of providing an adequate analgesic coverage, avoiding the complications and the sympathetic block associated with the conventional technique, as well as reducing the perioperative consumption of systemic opioids and the incidence of PONV. Recent scientific evidence suggests how IPP and PSP blocks block, when inserted in a multimodal approach, can provide a good anesthetic/analgesic option in the breast surgery extended to the armpit, especially in elderly patients or in patients with high anesthesiological risk due to the presence of coagulation disorders or associated comorbidities, which contraindicate the use of conventional locoregional techniques.

The use of IPP and PSP blocks turns out to be useful especially in day surgery, in accordance with the WAKE "zero tolerance criteria", as this allows an excellent control of the postoperative pain and a rapid discharge of the patient. Furthermore, these blocks, when integrated with an adequate intraoperative sedation, can be a rational choice in patients with an elevated anesthesiological risk and/or with comorbidity factors, thus allowing to avoid the risk connected to the execution of a general anesthesia (**Tables 5.1**, **5.2**).

Patients on whom the block should not be performed

Contraindications:

- patient's refusal
- allergy to AL
- infections in the site of injection

TABLE 5.1 SURGICAL INDICATIONS FOR IPP AND PSP

IPP	PSP
• Breast tissue expanders • Subpectoral prostheses • Traumatic chest injuries • Iatrogenic Dissections PMm, Pmm • Positioning of pacemakers and automatic cardiac defibrillators (ICD) • Port-a-caths • Thoracic drainages • Continuous postoperative analgesia in breast surgery	• Mastectomies • Large tumorectomies • Sentinel lymph node dissections • Axillary lymph node dissections • Surgeries that involve the intercostal nerves T2-T4 with extension up to T6

TABLE 5.2 MAIN LOCAL ANESTHETICS AND DOSES USED FOR IPP AND PSP BLOCKS

	IPP	PSP
Anesthesia (with or without GA)	• 10 ml of 0.5% levobupivacaine • 10 ml of 1.5% mepivacaine • 10 ml of 0.75% ropivacaine	• 20 ml of 0.5% levobupivacaine • 20 ml of 1.5% mepivacaine • 20 ml of 0.75% ropivacaine
Analgesia (with GA)	• 10 ml of 0.25% levobupivacaine • 10 ml of 0.375% ropivacaine	• 20 ml of 0.25% levobupivacaine • 20 ml of 0.375% ropivacaine
Adjuvants	Dexamethasone 4 mg Dexmedetomidine 1 mcg/kg	Dexamethasone 4 mg Dexmedetomidine 1 mcg/kg

GA, general anesthesia

COMPLICATIONS AND CONTRAINDICATIONS

Although the introduction of ultrasound systems in the clinical practice has allowed to improve the efficacy-safety combination connected to the implementation of locoregional techniques, the success of fascial blocks is strictly connected to the operator's experience. PSP block is a simple, superficial and relatively safe technique, but it might possibly involve rare complications that include pneumothorax, accidental intravascular injection, and the puncture of the axillary artery. A recent retrospective analysis has evaluated the incidence of complications in 498 PSP blocks performed in breast surgery, finding only 8 hematomas and no other complications among those previously indicated. The formation of hematoma remains a concern because of the proximity of vascular structures near the injection site. The intravascular injection in the pectoral branch of the acromiothoracic artery and the puncture of the axillary artery can probably be caused by a very high approach in the axillary cavity.

The indication for the execution of the blocks in patients with coagulation problems should be evaluated for each case on the basis of the risk/benefit ratio.

No absolute contraindication in the implementation of the PSP block is currently reported in the related literature.

Complications

- Vascular puncture (if performed by inexperienced operators)
- The formation of hematoma remains a concern because of the proximity of vascular structures near the injection site (for patients with coagulation problems, evaluate the risk/benefit ratio)
- Pneumothorax (if performed by inexperienced operators)
- Increased risk of LAST (connected to the high volumes of AL employed or the non-compliance of the maximum doses recommended)

RECOMMENDED READING

- Fusco P, Pizzorno L, Arcangeli V, Marinangeli F. Tube or not tube in COVID-19 positive patients: that is the question. Korean J Anesthesiol 2021 Dec;74(6):552-554
- Afsharimani B, Cabot P, Parat MO. Morphine and tumor growth and metastasis. Cancer Metastasis Rev. 2011 Jun;30(2):225-38.
- Andersen KG, et al. Persistent pain after breast cancer treatment: a critical review of risk factors and strategies for prevention. Journal of Pain. 2011;12:725-46.
- Andreae MH, Andreae DA. Regional anaesthesia to prevent chronic pain after surgery: a Cochrane systematic review and meta-analysis. British Journal of Anaesthesia. 2013;111(5):711-20.
- Apfelbaum JL, Chen C, Mehta SS, Gan TJ. Postoperative pain experience: results from a national survey suggest postoperative pain continues to be undermanaged. Anesth Analg. 2003;97:534-40.
- Bashandy GM, et al. Pectoral Nerves I and II Blocks in Multimodal Analgesia for Breast Cancer Surgery.A Randomized Clinical Trial. Reg Anesth Pain Med. 2015;40:68-74.
- Benyamin R, et al. Opioid complications and side effects. Pain Physician. 2008;11:S105-20.
- Blanco R, et al. Ultrasound description of Pecs II (modified Pecs I): a novel approach to breast surgery. Rev Esp Anestesiol Reanim. 2012 Nov;59(9):470-5.
- Blanco R. The 'pecs block': a novel technique for providing analgesia after breast surgery. Anaesthesia. 2011;66:847-8.
- Cancer Research UK. Breast Cancer incidence statistics, 2010. http://www.cancerresearchuk.org (accessed 01/03/2013)
- Coley KC, Williams BA, DaPos SV, Chen C, Smith RB. Retrospective evaluation of unanticipated admissions and readmissions after same day surgery and associated costs. J Clin Anesth. 2002;14: 349-53.
- Eti Z, Laçin T, Yildizeli B, Dogan V, Gögüs FY, Yüksel M. An uncommon complication of thoracic epidural anesthesia: pleural puncture. Anesth Analg. 2005;100:1540-1.
- Freise H, Van Aken HK. Risks and benefits of thoracic epidural anaesthesia. Br J Anaesth. 2011 Dec;107(6):859-68.
- Fusco P, De Sanctis F, Ruotolo F, Scimia P, Di Carlo S, Degan G, Marinangeli F. Pecs II and parasternal block for bilateral quadrantectomy and axillary surgery in a high anesthetic-risk patient. Regional Anesthesia and Pain Medicine. Volume 42, Number 5, Suppl 1, September-October 2017.
- Fusco P, Di Carlo S, Luciani A, Petrucci E, Degan G, Barattelli E, Marinangeli F. anesthetic use of pecs II block and parasternal block in radical mastectomy with prosthesis implant. Regional Anesthesia and Pain Medicine; Volume 42, Number 5, Suppl 1, September-October 2017.
- Fusco P, Scimia P, Petrucci E, Di Carlo S, Marinangeli F. The ultrasound-guided parasternal block: a novel approach for anesthesia and analgesia in breast cancer surgery. Minerva Anestesiol. 2017 Feb;83(2):221-2.
- Fusco P, Scimia P, Petrucci E, Luciani A, Danelli G, Pozone T, Marinangeli F. Ultrasound-guided Pecs II block in a high-anesthetic risk patient. Regional Anesthesia and Pain Medicine; Volume 40, Number 5, Suppl 1, September-October 2015. Abstracts and Highlight Papers of the 34th Annual European Society of Regional Anaesthesia & Pain Therapy (ESRA) Congress 2015 Ljubljana, Slovenia, 2-5 settembre 2015.
- Gan T J, et al. Consensus guidelines for the management of post-operative nausea and vomiting. Anesth Analg. 2014 Jan;118(1):85-113.
- Gray's Anatomy: The Anatomical Basis of Clinical Practice, 41 Ed. 2015 Elsevier.

- Hanna MN, Murphy JD, Kumar K, Wu CL. Regional techniques and outcome: what is the evidence? Curr Opin Anaesthesiol. 2009;22: 672-7.
- Kehlet H, Wilmore DW. Multimodal strategies to improve surgical outcome. Am J Surg. 2002;183(6):630-41.
- Lonnquist PA, Mackenzie SJ, Conacher ID. Paravertebral blockade: failure rate and complications. Anaesthesia. 1995;50:813-5.
- Office of National Statistics. Breast Cancer: Incidence, mortality and survival, 2010. http://www.ons.gov.uk (accessed 01/03/2013)
- Othman AH, El-Rahman AM, El Sherif F. Efficacy and Safety of Ketamine Added to Local Anesthetic in Modified Pectoral Block for Management of Postoperative Pain in Patients Undergoing Modified Radical Mastectomy. Pain Physician. 2016 Sep-Oct;19(7):485-94.
- Porzionato A, Macchi V, Stecco C, Loukas M, Tubbs RS, de Caro R. Surgical anatomy of the pectoral nerves and the pectoral musculature. Clinical Anatomy. 2012; 25: 559-75.
- Risdahl JM, Khanna KV, Peterson PK, Molitor TW. Opiates and infection. J Neuroimmunol. 1998 Mar 15;83(1-2):4-18.
- Sacerdote P, Franchi S, Panerai AE. Non-analgesic effects of opioids: mechanisms and potential clinical relevance of opioid-induced immunodepression. Curr Pharm Des. 2012;18(37):6034-42.
- Savoia G, Alampi D, Amantea B, et al. Postoperative pain treatment. SIAARTI Recommendations 2010 Short version. Minerva Anestesiol. 2010;76: 657-67.
- Scimia P, Fusco P, Petrucci E, Pozone T, Bafile A, Marinangeli F. Sindrome dolorosa cronica post-mastectomia. Dolore Aggiornamenti Clinici n° 1-2 / 2015, pp 22-30. Organo ufficiale della Associazione Italiana per lo Studio del Dolore.
- Shnabel A, Reichl SU, Kranke P, et al. Efficacy and safety of paravertebral blocks in breast surgery: a meta-analysis of randomized controlled trials. Br J Anaesth. 2010;105(6):842-52.
- Sinatra R. Causes and consequences of inadequate management of acute pain. Pain Med. 2010;11: 1859-71.
- Snyder GL, Greenberg S. Effect of anaesthetic technique and other perioperative factors on cancer recurrence. British Journal of Anaesthesia. 2010;105(2):106-15.
- Ueshima H, Hiroshi O. i Transcatheter aortic valve implantation performed with a PECS block and a TTP block. J Clin Anesth. 2017 May;38:1.
- Ueshima H, Otake H. Ultrasound-guided pectoral nerves (PECS) block: Complications observed in 498 consecutive cases. J Clin Anesth. 2017 Nov;42:46.
- Wallaert M, et al. Bloc interpectoral avec mise en place d'un cathéter pour analgésie postopératoire après chirurgie mammaire. Annales Françaises d'Anesthésie et de Réanimation. 2014; 33:269-71.
- Wang K, Zhang X, Zhang T, Yue H, Sun S, Zhao H, Zhou P. The Efficacy of Ultrasound-guided Type II Pectoral Nerve Blocks in Perioperative Pain Management for Immediate Reconstruction after Modified Radical Mastectomy. A Prospective, Randomized Study. Clin J Pain. 2017 Jun 16.
- White PF. The changing role of non-opioid analgesic techniques in the management of postoperative pain. Anesth Analg. 2005;101:15-22.
- Williams BA, Kentor ML.The WAKE Score: Patient-Centered Ambulatory Anesthesia and Fast-Tracking Outcomes Criteria. International Anesthesiology Clinics.2011; Volume 49, Number 3, 33-43.
- Yalamuri S, Klinger RY, Bullock WM, Glower DD, Bottiger BA, Gadsden JC. Pectoral Fascial (PECS) I and II Blocks as Rescue Analgesia in a Patient Undergoing Minimally Invasive Cardiac Surgery. Reg Anesth Pain Med. 2017 Nov/Dec;42(6):764-6.
- Pierfrancesco FUSCO, Emiliano PETRUCCI, Franco MARINANGELI, Paolo SCIMIA Block failure or lack of efficacy? The "DoubleV" Sign: a novel sonographic sign for a succesfull interfascial plane block. Minerva Anestesiologica 2019 August;85(8):917-8.
- Fusco P, Cofini V, Petrucci E, Pizzi B, Necozione S, Marinangeli F. The anaesthetic and analgesic effects of pectoral nerve and parasternal block combination for patients undergoing breast cancer surgery: A phase II study. Eur J Anaesthesiol 2019 Oct;36(10):798-801.
- F Costa, A Strumia, L M Remore, G Pascarella, R Del Buono, M Tedesco, G Sepolvere, P Scimia, P Fusco. Breast surgery analgesia: another perspective for PROSPECT guidelines. Anaesthesia 2020 Oct;75(10):1404-1405. doi: 10.1111/anae.15161. Epub 2020 Jun 11
- Karem El-Boghdadly et al. Standardizing nomenclature in regional anesthesia: an ASRA-ESRA Delphi consensus study of abdominal wall, paraspinal, and chest wall blocks. Reg Anesth Pain Med. 2021 Jul;46(7):571-580.

CLINICAL CASE 1 – SAFETY OF PSP (PECS BLOCK II) IN PATIENTS WITH HIGH ANESTHETIC RISK

Clinical history and anamnesis We reported the use of PCS II Block in a 65-year-old woman for external quadrantectomy with a recent (<30 days) ischemic heart attack with percutaneous coronary intervention (ASA III). She was under dual-antiplatelet therapy (clopidogrel and aspirin);

Technique description After IRB approval and written patient consent statement, in L'Aquila Academic Hospital an ultrasound-guided unilateral PSP Block was performed under aseptic conditions, using a linear probe in plane approach, a 22 G echogenic needle (SonoPlex stim cannula, Pajunk®) was directed towards the fascial plane and 20 ml of 0.5% Levobupivacaine were injected.

Materials and methods A light sleep with easy arousability was ensured with 1.5-3 mg/kg/h of propofol intravenously. Supplemental oxygen (2 l/min) was administered by nasal dispenser with $ETCo_2$ control. Heart rate, main blood pressure, arterial oxigen saturation and $ETCo_2$ greater or less than 30% of baseline were treated (**Figure 5.31**).

A good anesthesia and analgesia were obtained and no supplemental opiates were injected during surgery. No side effects were recorded and the patient, after PACU phases 1 and 2, was discharged and she came back in the ward without rest and incidence of pain. Only 1 g of acetaminophen every eight hours was systematically administered and no supplemental opioids were required. Postoperative nausea and vomiting and other complications were absent.
The day after surgery, the patient was discharged from the hospital and no side effects were recorded.

Conclusions This experience shows that PSP block is a good anesthetic alternative to ensure the possibility of surgery. PECS II block has proved to be a safe and effective alternative to conventional techniques, providing an adequate intraoperative hemodynamic stability and an excellent postoperative analgesia, avoiding the administration of additional systemic analgesics and the occurrence of complications in a patient at high anesthetic risk.

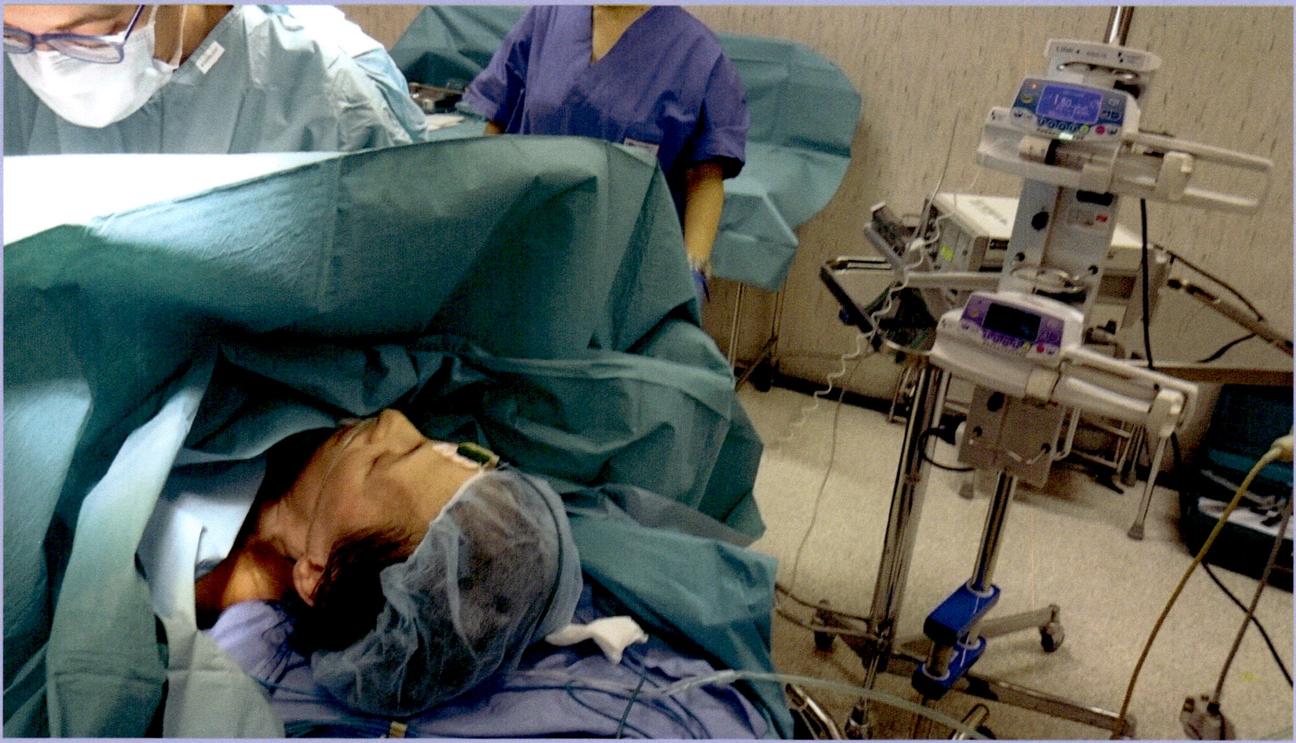

Figure 5.31 Patient undergoing external quandrantectomy and spontaneous breathing obtained by intravenous infusion of propofol at 1.5-3 mg/kg/h.

CLINICAL CASE 2 – FASCIAL PLANE BLOCK IN COVID-19 POSITIVE PATIENTS

Clinical history and anamnesis At San Salvatore Academic Hospital in L'Aquila, Italy, a 65-year-old woman, COVID-19 positive asymptomatic and negative for pneumonia, underwent a right supero-lateral quadrantectomy, with regional lymph node dissection that, according to the surgeon, was not postponable. She was 175 cm tall, weighed 140 kg (BMI 45 kg/m), and had an ASA physical status classification 3. She had a number of comorbidities: hypertension, OSA, respiratory insufficiency, diabetes mellitus type 2, dyslipidemia, peripheral neuropathy, empty saddle syndrome. Hemogasanalysis showed a paO_2 = 63 and pCO_2 = 51 with no oxygen implementation. The patient filled a lot of the criteria used to predict difficulty with intubation or ventilation: Mallampati = 3, STOP-Bang score = 7, El-Ganzouri score = 8, neck circumference of 43 cm.

Technique description In this patient, we decided to do PECS-2 (PSP) block and Parasternal Block (Superficial PIP) in sedation and spontaneous breathing, having in each moment everything we needed for anticipated airway management difficulty. PSP and Superficial PIP were conducted in a block room using a linear sound and a 50 mm needle (SonoPlex stim cannula, Pajunk®). The patient was placed in lateral position in order to keep away from operator the patient's droplets. PSP block was performed: the needle progresses up to below the Pectoralis minor and above the Serratus anterior, depositing local anesthetic (20 ml of ropivacaine 0.75%) in this anatomical space (in order to cover the medial pectoral nerve and the lateral branches of the intercostals), and Superficial PIP with ropivacaine 0.375% between pectoralis major and intercostal muscle (**Figure 5.32 A**, **B**).

Materials and methods A sedation with easy arousability was ensured with 3-4 mg/kg/h of intravenously propofol. Supplemental oxygen (8 l/min, 40% of inspired fraction of oxygen) is administered by Venturi mask under end tidal CO_2 control to ensure an oxygen saturation (O_2sa%) higher than 90%; heart rate, ECG, arterial blood pressure and O_2sa% were monitored during the surgery. A good quality anesthesia of the mammary and axillary regions was obtained with a good hemodynamic stability; at the end of surgical procedure, the patient was admitted in PacU phase 1 and phase 2, according to the PacU policy. In the first 24 hours after surgery the patient did not request opiates, and only 2000 mg of acetaminophen were administered without nausea, vomiting and cardiovascular and respiratory complications.

Conclusions The problem of the choice between general anesthesia and locoregional anesthesia, in this type of patient, is still today a challenge for the anesthetist. Literature suggests to use regional anesthesia for surgery in patients with difficult airway management, known or predicted, but we do not have enough data or indication about fascial block use in this type of patient. We propose this anesthesiologic approach in case of anticipated airway management difficulty especially in a COVID-19 positive patients, recommending the use of a fascial block, trusting in future works that could validate our anesthesiologic approach.

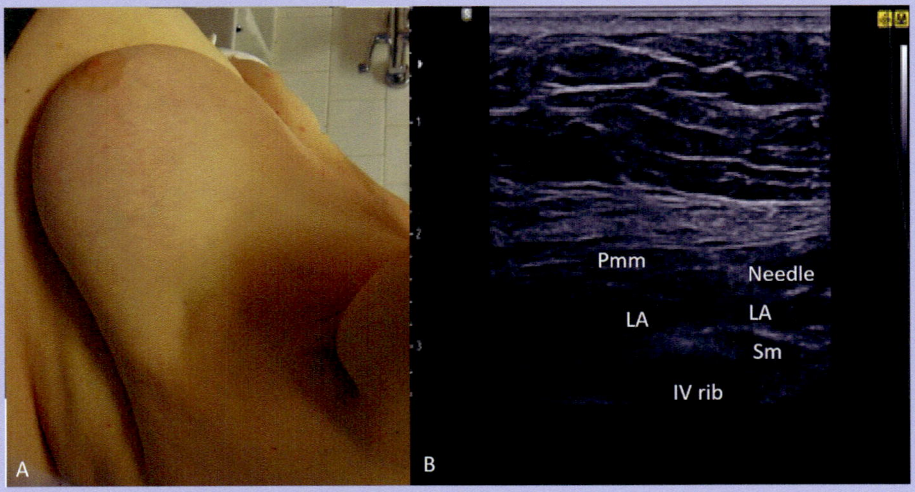

Figure 5.32 A Patient in lateral position to perform PSP block. **B** PSP Block. LA: local anesthetic; Pmm: pectoral minor muscle; Sm: serratus muscle.

CHAPTER 6

Superficial parasternal intercostal plane block (PIP)

Pierfrancesco Fusco, Giuseppe Paladini, Paolo Scimia, Luigi Tritapepe, Giuseppe Sepolvere

The surgery of the anterior chest wall often causes the onset of moderate-to-severe acute postoperative pain. Despite a multimodal approach, which requires the systemic administration of drugs such as opioids, anti-inflammatory drugs (NSAIDs), paracetamol, and dexamethasone, analgesic management is often unsatisfactory.

The related literature has recently shown the efficacy of the ultrasound-guided blocks of the chest walls – IPP, PSP, Serratus Anterior Plane Block (SAP superficial and deep), – ensuring a better postoperative pain management in breast surgery.

Furthermore, these blocks represent a valid alternative to the standard regional techniques, such as epidural anesthesia or paravertebral block, widely used in the chest wall and breast surgery, as they show many advantages in terms of efficacy and safety, especially in those patients with high anesthesiological risk.

Unfortunately, as indicated by Karmakar et al., these techniques do not allow to block the anterior cutaneous branches of the intercostal nerves T2-T6 near the sternum, and this in turn does not allow to achieve a complete antalgic cover, particularly in the medial region of the mammary gland. This observation has frequently led to the description of various techniques of locoregional anesthesia (LRA), aimed at blocking these nerve branches.

In 2005, a randomized-controlled trial by McDonald et al. (n = 20) showed the efficacy of parasternal infiltration in analgesic control after median sternotomy.

The literature describes several procedures named with different nomenclature. The principal factor that differentiates this constellation of techniques is where the nerves are targeted.

If local anesthetic is deposited deep to PMM and superficial to the external intercostal muscle (EIM) we describe the ultrasound parasternal block (PSB) or pecto-intercostal fascial block (PIFB), the anterior thoracic medial block or subpectoral interfascial plane block (PPB), the parasternal intercostal nerve block (PSI or PIB). If local anesthetic is injected between the internal intercostal muscle (IIM) and transversus thoracis muscle (TTM) we describe the transversus thoracis plane block (TTMPB). In 2014, de la Torre et al. described the pecto-intercostal fascial block, and subsequently, in 2016, Ueshima et al. described transverse thoracic muscle plane block (TTMPB) for post-median sternotomy analgesia and as adjuvant to PSP for breast surgery. However, as stated by the authors themselves, TTMPB is associated with an increased risk of pleural or vascular puncture, because the injection of the local anesthetic (AL) is done in a muscle plane situated deeper than the parasternal block target; for this reason, Ohgoshi et al. proposed as an alternative a technique for blocking the anterior branches of the intercostal nerves (parasternal intercostal nerve block, PSI block) that consists in injecting AL in the plane between the pectoralis major muscle and the external intercostal muscles.

As highlighted by Del Buono et al., this more superficial approach is comparable to TTMPB in terms of antalgic control, even though it is burdened by a lower morbidity. In 2016 Thomas et al described the parasternal block consisted in local anesthetic injection beyond the internal intercostal muscles, anterior to the transversus thoracic muscle to block the anterior branches of the intercostal nerves, in the same year Hansen et al. described the Parasternal PECS Block as support for PECS 1, PECS 2, and SPB block in breast surgery when the internal breast quadrants are involved.

Finally, in 2017, Fusco et al. described a superficial variant named the ultrasound guided parastenal block of the (PSB), which consists in depositing local anesthetic under the pectoralis major muscle, that is in the plane where the anterior branches of the intercostal nerves pierce the external intercostal muscle: therefore, if duly integrated with other interfascial blocks PSB can ensure the anesthetic/analgesic coverage of the entire anterior part of the chest wall and in the breast surgeries that require an incision of the medial quadrants of the breast.

Although several names have been coined, the recent first international consensus led by representatives of both ASRA and ESRA, on the nomenclature and anatomical descriptions of abdominal wall, chest wall, and paraspinal blocks established that there was a limited consensus on the various approaches described and which have been renamed as deep and superficial parasternal intercostal plane block (PIP)

For this reason in this chapter, we will use superficial parasternal intercostal plane blocks (PIP) instead of Parasternal block (PSB).

ANATOMY

To understand the anatomical targets of Superficial PIP, it is necessary to take into consideration the following reference lines that facilitate the subdivision in regions and the localization in medical reports:

- mediosternal line: divides the sternum in two halves and continues in the abdomen with the xipho-pubic line;
- marginal sternal line: tangentially follows the lateral margin of the sternum;
- parasternal line: runs parallel and laterally to the marginal sternal line, at about 2-3 cm from the latter;
- sternal angle line: horizontal, it passes through the joint between manubrium and sternum. Posteriorly, it corresponds to the T4 vertebra. The junction between manubrium and sternum forms an angle, easily identified by palpation and called sternal angle (or "the angle of Louis"), that corresponds to the second rib and, therefore, to the second intercostal space immediately below it.

Starting from the cutaneous surface, it is possible to identify the following muscles in the region between the marginal sternal and parasternal line, which is delimited by the second costal cartilage at the top and by the fourth costal cartilage at the bottom:

- Pectoralis major muscle – sternocostal part;
- External intercostal muscles and external intercostal membrane (connective aponeurosis placed between each external intercostal muscle and the sternum, on the same plane of the muscles themselves);
- Internal intercostal muscles;
- Innermost intercostal muscle;
- Transversus thoracic muscle.

The four intercostal spaces included in this area are occupied by the intercostal muscles. Below are the elements present in the costal sulcus, going from top to bottom along the inferior margin of the upper rib and passing through the plane between the two internal muscle layers:

- Intercostal vein: the intercostal veins drain into the systems of azygos veins or in the internal thoracic veins (or internal mammary veins) that join to the brachiocephalic veins in the neck.
- Anterior intercostal artery: the anterior intercostal arteries originate as lateral branches of the internal thoracic arteries (or internal mammary arteries). On each side, the internal thoracic artery lies posteriorly to the costal cartilages of the six upper ribs, at around 1 cm laterally from the sternum.
- Internal mammary artery: descends vertically about 1 cm lateral to the sternal border, behind the first 6 costal cartilages. It is accompanied by 2 mammary veins, which ascend medially and laterally, respectively (**Figure 6.1**) The IMA runs between internal intercostal muscle (IIM) and transversus thoracis muscle (TTM), which is a thin and hypoechogenic muscular layer close to the pleura (Pl) on the inner surface of the anterior thoracic wall.

- Intercostal nerve: the first six intercostal nerves run along the entire span of the corresponding intercostal space: once reaching the sternum, they perforate the chest wall and spread throughout the skin around the anterolateral thoracic area, as anterior cutaneous branches (**Figure 6.1**). The second, third, and fourth anterior cutaneous branches go to the medial part of the breast as medial mammary branches.

A layer of loose connective tissue called endothoracic fascia, containing variable quantities of adipose tissue, is situated at a deeper level in relation to the intercostal places and ribs, and is positioned in such a way as to separate these structures from the underlying pleura.

DESCRIPTION OF THE TECHNIQUE

The Superficial PIP is a locoregional technique for anterior thoracic wall analgesia, which consists in blocking anterior rami of intercostal nerve from T2 to T8. With the patient in supine decubitus position and both arms extended along the body, the operator places a high-frequency linear probe (12.5 MHz) at 2 or 3 cm laterally from the sternum in longitudinal position. Subsequently, the operator will proceed to the visualization: a) the short axis image of the ribs with the corresponding posterior shadow cone; b) the pectoralis major muscle; c) the intercostal muscles (external, internal, and innermost); d) the pleural sliding resulted from visceral pleural layer that slides over the parietal layer. The high echogenicity of the pleura and the characteristic sliding movements of the lung make the related anatomy easily recognizable.

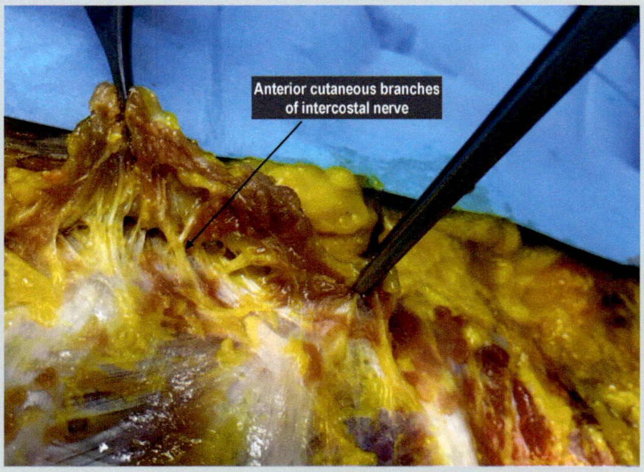

Figure 6.1 Dissection on fresh cadaver, anterior chest wall, parasternal region (courtesy of Prof. Carla Stecco, Department of Human Anatomy, University of Padua).

A characteristic image of sonoanatomy which can be kept in mind for performing Superficial PIP is the one called "bat sign", highlighted by the echo-reflecting convex surfaces of the ribs with the related shadow cone and the intercostal space with the underlying pleural line. This image generated by the sequence (rib-pleural line-rib) is called "bat sign" because of its resemblance to a bat.

A 22 G, 50-80 mm block echogenic needle (SonoPlex stim Pajunk®), is inserted "in-plane" to the ultrasonic beam in cranio-caudal direction, and directed towards the upper margin of rib II and, subsequently, towards the upper margin of rib IV, thus avoiding the vascular-nerve bundle and protecting the needle tip against pleural punctures.

Once reaching the block target, represented by the external intercostal membrane between the pectoralis major muscle and the external intercostal muscle, the operator administers 2-3 ml of physiological solution, in order to determine the correct localization of the needle tip (hydrolocation), attested by the correct opening of the target fascial plane (double V Sign), a total of 10 ml of the local anesthetic will be injected at the Rib II and RIB IV, in the fascial plane between the pectoral major muscle and the external intercostal muscle, 2 cm lateral to the sternal edge (**Figure 6.2 A**, **B**, **Video 6.1**) (**Flow chart 6.1 online**).

If the block is performed to obtain an anesthetic plan, it is recommended using a higher concentration of local anesthetic such as levobupivacaine 0.5%, ropivacaine 0.5%, mepivacaine 2%.

The authors recommend the use of Color Doppler to identify the internal mammary artery (**Figure 6.3**) and its branches, as well as the anterior intercostal arteries, which run along the intercostal spaces between the pectoralis major muscle and the internal intercostal muscles.

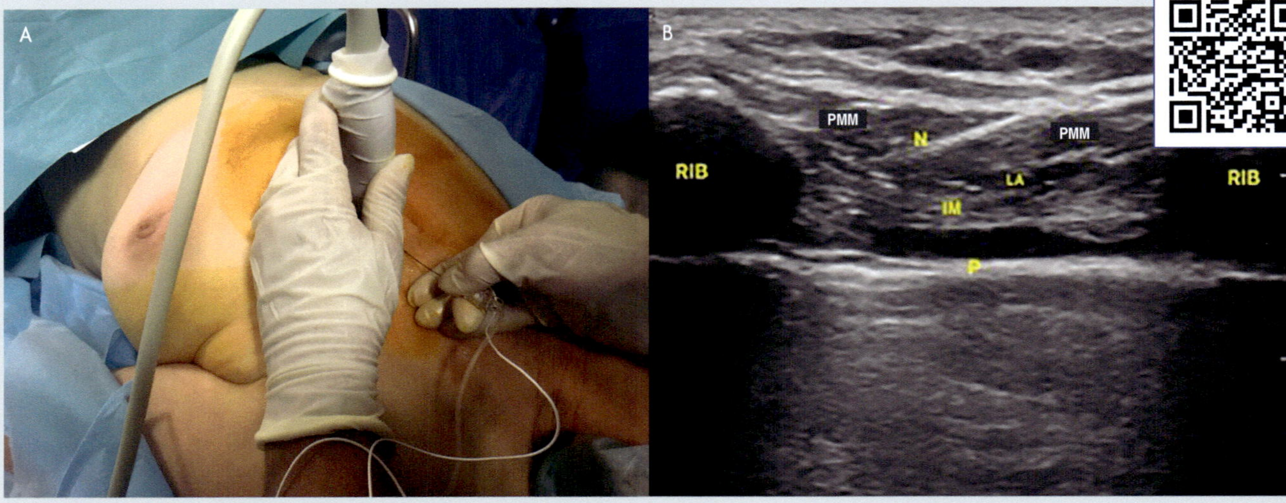

Figure 6.2 A Superficial PIP performed with atraumatic 22 G 50 mm SonoPlex stim Pajunk® needle using an in plane approach in cranial-caudal direction. **B** Superficial PIP. IM: intercostal muscle; LA: local anesthetic; N: needle; P: pleura; PMM: pectoralis major muscle; RIB: rib. The Superficial PIP target is the external intercostal membrane, located between the pectoralis major muscle and the intercostal muscle.

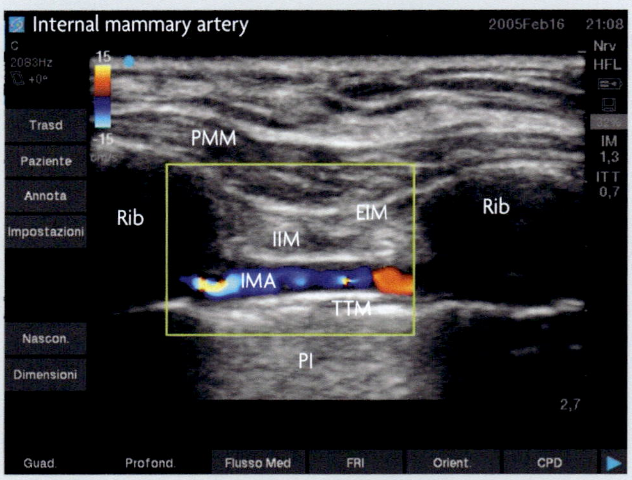

Figure 6.3 Ultrasound internal mammary artery landmarks. The internal mammary artery runs between the internal intercostal and tansversus thoracis muscles. EIM: external intercostal membrane; IM: intercostal muscle; IMA: internal mammary artery; Pl: pleura; PMM: pectoralis major muscle; TTM: transversus thoracis muscle.

It is also recommended to verify the presence of the pleural sliding at the end of block. The "seashore sign" is well-visible in M-Mode as a grainy image that indicates the rubbing between the pleural sheets that excludes the presence of pneumothorax.

The absence of sliding, which suggests the lack of contact between the visceral and parietal pleural sheets, can signal the interposition of air due to the presence of an iatrogenic pneumothorax. In this circumstance, the operator will find a pattern of parallel static lines called "barcode sign" in M-Mode.

INDICATIONS AND DOSAGES

Superficial PIP is indicated in all the operations of the anterior chest wall that involve the parasternal anterior branches of the intercostal nerves T2-T6, with potential applications in breast surgery, cardiac surgery, toracic surgery, and the treatment of the anterior chest wall deformities (pectus carinatum, pectus arcuatum, and pectus excavatum).

As to the doses, two separated 5 ml injections of long-acting or short-acting LA, at an adequate concentration based on the desired action at the level of the Rib II and Rib IV, are needed to obtain a successful block (**Table 6.1**).

TABLE 6.1 MAIN LOCAL ANESTHETICS AND DOSES USED FOR SUPERFICIAL PIP

	Local anesthetics
Anesthesia with or without GA:	Levobupivacaine 0.5% 10 ml
Anesthesia with or without GA:	Mepivacaine 1.5% 10 ml
Anesthesia with or without GA:	Ropivacaine 0.75% 10 ml
Analgesia with or without GA.	Levobupivacaine 0.375%
Adjiuvants	Dexamethasone 4 mg Dexmedetomidine 1 mcg/kg

GA, general anesthesia

Patients on whom the block should not be performed

Contraindications:

- patient's refusal
- allergy to AL
- infections in the injection site
- presence of subcutaneous implantable devices or costal fractures at the level of the target block site

COMPLICATIONS AND CONTRAINDICATIONS

Major complications after ultrasound thoracic wall blocks have not been reported. Superficial PIP is a simple, superficial, and relatively safe technique, especially due to the introduction of ultrasounds.

However, it is useful to remember that the success of the block is strictly linked to the operator's experience. Despite Superficial PIP having good safety profiles and reduced risk of complications, pneumothorax, and/or pericardial puncture, local anesthetic systemic toxicity, and IMA injury or hematoma especially in the case of poor visualization of the related anatomical structures and poor visualization of the needle point during the procedure should be considered. The indication for the execution of the blocks in patients with coagulation problems should be evaluated for each case on the basis of the risk/benefit ratio.

Absolute contraindications to Superficial PIP are not reported in the related literature, although the patient's refusal, a documented allergy to the local anesthetics used, the infections at the level of the injection site, the presence of implantable subcutaneous devices, or the presence of costal fractures obviously make this technique impractical.

Complications

- Accidental intravascular injection (LAST)
- Pneumothorax
- Pericardial puncture
- IMA injury or hematoma

APPLICATIONS TO THE PEDIATRIC SETTING

Superficial PIP is a technique that finds applications also in the pediatric setting, in all the superficial operations of the anterior chest wall that involve the anterior branches of the intercostal nerves T2-T6.

Consider the treatment of the chest wall deformities (pectus carinatum, pectus arcuatum, and pectus excavatum).

As to the doses employed in the pediatric setting, the recent ASRSA/ESRA recommendations suggest using the doses of 0.25- 0.75 mg/kg (Evidence B1) for bupivacaine or ropivacaine in fascial plane blocks.

With reference to other ALs, the maximum recommended doses based on the weight of the pediatric patients should not be exceeded.

Superficial parasternal intercostal plane (PIP) block and cardiac surgery

Cardiac surgery is commonly performed via median sternotomy which requires both muscle and bone division. Recent literature showed that the treatment of poststernotomy pain is often inadequate and associated with sympathetic nervous system activation and an increased hormonal stress response, which may lead to multiple adverse postoperative events, including myocardial ischemia, cardiac arrhythmias, hypercoagulability, dysfunctions of the respiratory system with a subsequent increased risk of delayed extubation and pulmonary infections, and increased rates of delirium and wound infection. Poorly controlled pain leading to the development of chronic pain that may compromise quality of life of patients with significant societal costs. Different approaches may be used in the treatment of acute poststernotomy pain, including thoracic epidural analgesia, spinal anesthesia, paravertebral and intercostal blocks, or opioids delivered via intravenous patient controlled analgesia (PCA). However, the use of neuraxial techniques for cardiac surgery remains controversial because of the possibility, although rare, of epidural hematoma in the setting of anticoagulation for cardiopulmonary bypass. Moreover, the use of opioids often provides minimal benefit to the patient and has significant adverse effects such as nausea, vomiting, ileus and respiratory depression. To further lower the risk of epidural hematoma and pneumothorax, regional techniques have been studied, including various fascial plane chest wall blocks, such as IPP, PSP, Serratus Anterior Plane Block (SAP superficial and deep), and erector spine plane blocks. These techniques are an important adjunct to optimal postoperative analgesia in cardiac surgery in order to provide enhanced postsurgical analgesia and facilitate faster functional recovery and earlier discharge.

Our experience with Superficial PIP (Parasternal block [PSB] described by Fusco et al.) began in breast surgery, using it with the rationale to provide anesthesia and analgesia for the medial part of the breast, which could not be covered by other thoracic wall blocks such as IPP, PSP, Serratus Anterior Plane Block (SAP superficial and deep). Since then, other authors have described the use of this block in different types of cardio-thoracic surgery in both adults and children.

Based on the result of recent literature, we could confirm that this block has three main characteristics. First, Superficial PIP block may be an effective technique in all interventions that involve the anterior rami of the intercostal nerves. Its effectiveness has been demonstrated for anesthesia and postoperative analgesia in cardiac surgery via median sternotomy, and in subcutaneous implantable cardioverter defibrillator (S-ICD) implantation.

Second, Superficial PIP Block may be a versatile and easy to perform technique. This block target a superficial fascial plane between Major Pectoral and intercostal muscles at level of external intercostal membrane, requires low doses of local anesthetic and has a rapid learing curve.

Third, Superficial PIP Block has an excellent safety profile. It represents a valid alternative to neuraxial technique and paravertebral block in patients with alterations of the preoperative coagulation profile, and presents a reduced risk of complications such as pneumothorax and local anesthetic systemic toxicity (LAST).

Many articles have been published describing the application of this technique for a wide cardiac surgery scenarios such as median sternotomy pain management, implantable cardioverter-defibrillator implantation, sternal resynthesis or steel sternal wire removal in spontaneous breathing. Current evidence suggests that Superficial PIP provide effective analgesia for breast and cardiac surgeries, cardiac device implantation, pericardiocentesis, and acute and chronic pain management. It is performed in the region of IMA and could be considered for the treatment of sternotomy pain and residual post-thoracotomy pain syndrome in cardiac surgery facilitating faster functional recovery, earlier discharge and fast track extubation reducing pulmonary complications and length of stay. On this basis, Superficial PIP became an integral part of Enhanced Recovery After Surgery (ERAS) protocols in cardiac surgery facilitate faster functional recovery and earlier discharge to achieve high-quality postoperative analgesia for sternotomy. It can be considered a safe technique for intra and postoperative pain relief in cardiac surgery and was used to obtain also an effective anesthetic plan for cardiac sternal resynthesis, steel sternal wire removal and sternal wound debridement in patients affected by severe chronic obstructive pulmonary disease, Covid-19 pneumonia or difficult predicted airway especially in patients with high anesthetic risk for whom general anesthesia and opioid administration could be harmful and increase intensive care unit length of stay, keeping them in spontaneous breathing. Furthermore, unlike neuraxial blocks, it can be used in patients who are anti-coagulated perioperatively and have deranged coagulation parameters.

RECOMMENDED READING

- Fusco P, DI Carlo S, Vespasiano M, Scimia P, Petrucci E, Panella L, Marinangeli F. Chest wall blocks and minimally invasive image-guide procedures: the meeting point between radiology and anesthesiology that could improve safety and patient outcomes in Nora. Minerva Anestesiologica 2018 August;84(8):993-4
- Abrahams MS, Horn JL, Noles LM, Aziz MF. Evidence-based medicine: ultrasound guidance for truncal blocks. Regional anesthesia and pain medicine. 2010;35:S36-42.
- Anastasi G, et al. Trattato di Anatomia Umana. 4th ed. Edi. Ermes; 2010.
- Blanco R. The 'pecs block': a novel technique for providing analgesia after breast surgery. Anaesthesia. 2011;66:847-8.
- Blanco R, Fajardo M, Parras Maldonado T. Ultrasound description of Pecs II (modified Pecs I): a novel approach to breast surgery. Revista espanola de anestesiologia y reanimacion. 2012;59:470-5.
- Blanco R, Parras T, McDonnell JG, Prats-Galino A. Serratus plane block: a novel ultrasound-guided thoracic wall nerve block. Anaesthesia. 2013;68:1107-13.
- Bouzinac A, Brenier G, Dao M, Delbos A. Bilateral association of pecs I block and serratus plane block for postoperative analgesia after double modified radical mastectomy. Minerva anestesiologica. 2015;81:589-90.
- de la Torre PA, Garcia PD, Alvarez SL, Miguel FJ, Perez MF. A novel ultrasound-guided block: a promising alternative for breast analgesia. Aesthetic surgery journal. 2014;34:198-200.
- Del Buono R, Costa F, Agro FE. Parasternal, Pecto-intercostal, Pecs, and Transverse Thoracic Muscle Plane Blocks: A Rose by Any Other Name Would Smell as Sweet. Regional anesthesia and pain medicine. 2016;41:791-2.
- Fusco P, Scimia P, Marinangeli F, Pozone T, Petrucci E. The association between the ultrasound-guided Serratus Plane Block and PECS I Block can represent a valid alternative to conventional anesthesia in breast surgery in a seriously ill patient. Minerva anestesiologica. 2016;82:241-2.
- Fusco P, Scimia P, Petrucci E, S DIC, Marinangeli F. The ultrasound-guided parasternal block: a novel approach for anesthesia and analgesia in breast cancer surgery. Minerva anestesiologica. 2017;83:221-2.
- Hansen CK, Dam M, Poulsen TD, Lönnqvist P-A, Bendtsen TF, Børglum J. Ultrasound-guided parasternal Pecs block: a new and useful supplement to Pecs I and serratus anterior plane blocks. Anaesthesia Cases. 2016:2016-0007.
- Huercio I, Abad-Gurumeta A, Gilsanz F. Regional blocks for breast surgery: is it enough? Minerva anestesiologica. 2016;82:369-70.
- Klein SM, Bergh A, Steele SM, Georgiade GS, Greengrass RA. Thoracic paravertebral block for breast surgery. Anesthesia and analgesia. 2000;90:1402-5.
- McDonald SB, Jacobsohn E, Kopacz DJ, et al. Parasternal block and local anesthetic infiltration with levobupivacaine after cardiac surgery with desflurane: the effect on postoperative pain, pulmonary function, and tracheal extubation times. Anesthesia and analgesia. 2005;100:25-32.
- Ohgoshi Y, Ino K, Matsukawa M. Ultrasound-guided parasternal intercostal nerve block. Journal of anesthesia. 2016;30:916.
- Scimia P, Basso Ricci E, Harizaj F, Cocconi A, Fusco P, Danelli F. The combination of ultrasound-guided pectoral nerves II and parasternal blocks as a valid alternative for anesthesia in breast surgery: an observational study. Interventional Pain Management Reports Volume 1, Number 4, pp175-179 2017, American Society of Interventional Pain Physicians©.
- Standrig S, Gray H. Gray's anatomy: the anatomical basis of clinical practice. 41 ed. Churchill Livingstone/Elsevier; 2015.
- Suresh S, Ecoffey C, Bosenberg A, et al. The European Society of Regional Anaesthesia and Pain Therapy/American Society of Regional Anesthesia and Pain Medicine Recommendations on Local Anesthetics and Adjuvants Dosage in Pediatric Regional Anesthesia. Reg Anesth Pain Med. 2018;43: 211-6.
- Tighe SQ, Karmakar MK. Serratus plane block: do we need to learn another technique for thoracic wall blockade? Anaesthesia. 2013;68:1103-6.
- Ueshima H, Hara E, Marui T, Otake H. The ultrasound-guided transversus thoracic muscle plane block is effective for the median sternotomy. Journal of clinical anesthesia. 2016;29:83.
- Karem El-Boghdadly et al. Standardizing nomenclature in regional anesthesia: an ASRA-ESRA Delphi consensus study of abdominal wall, paraspinal, and chest wall blocks. Reg Anesth Pain Med. 2021 Jul;46(7):571-580.
- Sepolvere G, Tedesco M, Cristiano L. Ultrasound Parasternal Block as a Novel Approach for Cardiac Sternal Surgery: Could it Be the Safest Strategy? J Cardiothorac Vasc Anesth. 2020 Aug;34(8):2284-2286. doi: 10.1053/j.jvca.2020.03.014. Epub 2020 Mar 19. PMID: 32360012
- Sepolvere G, Fusco P, Tedesco M, Scimia P. Bilateral ultrasound-guided parasternal block for postoperative analgesia in cardiac surgery: could it be the safest strategy? Reg Anesth Pain Med. 2020 Apr;45(4):316-317. doi: 10.1136/rapm-2019-100872. Epub 2020 Jan 20. PMID: 31964853.

CLINICAL CASE 1 – CHEST WALL BLOCKS AND MINIMALLY INVASIVE IMAGE-GUIDE PROCEDURES: THE MEETING POINT BETWEEN RADIOLOGY AND ANESTHESIOLOGY THAT COULD IMPROVE SAFETY AND PATIENT OUTCOMES IN NORA

Clinical history and anamnesis We report the use of superficial PIP Block (Parasternal Block) for computerized tomography-guided biopsy (CT-G B) for sternal manubrium metastasis in a 56-year-old (height 1.65 m, weight 75 kg, BMi 27.55), suffering from hypertension, severe chronic obstructive pulmonary disease (COPD) and metastatic colorectal cancer with neuropathic chest disturbances.

Technique description Under aseptic conditions, using a linear probe and a 22 G echogenic needle in plane approach (SonoPlex stim cannula, PaJunk®) a bilateral superficial PIP Block was performed at the II rib level; 10 ml of levobupivacaine 0.375% for each side were injected to open the fascial plane between the pectoralis major muscle (PMm) and the intercostal muscle (IM) administered. (**Figure 6.4 A**, **B**)

Materials and methods Written informed consent was obtained. A peripheral venous access (18 g) was obtained and standard monitoring were applied. Supplemental oxygen was administered by Venturi-mask (8 l/min of oxygen flow) with continuous expired CO_2 ($CECO_2$) monitoring; midazolam 0.05 mg·kg-1 and sufentanil 0.1 μg·kg-1 were administered by intravenous (iV) injection prior to anesthesia. Vital and respiratory parameters (Hr, MaP, SaO_2% and $CECO_2$) were monitored. No advanced airway control was required. No supplementary opiates nor other local anesthetic agents were administered. additionally, no complications of the block were recorded; the needle for biopsy was inserted through the skin and up to the cortical bone of the sternal manubrium without the patient's discomfort.

Conclusions Collaboration and communication between radiologist and anesthetists play a central role for an excellent patient outcome, and the new chest wall blocks, like PIP Block could be considered an important meeting point between the interventional radiology and anesthesiology to ensure the best comfort especially in high risk patients.

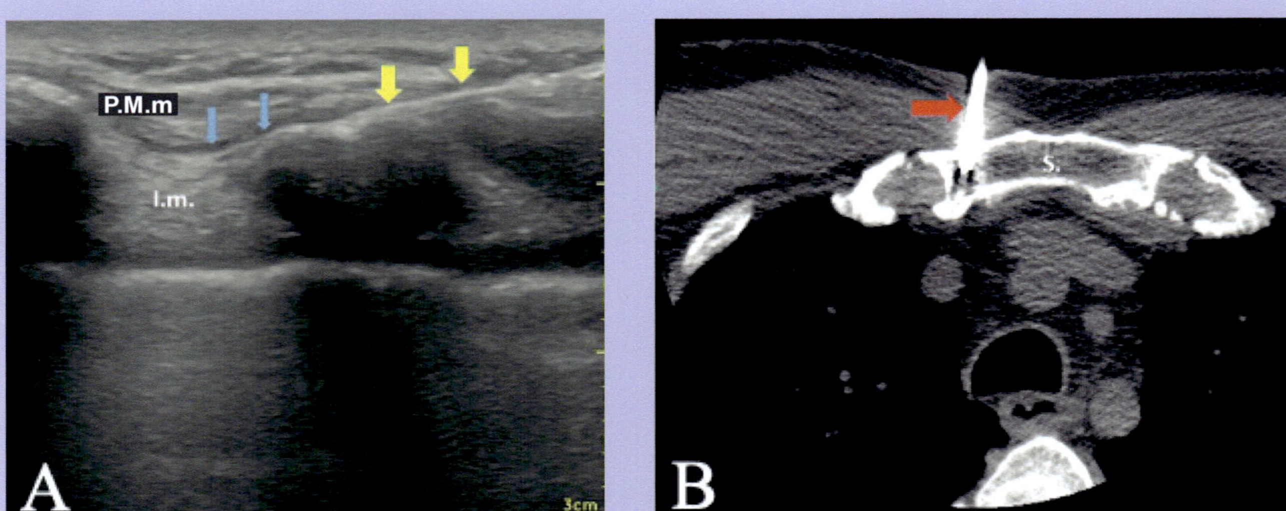

Figure 6.4 A Execution of the block at the level of the second rib, the ticker arrows show the needle and the thinner arrows the spread of local anesthetic in the fascial plane between intercostal muscles (I.m.) and pectoralsi major muscle (P.M.m.). **B** CT scan that shows the biopsy needle (arrow) after insertion into the sternum (s).

CLINICAL CASE 2 – ULTRASOUND PARASTERNAL BLOCK (PIP BLOCK) AS A NOVEL APPROACH FOR CARDIAC STERNAL SURGERY: COULD IT BE THE SAFEST STRATEGY?

Clinical history and anamnesis We report a patient with previous laryngectomy with severe COPD treated with oxygen therapy and scheduled to undergo cardiac sternal resynthesis and vacuum-assisted closure therapy (VACT).

Technique description Written informed consent for the procedures and patient approval for the publication were obtained. An airway tracheostomy cannula was inserted for the laryngectomized patient. Under aseptic conditions, via an in-plane approach, using a linear probe and a 22 G echogenic SonoPlex stim Pajunk® needle, a bilateral PIP Block was performed 30 minutes before surgical incision. The blocks were performed bilaterally via 2 separate injections of 20 ml of 0.5% levobupivacaine and dexamethasone, 2 mg, at the second and fourth intercostal spaces into the interfacial compartment between the pectoralis major and intercostal muscles to manage cutaneous and bone sternal pain (**Figure 6.5 A**, **B**, **Video 6.2**). No complications, such as pneumothorax, infections, and local anesthetic systemic toxicity, were recorded.

Materials and methods The patient received light sedation via continuous intravenous dexmedetomidine (0.7 mg/kg/h) and supplemental oxygen was administered (8 l/min of oxygen flow). Vital and respiratory parameters (Hr, MaP, SaO_2%) were monitored. Spontaneous ventilation was maintained, and the patient was cooperative (Richmond Agitation Sedation Scale 1) and reported no pain (numerical rating scale 0) during surgery. No respiratory depression or pulmonary complications were recorded. Good pulmonary capacity was demonstrated; the patient had a partial pressure of arterial oxygen-to-fraction of inspired oxygen ratio of 300 mmHg. Oxygen saturation was >96%, partial pressure of arterial oxygen was >90 mmHg, and partial pressure of arterial carbon dioxide was 35 mmHg on average. In the first 24 postoperative hours, the patient reported good analgesia (numerical rating scale <3) and was very satisfied with their level of anesthesia. In total, acetaminophen, 3 g, was administered without the need for nonsteroidal anti-inflammatory agents or opioids

Conclusions Bilateral superficial PIP Block may be an effective and safe alternative anesthetic technique to manage cardiac sternal disease in patients with severe COPD for whom general anesthesia and opioid administration could be harmful and increase intensive care unit length of stay.

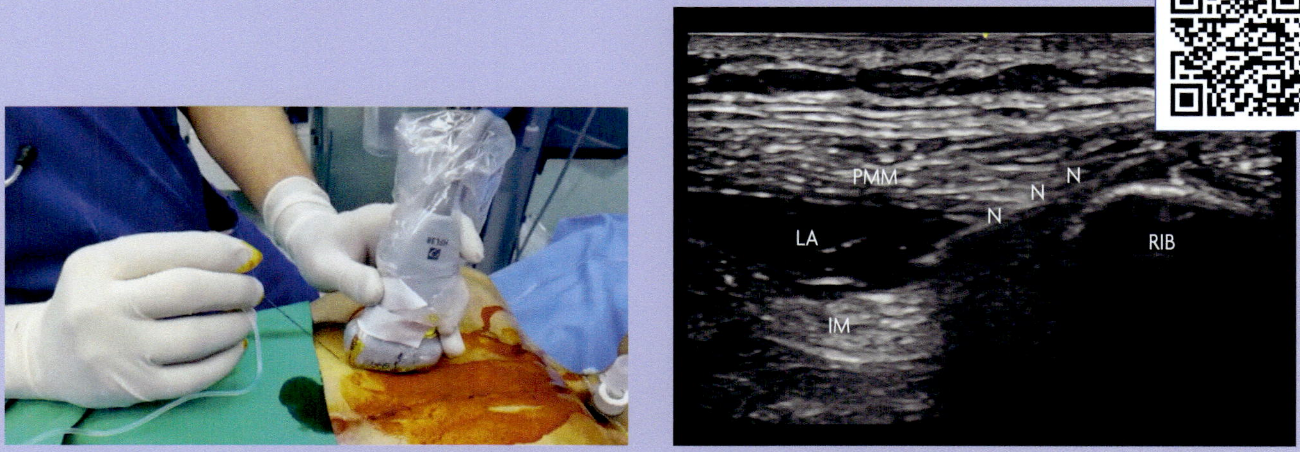

Figure 6.5 A A linear probe is positioned in the parasternal region. The block is first performed at the second then at the fourth intercostal space bilaterally. **B** Superficial PIP Block. Local anesthetic is injected into the interfacial compartment between the pectoralis major and the intercostal muscles. IM: intercostal muscle; LA: local anesthetic; N: needle; PMM: pectoralis major muscle.

CHAPTER
7

Trasversus abominis plane block (TAP)

Pierfrancesco Fusco, Raffaele Perna, Fabio Gobbi, Paolo Scimia, Walter Ciaschi, Andrea Luigi Ambrosoli, Fabrizio Fattorini

Major abdominal surgery is often associated with significant acute postoperative pain, which, if not adequately treated, can lead to increased perioperative morbidity, hospitalization length and costs.

The literature shows that postoperative pain in abdominal surgery is still a problem that has not been completely resolved, since it has a somatic component, originating from the surgical incision, and a visceral component. Epidural analgesia is currently the gold standard for the treatment of acute postoperative pain in major abdominal surgery and, although it allows adequate analgesia, it is not always easy to perform or to implement, and above all it is not free from risks and complications. An alternative is intravenous opioid analgesia which, although providing good control of pain at rest is not as effective in the treatment of pain on movement (incident) and has dose-dependent side effects.

These observations suggest that alternative analgesic techniques are needed to reduce the use of opioids and their associated side-effects.

The Transversus abdominis plane (TAP) block is a compartmental or neurofascial block technique that allows analgesia of the whole abdominal wall. It is mainly used in abdominal surgery.

Recent international guidelines strongly recommend echo-guided TAP block as part of a multimodal analgesic regimen to reduce opioid consumption, improve pain control, patient satisfaction and accelerate recovery of bowel function.

The use of this technique, in the context of a multimodal therapeutic strategy, if correctly performed by experienced operators and with an adequate approach, can provide an extension of the analgesic blockade, which is potentially able to exert its action also on the visceral component of postoperative pain, thus allowing to limit or avoid the use of intrathecal or systemic opioids.

ANATOMY AND SONOANATOMY

The anatomy of the abdominal wall is made up of the following elements: the rectus abdominis muscle with its fascia in the middle, and three muscle layers in its antero-lateral part, i.e. the external oblique (EO), internal oblique (IO) and transverse abdominis (TA) muscle, with their respective fascia. The abdominal wall (skin, muscles, and parietal peritoneum) is innervated by the anterior rami of the spinal nerves T7 to L1.

The terminal rami of these somatic nerves run in the lateral wall of the abdomen within a plane between the IO and TA above the TA. This interfascial plane is called the transversus abdominis plane (TAP).

The anterior divisions T7 to T11 cross the intercostal space to enter the abdominal wall between the internal oblique and transverse muscles of the abdomen, until they reach and innervate the rectus abdominis muscle, ending as anterior cutaneous rami innervating the skin of the anterior abdominal wall (**Figure 7.1**).

On their way, these nerve roots cross the external oblique muscle, giving off lateral cutaneous rami, which in turn divide into anterior and posterior cutaneous rami, which innervate the external oblique and the great latissimus dorsi muscle, respectively. The ilio-hypogastric nerve (L1) divides between the inter-anterior oblique and transverse abdominal muscles near the iliac crest into anterior and lateral cutaneous rami; the former innervate part of the skin of the gluteal re-

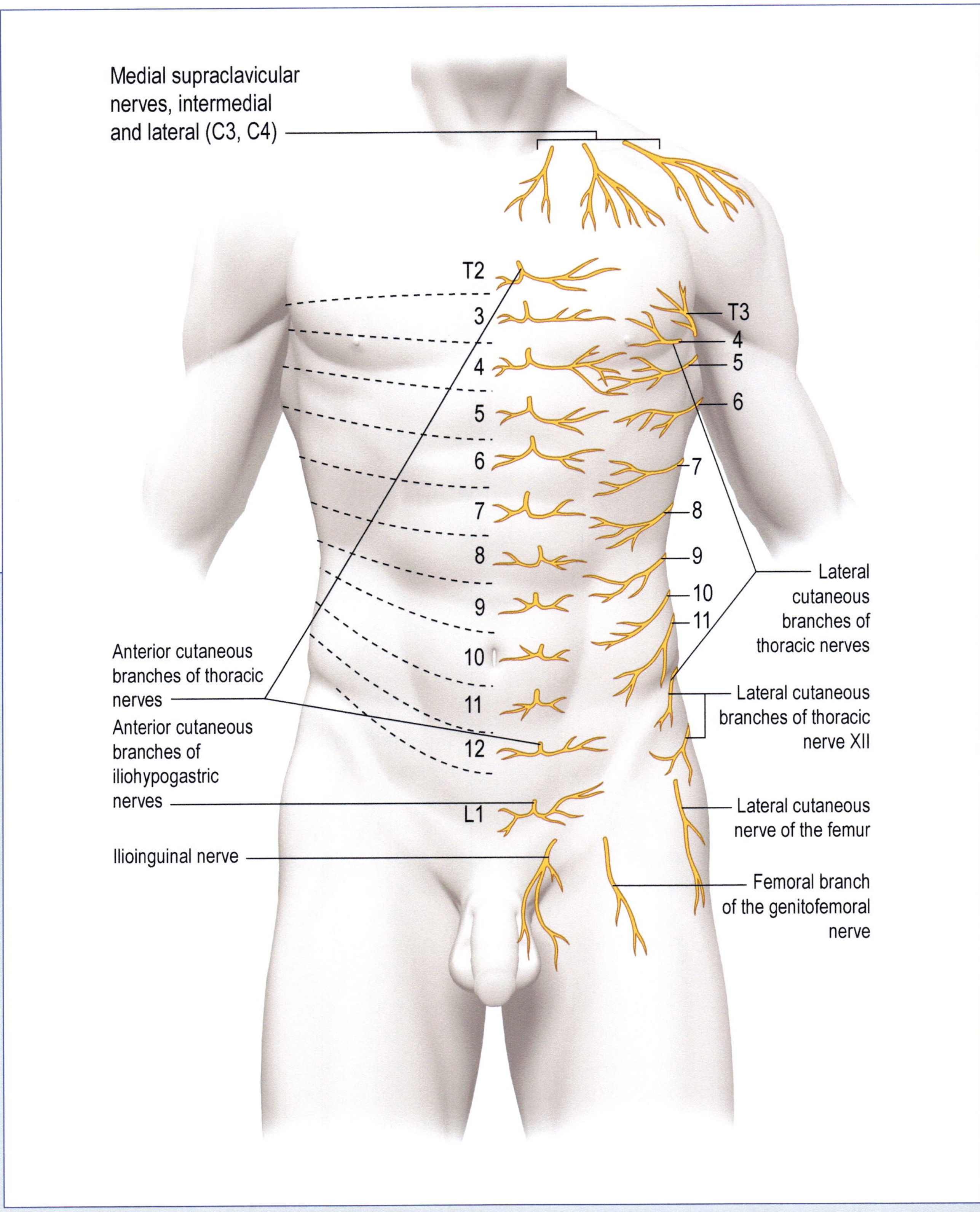

Figure 7.1 Diagram of the distribution of the cutaneous nerves in the anterior trunk wall.

gion, while the latter innervate the hypogastric region. The ileo-inguinal nerve (L1) innervates the upper and medial part of the thigh and part of the skin covering the genitals. In addition, as demonstrated by anatomical dissections on cadavers, the nerves T6 to L1 ramus and communicate with each other, forming two distinct plexuses: the rami T6 to T9 form a high plexus called "intercostal plexus", while the rami T10 to L1 form the so-called "TAP plexus". From this it follows, as shown in cadaveric and in vivo studies, that the dermatome extent of the blockage may depend on the type of approach used, irrespective of the concentration and volumes of LA (**Figure 7.2**).

The sonoanatomy of the abdominal wall, in the classic approach between the costal margin and the iliac crest at the middle axillary line, is characterized, starting from the skin and subcutis, by the presence of three muscle layers separated by a hyperechogenic band: external oblique muscle (EO), internal oblique muscle (IO), and transverse abdominal muscle (TA). Below the TA is the peritoneum and the loops of bowel. The nerves of the abdominal wall are not ultrasound visible in the TAP, although their identification is not necessary for the execution of the block (**Figure 7.3**).

TARGET AND TIMING OF THE BLOCK

The aim of the block is to place the tip of the needle between the IO and TA muscles and inject the local anesthetic into the interfascial plane between the two muscle layers (tranversus abdominis plane), in order to block the anterior spinal nerve roots that run within it (**Figure 7.4 A, B**).

The blockage can be carried out by blind technique or with the aid of ultrasound, which allows the deposition of LA in the TAP to be visualized. Considering that the onset time for adequate analgesic efficacy is 30

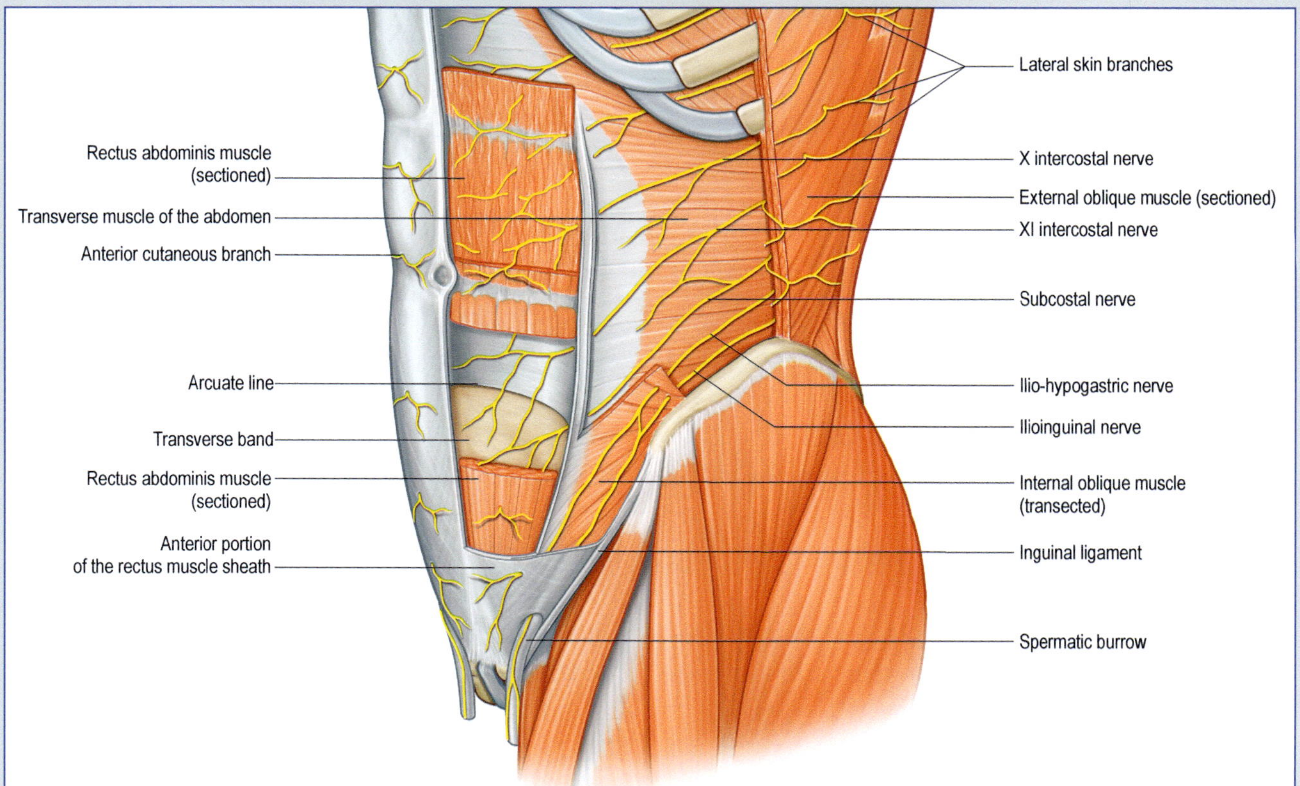

Figure 7.2 Structures and sensory innervation of the anterior abdominal wall. Parts of the muscles of the anterolateral abdominal wall were excised, including most of the anterior portion of the rectus muscle sheath and part of the belly of the rectus muscle of the abdomen.

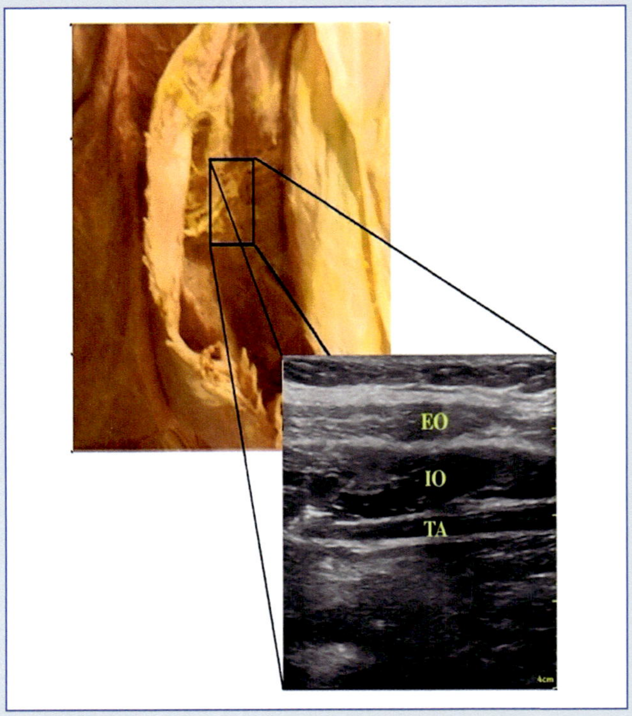

Figure 7.3 Cadaveric dissection of the abdomen after removal of the external and internal oblique muscles with opening of the TAP of the anterior abdominal wall. EO: external oblique muscle; IO: internal oblique muscle, TA: transverse abdominal muscle (bottom picture) (courtesy of Dr. Astrid Ursula Behr and Prof. Carla Stecco).

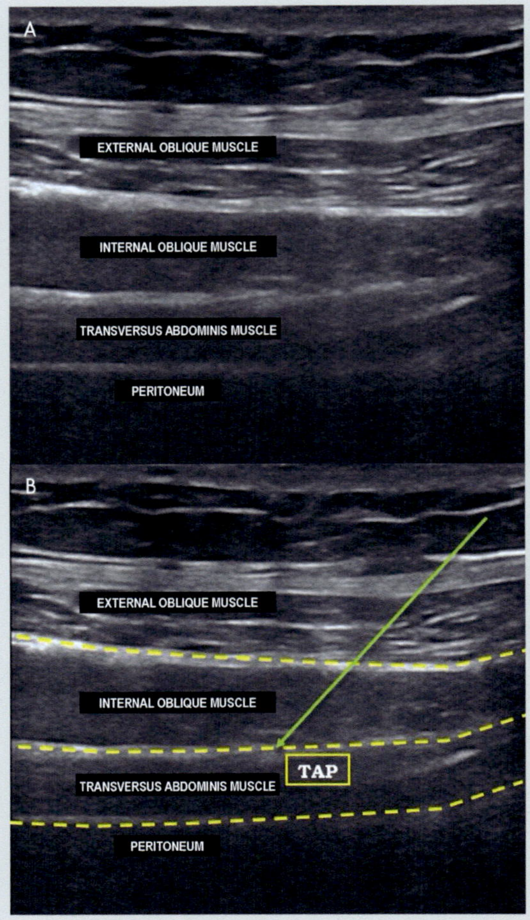

Figure 7.4 A, B Sonoanatomy of the anterior abdominal wall.

minutes, blockade should be performed after induction of anesthesia and before surgical incision in order to exploit the intraoperative analgesic effect.

DESCRIPTION OF TECHNIQUES

The following equipment is required to perform the block:

- ultrasound scanner equipped with a high-frequency linear probe (6-12 MHz);
- sterile probe cover and sterile gel (in obese patients or in case of posterior approach, a convex probe may be required);
- standard nerve block trolley;
- antiseptic for skin disinfection and sterile gloves;
- TAP block needle (Sonotap®) 50-100 mm, 20-21 G diameter;
- two 20 ml syringes containing local anesthetic and one 10 ml syringe containing saline and a three-way stopcock (**Figure 7.5**).

The presence of an assistant to perform the injection of the local anesthetic is considered useful.

Blind technique

The "blind technique" involves inserting the needle within the Petit triangle, with a perpendicular approach to the skin, just cranially of the iliac crest and behind the mid axillary line (**Figure 7.6**).

The path of the needle through the abdominal myofascial structures allows the operator to perceive a sensation of loss of resistance twice and is most appreciable when using a blunt-tipped needle felt as a pop. The first "pop" indicates penetration of the EO

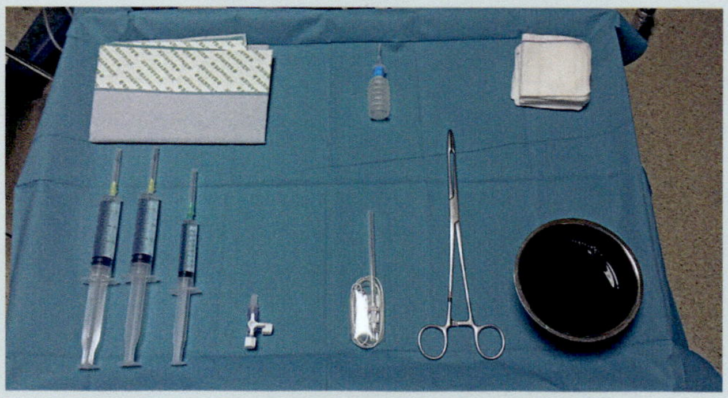

Figure 7.5 Material needed for the block.

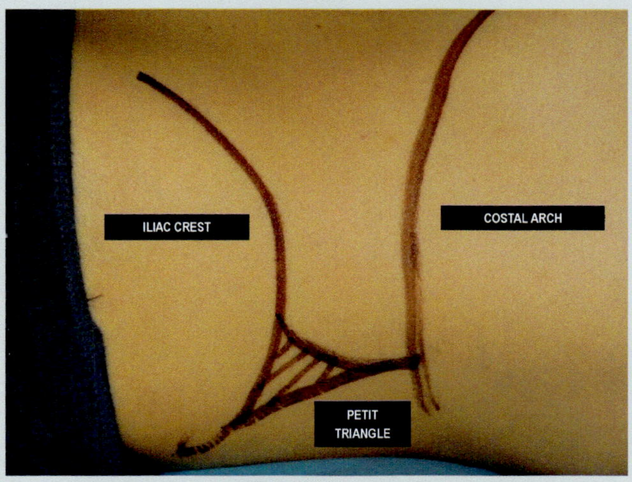

Figure 7.6 TAP block. Identification of anatomical landmarks on the skin.

band, the second "pop" indicates penetration of the IO band, and thus entry into the TAP. After aspiration, 20 ml of local anesthetic is injected on each side.

Echo-guided technique

The ultrasound-guided technique, initially described by Hebbard, allows the placement of the needle tip and the injection of local anesthetic into the TAP, confirming the opening of the interfascial target plane by ultrasound.

The authors recommend using a three-way tap, connecting the main way to the syringe containing saline and the second way to the syringe containing local anesthetic. The operator places the ultrasound monitor in front of him/her, opposite the chosen side, and should adopt the most comfortable position to allow proper needle-probe alignment. With the patient in the supine position, after carefully disinfecting the skin, a high-frequency (6-18 MHz) linear probe is positioned, with variable orientation depending on the type of approach used. The three muscle layers are then identified, separated by a hyperechoic band: EO, IO (generally the most represented) and TA (the thinnest). The peritoneal cavity and peritoneum are located below the transverse muscle.

If identification of the three muscle layers is difficult, the authors consider it useful to first visualize the intestinal loops and peritoneum and then, starting from the bottom upwards, find the first hyperechogenic line above the peritoneum, which corresponds to the target interfascial plane of the block (transversus abdominis plane). Once optimal visualization is achieved, the needle is inserted, using an in-plane technique, through the subcutaneous tissue and advanced through the EO and IO muscles. In order to optimize needle-probe alignment, it is recommended to insert the needle in a sagittal plane, at a distance of 3-4 cm from the probe itself, increasing this distance further especially in obese patients where the TAP may be deeper (**Figures 7.7, 7.8**).

Once the first resistance encountered when passing the needle between the EO and IO muscles has been overcome, the needle is advanced and the penetration of the needle tip into the TAP is perceived as a second "pop" (**Figure 7.9**, **Video 7.1**, **Figure 7.10**, **Video 7.2**, **Figure 7.11**, **Flow chart 7.1 online**).

Only after correct positioning of the needle tip in the TAP, after aspiration and resistance test, will the saline solution be injected through the three-way tap, confirming ultrasound "opening" of the target interfascial plane with diffusion of the LA along the plane itself. It is also recommended that any air bubbles inside the syringe or needle connection circuit be removed to prevent air from obstructing the sound. Subsequently, local anesthetic is injected, trying to move the tip of the needle inside the TAP to favor its "opening", verifying the downward ablation of the TA muscle and of the peritoneum and checking at the end of the injection the dis-

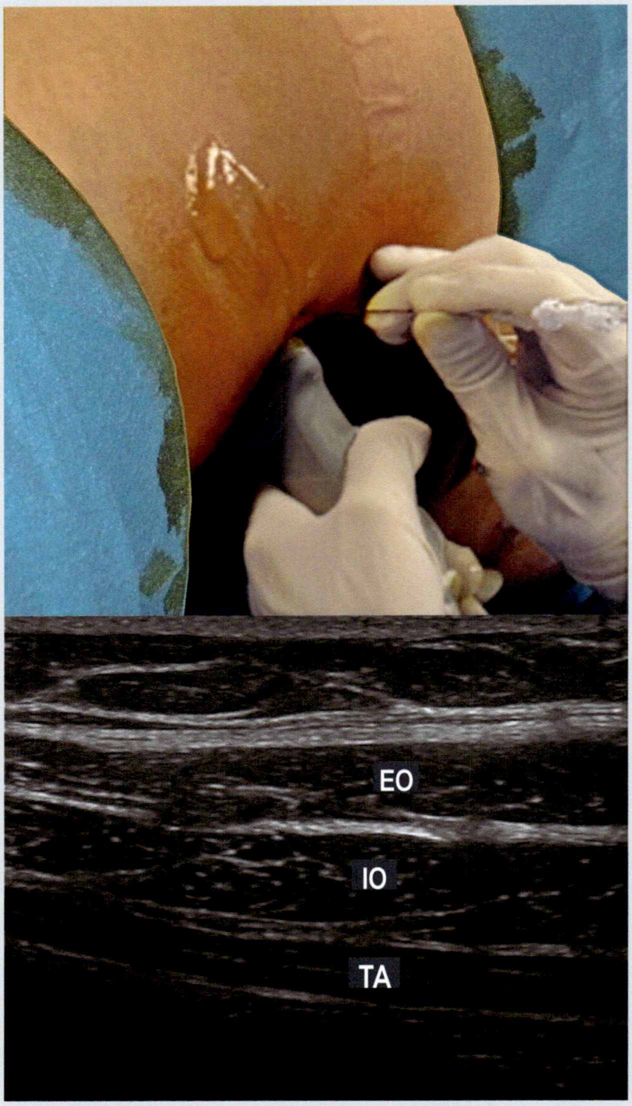

Figure 7.7 Position of the probe and ultrasound visualization of the abdominal wall. EO: external oblique muscle; IO: internal oblique muscle; TA: transverse muscle of the abdomen.

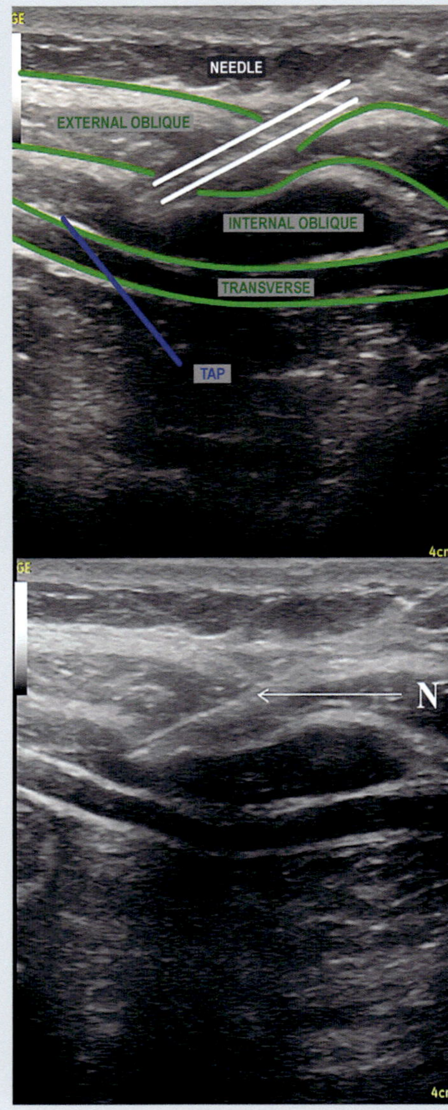

Figure 7.8 Needle tip (Sonotap®) at the fascia between the external oblique and internal oblique muscles. N: needle.

tribution of the anesthetic in the cranio-caudal and latero-medial sense.

Based on studies using contrast-enhanced MRI in both healthy volunteers and cadavers, several different ultrasound-guided approaches to TAP have been described in the literature, resulting in different cranio-caudal and latero-medial dermatome extension of the block. The approaches described include the classic mid-axillary, the oblique subcostal, and the more recent posterior approach. These clinical observations show that the dynamics of anesthetic solution diffusion can vary widely depending on the site of injection into the TAP. The availability of multiple approaches allows the operator to use the ultrasound-guided TAP block for postoperative analgesia in a variety of abdominal surgical procedures: the posterior and mid-axillary ultrasound approaches are indicated for sub-umbilical incisions; the subcostal and

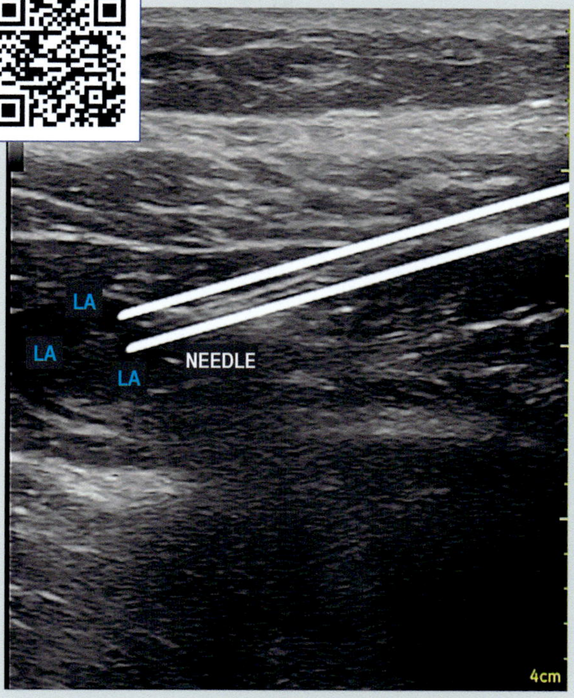

Figure 7.9 Sonoanatomy of the anterior abdominal wall. Local anesthetic injected between the internal oblique and transverse muscle with "opening" of the TAP. LA: local anesthetic.

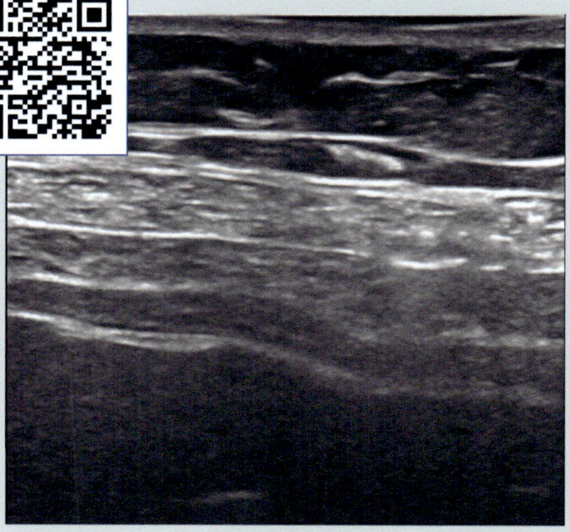

Figure 7.10 Sonoanatomy TAP.

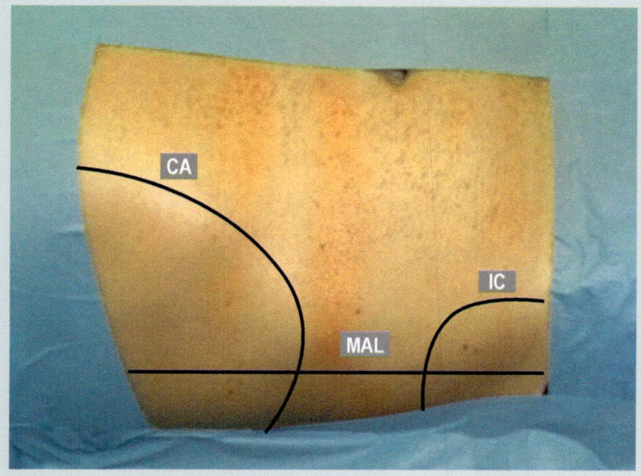

Figure 7.11 Anatomical findings in the mid-axillary approach. CA: costal arch; IC: iliac crest; MAL: mid axillary line.

oblique subcostal ultrasound approaches are indicated for peri- and supra-umbilical surgery. Therefore, in order to achieve adequate analgesic coverage of the abdominal wall from T6/T7 to L1, a double approach (subcostal or oblique subcostal + mid-axillary or posterior) should be performed. For complete analgesic coverage of the abdominal wall, Borglum et al. suggest a dual bilateral approach.

APPROACHES TO TAP BLOCK EXECUTION

Mid-axillary approach (before "Lateral TAP BLOCK")

With the patient in the supine position, after thorough skin disinfection, a high-frequency linear probe is placed in the space between the iliac crest and the inferior costal margin; on the mid-axillary line, the presence of three muscle layers, represented by the EO, IO and TA muscles, with the peritoneum and the intestinal loops underneath, will be evident from the skin and the subcutis (**Figure 7.12**).

Once the TAP has been identified, a 100 mm needle (Sonotap®) will be inserted in-plane with respect to the probe, in a sagittal plane, medial-to-lateral orientation, 2-3 cm away from the probe.

Constant ultrasound visualization of the needle tip is always recommended for the correct positioning of the needle in the TAP where, after aspiration, 2-3 ml of physiological solution will be injected in order to verify the correct localization of the needle tip in the TAP.

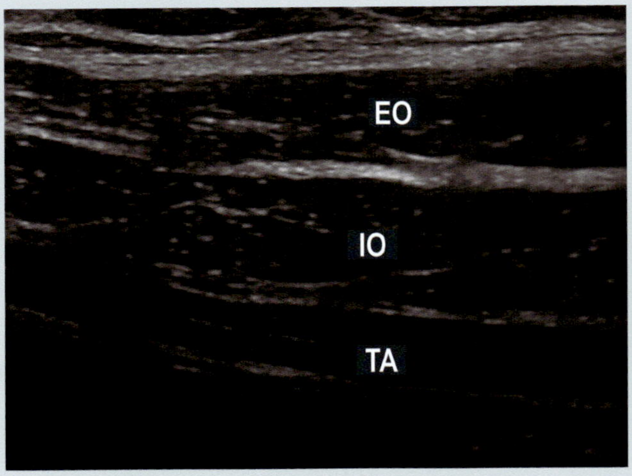

Figure 7.12 Sonoanatomy of the abdominal part at the mid-axillary line. EO: external oblique muscle; IO: internal oblique muscle; TA: transverse muscle of the abdomen.

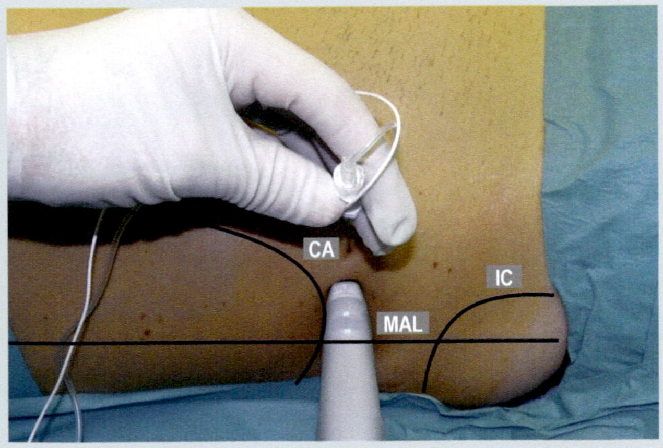

Figure 7.13 Probe and needle position in the mid-axillary approach. CA: costal arch; IC: iliac crest; MAL: mid axillary line.

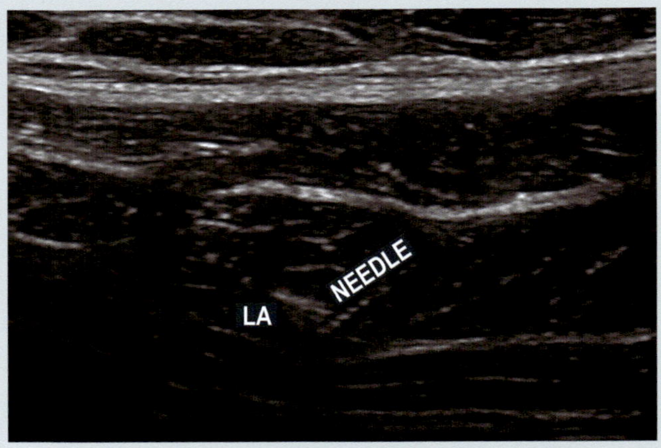

Figure 7.14 Local anesthetic injection and TAP opening. Note the diffusion of local anesthetic along the TAP. LA: local anesthetic.

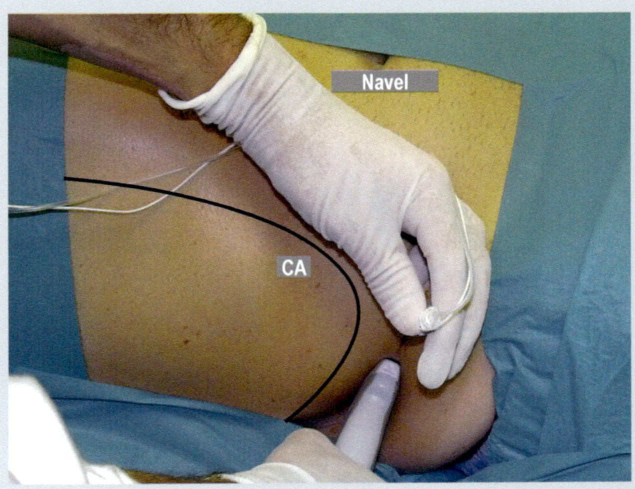

Figure 7.15 Position of the probe and needle in the posterior approach. CA: costal arch.

After the ultrasound confirmation of the "opening" of the target interfascial plane, which will appear as a "hypoechogenic pocket", the local anesthetic will be injected, 20 ml for each side, verifying, at the end of the injection, the distribution in cranio-caudal and latero-medial sense (**Figures 7.13**, **7.14**).

Lateral QLB (before "Posterior approach")

The ultrasound-guided posterior approach to the TAP (quadratus lumborum or quadratus plane block), recently described by Blanco, represents an extension of the TAP block to the dorsal region.

With the patient in a lateral or supine position, the probe is always positioned in the space between the iliac crest and the costal margin on the mid axillary line. From here the probe is slid posteriorly until the aponeurosis of the EO, IO and TA muscles are visualized, close to the quadratus lumborum muscle (**Figures 7.15**, **7.16**, **7.17**).

Once an optimal image has been obtained, the tip of the needle will be directed towards the aponeurosis of the transverse muscle towards the latero-lateral aspect of the quadratus lumborum, which is the target for local anesthetic injection. This approach allows a more posterior distribution of local anesthetic, with diffusion towards the paravertebral space.

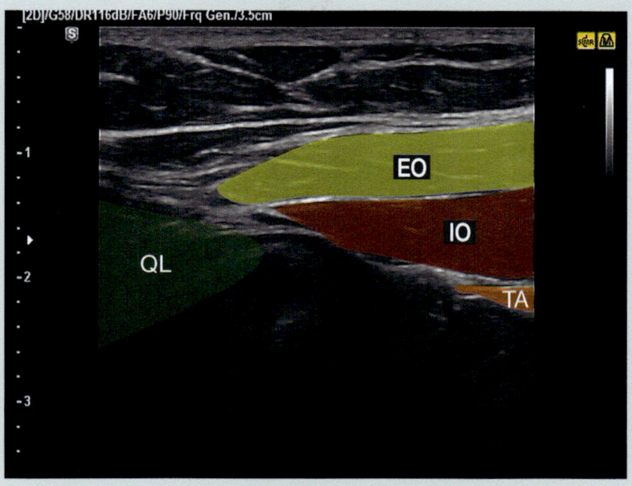

Figure 7.16 Sonoanatomy in the posterior approach. EO: external oblique muscle; IO: internal oblique muscle; QL: quadratus lumborum muscle; TA: transverse abdominis muscle.

Oblique subcostal approach

With the patient in the supine position, a linear probe is used, placing it parallel to the costal margin, a few cm lateral to the xiphoid process. It is important to remember that the superior epigastric artery emerges below the costal margin, lateral to the xiphoid process, and runs within the TAP before entering the rectus fascia. Therefore, it is always advisable to use colour-echo-Doppler in order to avoid accidental intravascular injection. At this level, the rectus muscle of the abdomen will be visualized. From this point, the probe is moved laterally until the medial part of the TA muscle, located sometimes below the rectus muscle, is detected (**Figures 7.18**, **7.19**, **7.20**).

A 5 cm needle is introduced with in-plane approach, in the mid-lateral direction, directing the tip of the needle between the IO muscle and the rectus abdominis. As described for the other approaches, once the target plane has been opened by injection of saline, the LA injection will be performed.

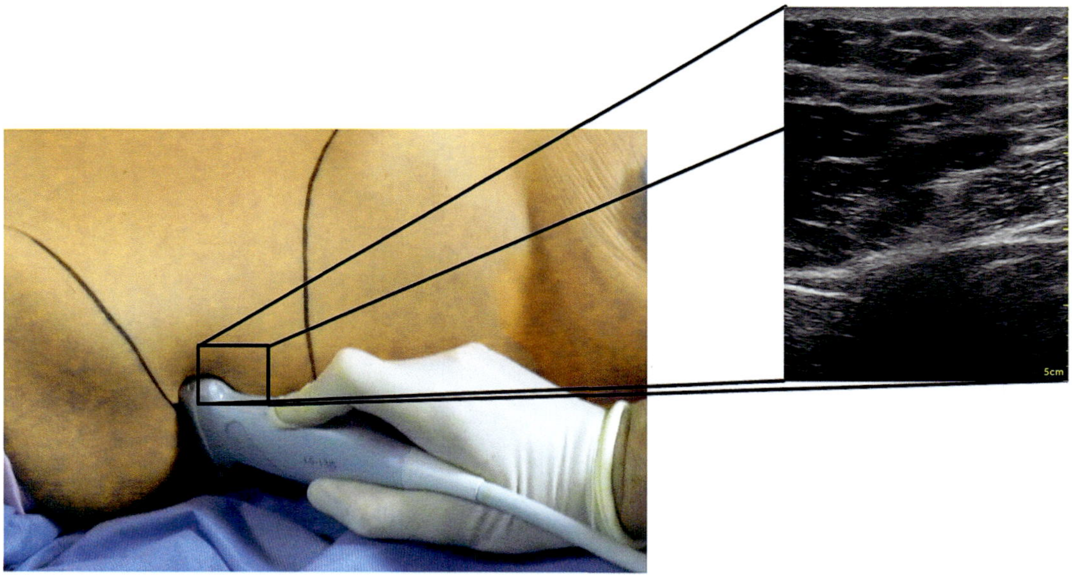

Figure 7.17 Posterior approach (QLB I) and its sonoanatomy.

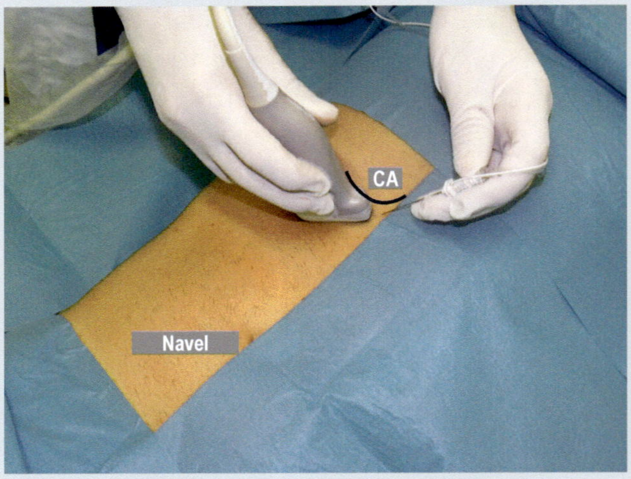

Figure 7.18 Probe and needle position in the subcostal oblique approach. CA: costal arch.

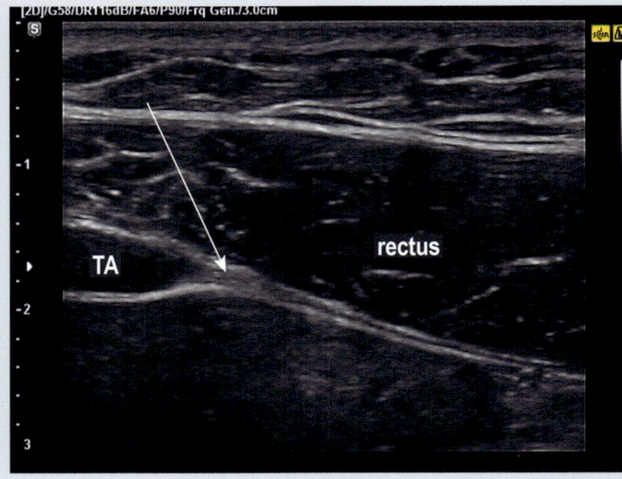

Figure 7.19 Sonoanatomy in the oblique subcostal approach. Note the injection point of LA between the rectus muscle and the transverse muscle of the abdomen. TA: transverse muscle of the abdomen.

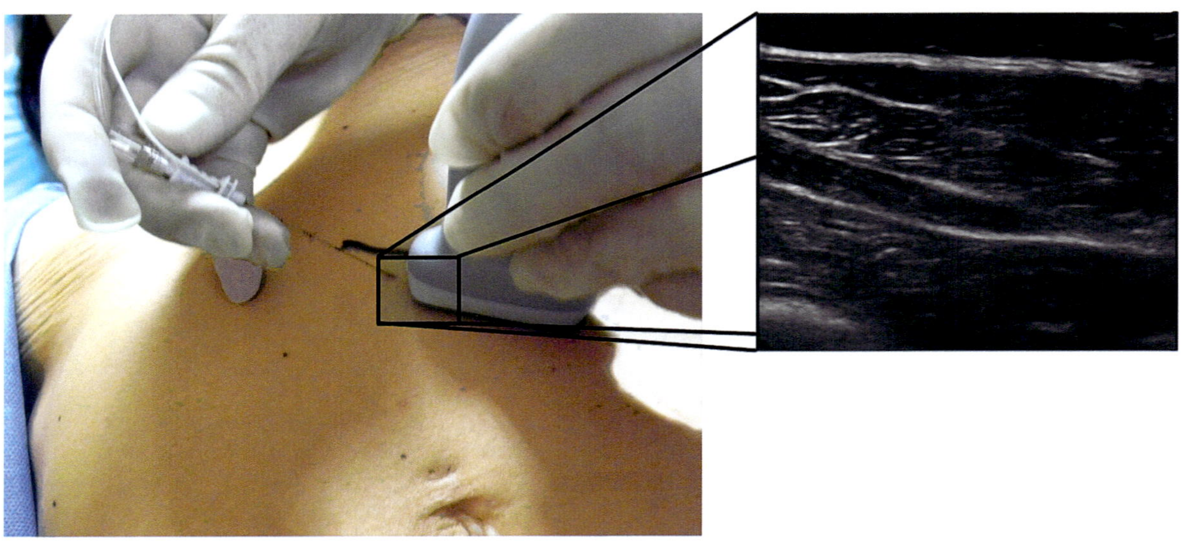

Figure 7.20 Subcostal oblique approach and its sonoanatomy.

Subcostal approach

The subcostal approach, described by Hebbard in 2007, is also indicated in supra-umbilical surgery. The supine position of the patient also makes it easy to perform the block. With the linear probe positioned close to the midline, the rectus abdominis muscle is identified from which the patient is directed laterally until the point where the rectus muscle ends and the EO, IO, and TA muscles begin is identified (**Figures 7.21**, **7.22**).

At this point, the needle is inserted, using an in-plane approach, in a medial-lateral orientation, directing the tip of the needle between the IO and TA muscles.

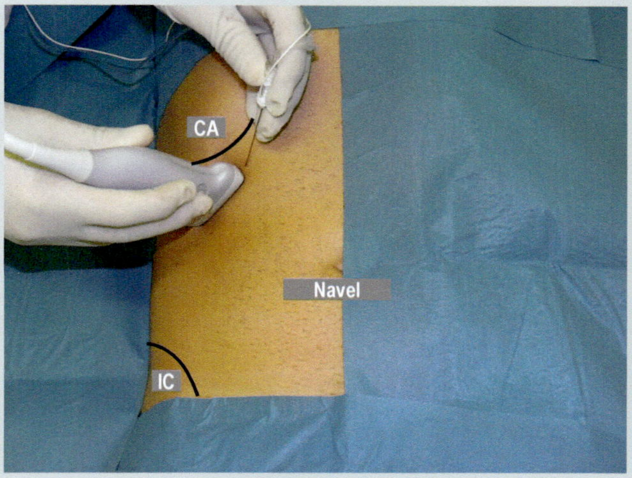

Figure 7.21 Probe and needle position in the subcostal approach. CA: costal arch; IC: iliac crest.

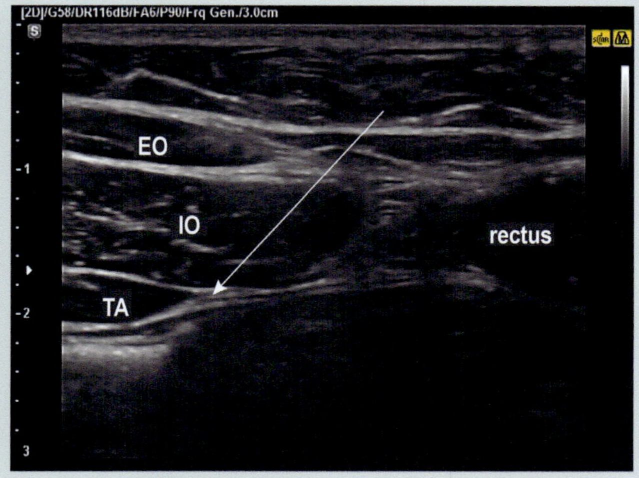

Figure 7.22 Sonoanatomy in the subcostal approach. Note the injection point of LA between the internal oblique and transverse muscle. EO: external oblique muscle; IO: internal oblique muscle; TA: transverse muscle of the abdomen.

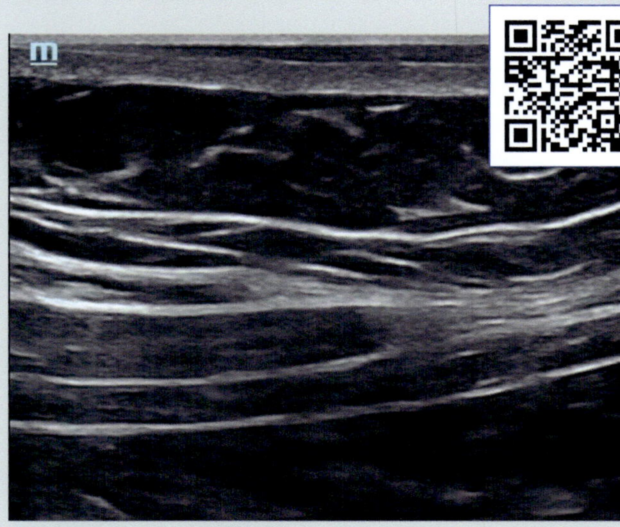

Figure 7.23 Sonoanatomy subcostal approach.

Bilateral dual TAP block

In order to achieve greater extension of the block not only bilaterally, but also to the upper and lower abdominal wall, Borglum et al. introduced the bilateral dual TAP block using a four-point single-shot technique, i.e. bilateral subcostal combined with the bilateral mid-axillary approach. The aim of the four-point approach is to anesthetize both the high subcostal plexus and the TAP plexus located inferiorly, to allow coverage of the surgical wound above and below the abdomen (**Figure 7.23**, **Video 7.3**).

CONTINUOUS TAP BLOCK

Data from the international literature confirm that single-shot TAP block, placed in a multimodal setting, can provide effective pain control between 12 and 48 hours postoperatively. As demonstrated in a recent meta-analysis, the placement of a continuous infusion catheter in the TAP plane after adult abdominal surgery has demonstrated non-infrequent pain control beyond 24 to 48 hours postoperatively.

The catheter can be inserted into the TAP plane by the approaches described above. The literature is unclear as to which approach is most advantageous for delivery of the continuous infusion catheter into the TAP plane, but it is clear that the decision to use a specific approach is sub-ordinate to the site of the surgical wound. The technique is essentially the same as that described for single-shot and, therefore, once the plane of the TAP has been ultrasounded, the fascial plane is "opened", followed by injection of LA, followed by insertion of the catheter, visualizing the progression of the tip, and encouraging its release within the plane. Tunnelling may be indicated to ensure better stability and in anticipation of prolonged catheter stay, but its utility remains controversial in the literature. Continuous infusion of local anesthetic can be achieved either by preprogrammed PCA pump, or by elastomer prefilled at 5 ml/h with ropivacaine 0.2% or other anesthetic solutions such as levobupivacaine 0.375%, as reported by Niraj et al. There are still few reports in the literature that give a central role to continuous TAP block as the analgesic postoperative technique of first choice in major abdominal surgery, where the peridural technique is currently the gold standard.

TAP BLOCK AND ADJUVANT USE

The few data available in the literature allow us to hypothesize how the use of adjuvant drugs to be infused in the TAP plane in addition to the local anesthetic, in the context of a multimodal therapeutic strategy, can provide a prolongation of the analgesic block, allowing to reduce the use of opiates. Dexamethasone is one of the most widely used adjuvants in peripheral nerve blocks, but currently only three clinical trials have reported prolongation of analgesia duration when used in combination with levobupivacaine in TAP block, with reduced opioid and NSAID consumption postoperatively. Clonidine, used as an adjuvant in TAP block after caesarean section, does not appear to increase the analgesic effect of LA and does not prevent control of hyperalgesia related to the presence of the surgical wound.
Recently, several RCTs have tested the efficacy of magnesium sulphate and dexmedetomidine as adjuvants in TAP block, with promising results in terms of prolongation of analgesic effect, reduction in VAS score, postoperative opioid consumption and PONV episodes.

INDICATIONS AND DOSAGES OF LOCAL ANESTHETIC

The TAP block is only indicated for the treatment of the somatic component of postoperative pain and should therefore always be included in a multimodal analgesic scheme.
For complete analgesic coverage of the abdominal wall, a dual bilateral approach is required. Ultrasound-guided TAP block may be a valid alternative in cases where epidural analgesia is contraindicated, impractical, or refused by the patient.
The mid-axillary approach seems to be more appropriate for lower abdominal surgery, in contrast to the subcostal approach which provides better analgesia results in supraumbilical abdominal surgery.
Randomized clinical trials have documented the analgesic efficacy of ultrasound-guided TAP block in different types of surgery: colorectal surgery, caesarean section, umbilical surgery, cholecystectomy, hysterectomy, and gynecological surgery, inguinal herniorrhaphy, appendectomy, nephrectomy, kidney and liver transplantation, prostatectomy, anterior iliac crest removal, gastrectomy, bariatric surgery, or laparoscopic surgery.
Although the TAP block can be performed unilaterally (e.g., appendectomy), in the case of midline incisions (e.g., Pfannenstiel) or laparoscopic surgery, a bilateral block should be performed. Several authors recommend the use of the posterior approach, which may partly justify the coverage of visceral pain, due to the diffusion of the anesthetic solution towards the para-vertebral space.
Table 7.1 summarizes the indications that the scientific literature suggests regarding the application of TAP block for different types of abdominal surgery.
Recent clinical trials highlight the usefulness of the ultrasound-guided TAP block as an analgesic option in other types of surgery and clinical situations, as shown in **Table 7.2**.
Regarding the timing of the procedure, the literature recommends that the TAP block should be performed under general anesthesia, prior to the surgical incision, to exploit the intraoperative analgesic effect and to have a longer duration of postoperative analgesia, both in adult and pediatric patients.
The efficacy of the block is related to the spread of the local anesthetic rather than its concentration and is volume dependent. A dosage of 0.3-0.6 ml/kg on each side can be used to calculate the volume to be used.
Table 7.3 shows the dosages and volumes of local anesthetic to be used when performing TAP block in both adult and pediatric patients.

TABLE 7.1 INDICATIONS FOR PERFORMING TAP BLOCK IN DIFFERENT TYPES OF ABDOMINAL SURGERY

Type of approach for TAP Block	Anatomical landmarks	Target	Needle-to-probe ratio	Needle orientation	Type of intervention
Mid-axillary	Iliac crest, costal margin along middle axillary line	Myofascial plan between IOM and TAM	"In-plane"	"Medial-to-lateral"	Sub-umbilical surgery
Posterior	Iliac crest, costal margin along middle axillary line	Myofascial plane between IOM aponeurosis and quadratus lumborum	"In-plane"	"Medial-to-lateral"	Sub-umbilical surgery
Oblique subcostal	Costal margin, near the xiphoid process (need to visualise the epigastric artery by means of echo-color and power-doppler)	Myofascial plane between TAM and rectus abdominis	"In-plane"	"Medial-to-lateral"	Supra- and peri-umbilical surgery
Sub-costal	Costal margin, near the midline	Myofascial plane at the point where the rectus muscle ends and the IOM aponeurosis begins	"In-plane"	"Medial-to-lateral"	Supra- and peri-umbilical surgery

Contraindications to the block

Contraindications:

- patient refusal
- allergy to LA
- injection site infections

Surgery at the injection site and coagulopathy are relative contraindications.

COMPLICATIONS AND CONTRAINDICATIONS

TAP block, when performed by experienced operators and with the aid of ultrasound guidance, is a relatively simple technique with an excellent safety profile for all approaches and a very low incidence of complications. The "blind" technique, on the other hand, is not entirely free of risks and complications. The Petit Triangle may be difficult to palpate in some patients, such as the obese, and the literature reports a case of accidental liver trauma in a patient undergoing total hysterectomy. In addition to liver puncture injury, other complications described in the literature include intraperitoneal injection, intestinal injury, colon puncture, haematoma formation at the injection site, transient femoral nerve palsy, and failure of systemic local anesthetic toxicity. Local anesthetic toxicity may occur due to improper technique when using large volumes of local anesthetic to perform the block, especially when performed bilaterally. In addition, improper deposition of local anesthetic at analgesic doses within a muscle belly, and thus outside the TAP, can also lead to symptoms of local anesthetic neurotoxicity.

There are few contraindications to performing TAP block. Absolute contraindications include the patient's failure to consent to the procedure, a history of allergy to local anesthetics, infection of the abdominal wall, and localized abnormalities at the site of injection. Relative contraindications are surgery at the injection site and the presence of coagulopathy, although there is currently no evidence that coagulation disorders contraindicate the technique.

TABLE 7.2 OTHER INDICATIONS FOR THE EXECUTION OF THE TAP BLOCK

Type of intervention	Application of TAP Block	Type of approach	Adult	Pediatric
Analgesia after abdominal aortic surgery (Minami et al.)	Repair of abdominal aortic aneurysm	Mid-axillary, posterior, subcostal and subcostal oblique	Ropivacaine 0.25% Levobupivacaine 0.25% or 0.375% 1 mg/kg each side	No scientific evidence
Biopsy and bone harvesting (Tanaka et al.)	Paediatric patients undergoing bone harvesting from the iliac crest	Mid-axillary, posterior, subcostal and subcostal oblique	Ropivacaine 0.25% Levobupivacaine 0.25% or 0.375% 1 mg/kg each side	Ropivacaine 0.25%; Levobupivacaine 0.25% or 0.375% 0.4-1 mg/kg each side
Neurolysis with alcohol or phenol (Hung et al.)	Long-term control of cancer pain in neoplasms or neoplasms or metastatic infiltration of the abdominal wall, in cases of pain refractory to systemic opioid therapy	Mid-axillary, posterior, subcostal and subcostal oblique, in relation to reported algic irradiation and anatomical site of lesion	Ropivacaine 0.25% Levobupivacaine 0.25% or 0.375% 1 mg/kg each side	Ropivacaine 0.25 Levobupivacaine 0.25% or 0.375% 0.4-1 mg/kg for each side (no solid scientific evidence)
Treatment of algic flare-ups (Smith et al.)	Acute chronic pancreatitis	Subcostal Oblique and posterior subcostal, predominantly	Ropivacaine 0.25% Levobupivacaine 0.25% or 0.375% 1 mg/kg each side	Ropivacaine 0.25 Levobupivacaine 0.25% or 0.375% 0.4-1 mg/kg for each side (Beware! No scientific evidence)
Analgesia in hepatopathic patients (Eldin et al.)	Cirrhotic patients undergoing liver resection	Subcostal Oblique and posterior subcostal, predominantly	Ropivacaine 0.25% Levobupivacaine 0.25% or 0.375% 1 mg/kg each side (Beware of increased plasma levels of local anesthetic in case of continuous TAP Block!)	No scientific evidence
Emergency intra-abdominal surgery (Vuong et al.)	Elderly patient for emergency abdominal surgery	Mid-axillary, posterior, subcostal and subcostal oblique		No scientific evidence

TABLE 7.3 DOSAGES AND VOLUMES OF LOCAL ANESTHETIC TO BE USED IN TAP BLOCK

	Volume of local anesthetic	Concentration and recommended local anesthetic	Maximum permitted dosage of local anesthetic
Adult	0.3-0.6 ml/kg each side (20 max. 30 ml per side)	Ropivacaine 0.25% Levobupivacaine 0.25% or 0.375%	1 mg/kg each side
Child	0.2-0.3 ml/kg each side	Ropivacaine 0.25% Levobupivacaine 0.25% or 0.375%	Up to a maximum of 3 mg/kg total

Complications

- Vascular puncture
- Intraperitoneal injection
- Colon puncture
- Liver puncture
- Increased risk of LAST (related to high volumes of LA used or failure to meet maximum recommended dosages)

PEDIATRIC SETTING

The anatomy and sonoanatomy of the TAP are superimposable in children and adults.

Briefly, it is recalled that the aim of the technique is to deposit the LA in the fascial plane between the internal oblique (IO) and transverse muscle, in order to block the nerve structures that cross it (anterior rami of the intercostal nerves T6 to T12 and the first lumbar nerve L1), with consequent anesthesia/analgesia of the skin, muscles and parietal peritoneum of the anterior abdominal wall.

The ultrasound-guided technique in children involves the use of the following equipment: a high-frequency (7-12 MHz) linear probe, sterile probe cover, sterile gel, short-bevel needle (50 mm, 22-25 G), sterile drapes and antiseptic solution to make up a sterile field.

With the patient supine, the probe is placed transversely on the anterior or mid axillary line between the costal margin and the iliac crest to visualize the three muscle layers – external oblique (EO), internal oblique (IO), transverse abdomen (TA) – separated by their respective hyperechogenic fasciae.

The technique and approaches are the same as described for adults.

It is recommended to use a volume of 0.2-0.3 ml/Kg of levobupivacaine 0.25% or ropivacaine 0.2% per side, without exceeding the safe doses of local anesthetics (3 mg/kg for levobupivacaine and ropivacaine).

In children, the TAP block is indicated for the treatment of postoperative pain following abdominal or pelvic surgery and as an alternative to peridural analgesia in subjects with contraindications to neuraxial blocks. There are no absolute contraindications to this block, other than the presence of infection at the puncture site.

The main complication is systemic toxicity from local anesthetics, which can be caused either by an accidental intravascular injection or by a miscalculated overdose.

However, the Pediatric Regional Anaesthesia Network (PRAN) has recently reported only two minor complications out of 1994 cases: a vascular puncture and a peritoneal puncture.

CHRONIC PAIN

It is estimated that approximately 10% of patients with idiopathic chronic abdominal pain are specifically affected by abdominal wall pain (CAWP).

CAWP is mainly caused by degenerative diseases, but in a high percentage of patients it is almost always the result of surgical procedures. Indeed, it is believed that in most cases peripheral nerve injury can lead to persistent changes in the central nervous system, resulting in central sensitization, which in turn can lead to chronic pain syndromes.

In the face of chronic abdominal pain of uncertain origin, the TAP block allows an easy differential diagnosis, providing a valuable aid in differentiating between somatosensory and visceral pain. In the case of pain reduction of more than 50% after LA injection, the parietal and neuropathic origin of the pain symptoms can be established with almost absolute certainty.

On the other hand, with regard to the therapeutic role, the data provided by the literature are currently scarce. Promising results have been obtained using corticosteroids as adjuvants.

In addition, the injection of a large volume (10-20 ml) of local anesthetic can determine a mechanical action of lysis of any adhesions, responsible for the abdominal pain; while the topical deposition of glucocorticoid can exert an anti-inflammatory and, more generally, inhibitory effect on fibroblasts, with the ultimate result of reducing the formation of new adhesions.

The use of TAP block has also been described in patients with cancer pain. When combined with phenol neurolysis, it has been used as a therapeutic approach in patients with abdominal pain of oncological origin, which is not responsive to common therapies.

RECOMMENDED READING

- Abdallah FW, Laffey JG, Halpern SH, Brull R. Duration of analgesic effectiveness after the posterior and lateral transversus abdominis plane block techniques for transverse lower abdominal incisions: a meta-analysis. British journal of anaesthesia. 2013;111:721-35.
- Abd-Elsalam KA, Fares KM, Mohamed MA, Mohamed MF, El-Rahman AMA, Tohamy MM. Efficacy of Magnesium Sulfate Added to Local Anesthetic in a Transversus Abdominis Plane Block for Analgesia Following Total Abdominal Hysterectomy: A Randomized Trial. Pain physician. 2017;20:641-7.
- Baciarello M, Migliavacca G. TAP block e dolore cronico addominale. In: Fusco P, Marinangeli F. Blocchi nervosi ecoguidati del tronco e della parete addominale, Edizioni Edra, Milano 2016; 87-92.
- Blanco R. Tap block under ultrasound guidance: the description of a "no pops" technique: 271. Regional Anesthesia and Pain Medicine. 2007;32:130.
- Børglum J, Maschmann C, Belhage B, Jensen K. Ultrasound-guided bilateral dual transversus abdominis plane block: a new four-point approach. Acta anaesthesiologica Scandinavica. 2011;55:658-63.
- Carney J, Finnerty O, Rauf J, Bergin D, Laffey JG, Mc Donnell JG. Studies on the spread of local anaesthetic solution in transversus abdominis plane blocks. Anaesthesia. 2011;66:1023-30.
- Carney J, McDonnell JG, Ochana A, Bhinder R, Laffey JG. The transversus abdominis plane block provides effective postoperative analgesia in patients undergoing total abdominal hysterectomy. Anesthesia and analgesia. 2008;107:2056-60.
- Chou R, Gordon DB, de Leon-Casasola OA, et al. Management of Postoperative Pain: A Clinical Practice Guideline From the American Pain Society, the American Society of Regional Anesthesia and Pain Medicine, and the American Society of Anesthesiologists'Committee on Regional Anesthesia, Executive Committee, and Administrative Council. The Journal of Pain. 2016;17(2):131-57.
- Deshpande JP, Ghodki PS, Sardesai SP. The Analgesic Efficacy of Dexamethasone Added to Ropivacaine in Transversus Abdominis Plane Block for Transabdominal Hysterectomy under Subarachnoid Block. Anesthesia, essays and researches. 2017;11:499-502.
- Fusco P, Cofini V, Petrucci E, et al. Transversus Abdominis Plane Block in the Management of Acute Postoperative Pain Syndrome after Caesarean Section: A Randomized Controlled Clinical Trial. Pain physician. 2016;19:583-91.
- Fusco P, Scimia P, Paladini G, et al. Transversus abdominis plane block for analgesia after Cesarean delivery. A systematic review. Minerva anestesiologica. 2015;81:195-204.
- Fusco P, Scimia P, Petrucci E, Di Carlo S, Paladini G, Marinangeli F. Transversus Abdominis Plane Block as Analgesic Technique for Postoperative Pain Management After Cesarean Section: No More? Reg Anesth Pain Med. 2017;42:541.
- Griffiths JD, Le NV, Grant S, Bjorksten A, Hebbard P, Royse C. Symptomatic local anaesthetic toxicity and plasma ropivacaine concentrations after transversus abdominis plane block for Caesarean section. British journal of anaesthesia. 2013;110:996-1000.
- Hebbard P, Fujiwara Y, Shibata Y, Royse C. Ultrasound-guided transversus abdominis plane (TAP) block. Anaesthesia and intensive care. 2007;35:616-7.
- Hebbard P. Subcostal transversus abdominis plane block under ultrasound guidance. Anesthesia and analgesia. 2008;106:674-5.
- Hung JC, Azam N, Puttanniah V, Malhotra V, Gulati A. Neurolytic transversus abdominal plane block with alcohol for long-term malignancy related pain control. Pain physician 2014;17:E755-60.
- Lancaster P, Chadwick M. Liver trauma secondary to ultrasound-guided transversus abdominis plane block. British journal of anaesthesia. 2010;104:509-10.
- Long JB, Birmingham PK, De Oliveira GS, Jr., Schaldenbrand KM, Suresh S. Transversus abdominis plane block in children: a multicenter safety analysis of 1994 cases from the PRAN (Pediatric Regional Anesthesia Network) database. Anesthesia and analgesia. 2014;119:395-9.
- McDonnell JG, O'Donnell B, Curley G, Heffernan A, Power C, Laffey JG. The analgesic efficacy of transversus abdominis plane block after abdominal surgery: a prospective randomized controlled trial. Anesthesia and analgesia. 2007;104:193-7.
- Mukhtar K, Singh S. Transversus abdominis plane block for laparoscopic surgery. British journal of anaesthesia. 2009;102:143-4.
- Nelson G, Altman AD, Nick A, et al. Guidelines for postoperative care in gynecologic/oncology surgery: Enhanced Recovery After Surgery (ERAS(R)) Society recommendations-Part II. Gynecologic oncology. 2016;140:323-32.
- Niraj G, Kelkar A, Darbar A, Hart E. Posterior transversus abdominis plane (TAP) catheters in lower abdominal surgery. International Journal of Ultrasound & Applied Technologies in Perioperative Care. 2010;1:79-81.
- Rafi AN. Abdominal field block: a new approach via the lumbar triangle. Anaesthesia. 2001;56:1024-6.

- Rozen WM, Tran TM, Ashton MW, Barrington MJ, Ivanusic JJ, Taylor GI. Refining the course of the thoracolumbar nerves: a new understanding of the innervation of the anterior abdominal wall. Clinical anatomy (New York, NY). 2008;21:325-33.
- Sanderson BJ, Doane MA. Transversus Abdominis Plane Catheters for Analgesia Following Abdominal Surgery in Adults. Reg Anesth Pain Med. 2018;43:5-13.
- Tanaka M, Mori N, Murakami W, et al. The effect of transversus abdominis plane block for pediatric patients receiving bone graft to the alveolar cleft. Masui, The Japanese journal of anesthesiology. 2010;59:1185-9.
- Tran TM, Ivanusic JJ, Hebbard P, Barrington MJ. Determination of spread of injectate after ultrasound-guided transversus abdominis plane block: a cadaveric study. British journal of anaesthesia. 2009;102:123-7.
- Vuong J, McQuillan P, Messaris E, Adhikary S. Transversus abdominis plane block as the primary anesthetic for laparotomy. Journal of Anaesthesiology. Clinical Pharmacology. 2014;30:419-21.
- Xu L, Hu Z, Shen J, McQuillan PM. Efficacy of US-guided transversus abdominis plane block and rectus sheath block with ropivacaine and dexmedetomidine in elderly high-risk patients. Minerva anestesiologica. 2018;84:18-24.

CLINICAL CASE 1 – SUBCOSTAL TAP BLOCK FOR POSTOPERATIVE ANALGESIA IN LAPAROSCOPIC CHOLECYSTECTOMY

Clinical history and anamnesis A 62-year-old woman with anamnesis: hypertension, hysterectomy, kidney transplant, to submit intervention by laparoscopic cholecystectomy.

Technique description Following the end of surgery, the skin was prepared with 2% chlorhexidine solution. Bilateral subcostal approach TAP blocks were performed using ultrasound imaging with a linear 5-13 MHz transducer (**Figure 7.24**). We used a 22 G echogenic needle in plane approach (SonoPlex II, Pajunk®). The neurofascial plane between the internal oblique and TAP was identified. Following the demonstration of negative aspiration, 20 ml of 0.25 % levobupivacaine was injected bilaterally (**Figure 7.25**). At the end of the procedure, the patient is awakened. No advanced airway control was required. No supplementary opiates nor other local anesthetic agents were administered additionally, no complications of the block were recorded. After 15 minutes of waking up, the patient does not report any pain (VAS 0). After 6 h = VAS 2.

Materials and methods Written informed consent was obtained. General anesthesia was induced with fentanyl 100 μg, propofol 130 mg and rocuronium 40 mg.
The airway was secured with an endotracheal tube and mechanical ventilation.
General anesthesia was maintained with sevoflourane. No further analgesics were administered intraoperatively. Duration of anesthesia 35 m.

Conclusions Our results indicate that the BD-TAP block improve the quality of recovery or analgesic outcomes, if correctly performed, following laparoscopic cholecystectomy.
Further studies are needed, especially with other methods (e.g. ESP).

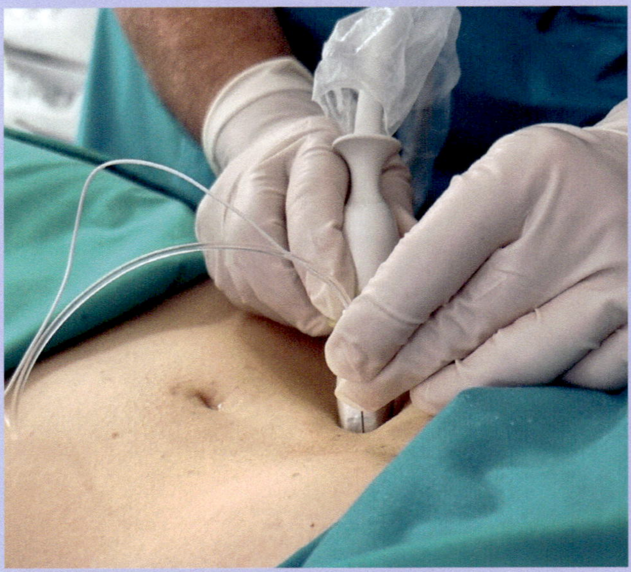

Figure 7.24 Probe and needle position in the subcostal oblique approach.

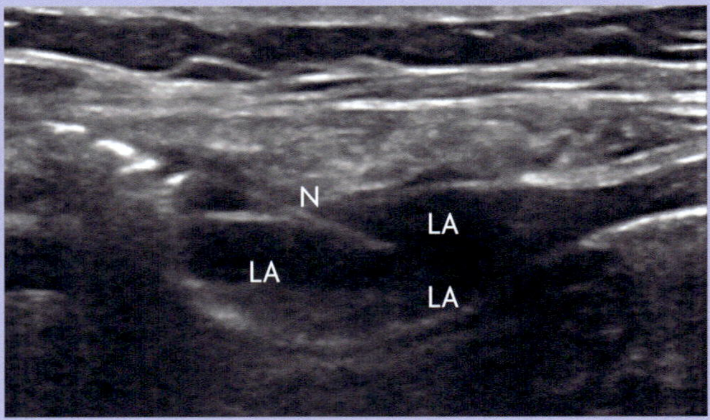

Figure 7.25 Local anesthetic injected between the internal oblique and transverse muscle with "opening" of the TAP. LA: local anesthetic; N: needle (Sonotap®).

CLINICAL CASE 2 – SUBCOSTAL AND MID-AXILLARY TAP BLOCK APPROACH (FOUR-POINTS) FOR POSTOPERATIVE ANALGESIA IN CHOLECYSTECTOMY WITH XIFO-UMBILICAL LAPAROTOMY TECHNIQUE

Clinical history and anamnesis A 82-year-old man with anamnesis: hypertension, diabetes mellitus, to submit intervention by laparoscopic cholecystectomy. Subsequently, given the impossibility of continuing, the intervention is converted with xifo-umbilical laparotomy technique

Technique description Following the end of surgery, the skin was prepared with 2% chlorhexidine solution. Bilateral subcostal and mid-axillary TAP blocks were performed using ultrasound imaging with a linear 5-13 MHz transducer. We used a 22 G echogenic needle in plane approach (SonoPlex II, Pajunk®) (**Figure 7.26**).
The neurofascial plane between the internal oblique and TAP was identified in the four points. Following the demonstration of negative aspiration, 15 ml of 0.25 % levobupivacaine was injected bilaterally subcostal and bilaterally mid-axillary TAP (four-points). At the end of the procedure, the patient is awakened. No advanced airway control was required. We were administered, additionally, Paracetamol 1gr. No complications of the block were recorded.

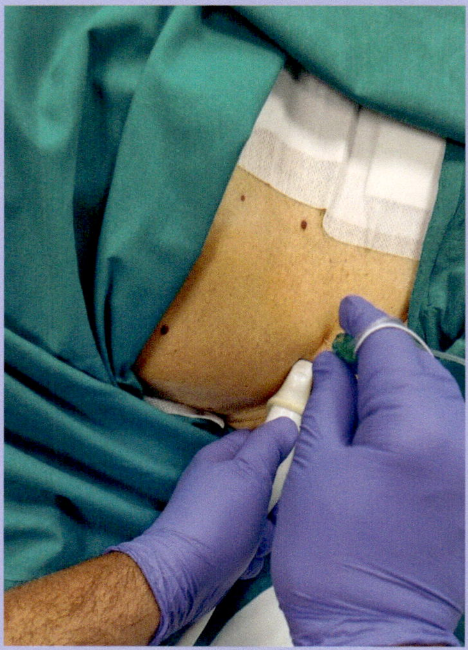

Figure 7.26 Probe and needle position in the mid-axillary approach.

After 30 minutes of waking up, the patient reports mild pain (VAS 2).
After 6 h we administered additionally paracetamol 1 g. The patient does not report any pain.

Materials and methods Written informed consent was obtained.
General anesthesia was induced with fentanyl 100 µg, propofol 150 mg and rocuronium 40 mg.
The airway was secured with an endotracheal tube and mechanical ventilation.
General anesthesia was maintained with Sevoflourane. Fentanyl 100 µg (50+50), rocuronium 20 mg.
Duration of anesthesia is 75 m.

Conclusions Our results indicate that the BD-TAP block at four points improve the quality of recovery or analgesic outcomes, if correctly performed, following xifo-umbilical laparotomy technique.
This four-point technique also reduces (or completely abolishes) the use of opioids in the postoperative period.

Iliohypogastric (IH), Ilioinguinal (II), and Genitofemoral (GF) nerve block

Paolo Scimia, Claude Thierry Bagaphou, Roberta Monzani, Pierfrancesco Fusco

The iliohypogastric (IH), ilioinguinal (II), and genitofemoral (GF) nerves are the terminal branches of the lumbar plexus and represent the main nerves providing sensory innervation to the skin bordering the region between the root of the thigh and the abdomen. Due to this feature, they are collectively defined as "border nerves" (**Figure 8.1**). Blocking these nerves can generally provide a reliable anesthesia/analgesia to the hypogastric region, the inguinal fold, the upper medial thigh region, the mons pubis, part of the labia majora

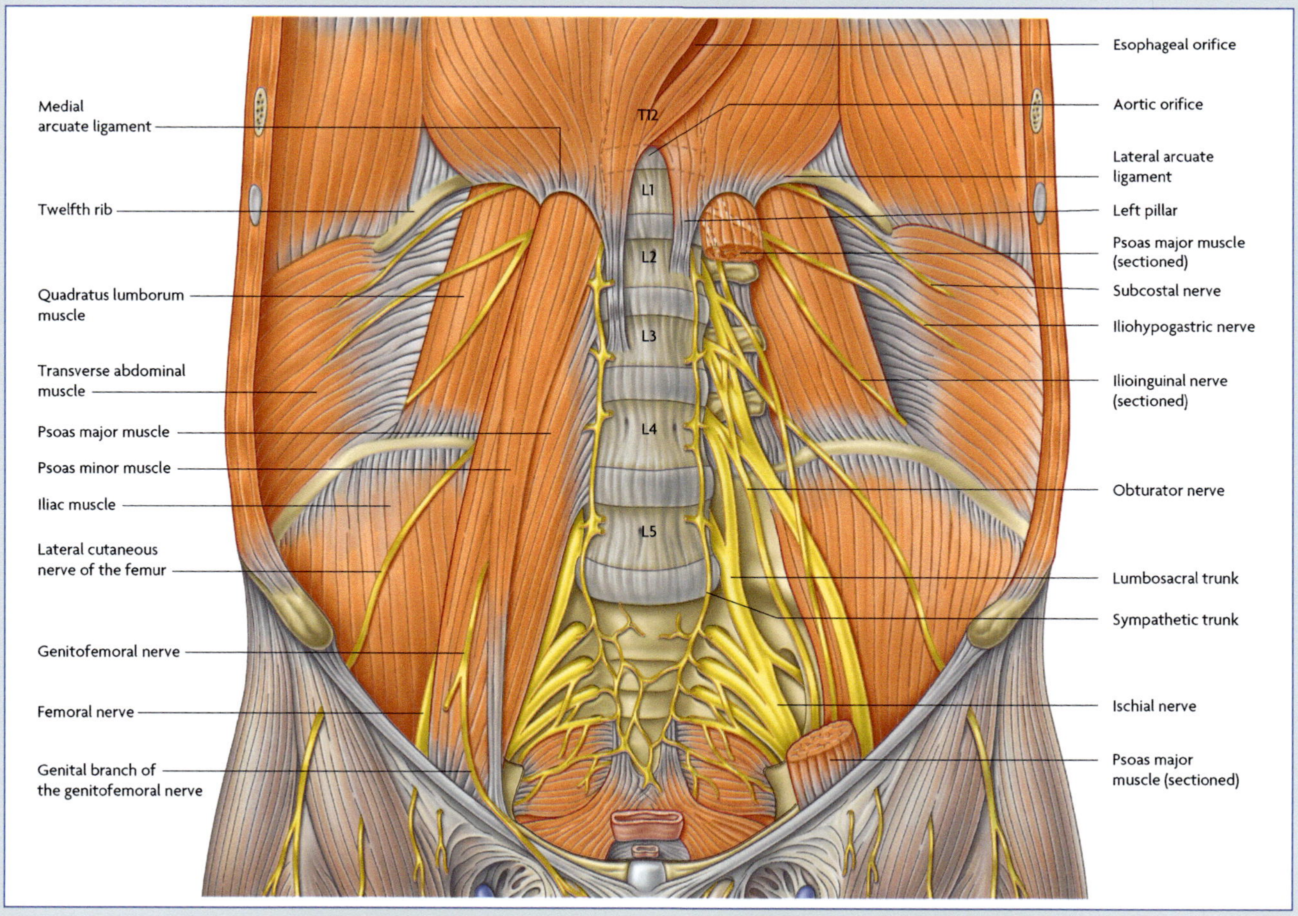

Figure 8.1 Anatomy of the "border nerves".

in women, the root of the penis, and the anterior part of the scrotum, with considerable individual variability in terms of sensory distribution. These techniques of locoregional anesthesia/analgesia (LRA) find a wide field of applications, with indications both in anesthesiology and in acute and chronic pain management. IH and II nerve block, sometimes associated with GF nerve block, is commonly used in pediatric anesthesia, as it has shown an analgesic efficacy equal to the caudal block in surgeries such as inguinal hernia repair, orchidopexy, and hydrocelectomy. Even in adult patients, the use of these techniques has shown a proven clinical efficacy, as part of a multimodal analgesic regimen, in caesarean section, inguinal hernia repair, and the surgeries that require transversal incisions in the lower abdominal region. Unfortunately, due to their superficial course, these nerve structures are not free from risk of iatrogenic lesions that might occur in different types of surgeries involving the abdominal or pelvic areas. Injury of IH, II, and GF nerves could favor the onset of chronic neuropathic pain syndromes at the level of the abdominal wall with variable extension to the inguinal and pelvic region. In this context, blocking these nerves can play a key role not only for the treatment of painful symptoms reported by the patient, but the treatment of painful symptoms reported by the patient, but especially in differential diagnosis helping the clinicians to identify the etiology of the chronic inguinal pain which is frequently difficult to understand due to the extreme anatomical variability characterizing the sensory innervation of the region involved.

ANATOMY AND SONOANATOMY

The lumbar plexus is formed by the ventral rami of nerves L1 to L3 and majority of the ventral ramus of L4, with a contribution from the T12 (subcostal) nerve. The II, IH, and GF nerves are the terminal branches of the lumbar plexus together with lateral femoral cutaneous nerve of the thigh, femoral and obturator nerves. Border nerves provide innervation to the muscle structures of the abdomen, the skin of the hypogastric region, the buttocks, the external genitalia, and the medial and antero-superior surface of the thigh (**Figure 8.2**).

The II and IH nerves originate from the anterior branch of L1 and a branch of T12 and emerge near the lateral margin of the psoas major muscle, in front of the quadratus lumborum muscle and posteriorly to the kidneys. They subsequently extend diagonally towards the iliac crest bone. At this level, the two nerves penetrate the lumbar fascia, reaching in 90% of the cases the plane between the internal oblique muscles (IOM) and the transverse abdominal muscle (TAM), also known as transversus abdominis plane (TAP) (**Figure 8.3**).

The IH nerve runs superiorly to the II nerve, proceeds centrally between the IOM and the external oblique muscle (EOM) and, after reaching the iliac crest bone just above the inguinal ligament, splits into two terminal branches: the genital branch, which provides innervation to the skin of the external genitalia, and the anterior cutaneous branch, which provides innervation to the skin of the hypogastric region. Furthermore, before splitting into the terminal branches, it gives rise to the muscular branches and a lateral cutaneous branch, which provides innervation to the skin of the ventral region of the buttocks.

The II nerve runs below the IH nerve, crosses TAM at the level of the iliac crest bone and continues ventrally by perforating the abdominal oblique muscles (IOM and EOM), until it reaches the interior margin of the round ligament of the uterus in women and the spermatic cord in men, before entering the inguinal canal. Along its course, it gives rise to secondary sensory nerves that provide innervation to the skin of the following areas: upper medial portion of the thigh, scrotum, root of the penis, and labia majora.

The GF nerve arises from the L1 and L2 spinal nerve roots as part of the lumbar plexus. However, it is a nerve of huge anatomical variation which could also be originating from T12 or L3, although L2 contribution tends to be more consistent. It is It is mainly a sensory nerve except for motor fibers of the cremasteric muscle. At the level of the disk of the third intersomatic space, it perforates the psoas muscle and starts running, as a single trunk, over its ventral surface until it reaches the inguinal ligament, where it splits into two terminal branches: the femoral and the genital branches. The division of the genital and femoral branches is very variable and can happen anywhere during the course of the nerve.

The femoral branch runs together with the external iliac artery (EIA), passes below the inguinal ligament, crosses the fascia lata, and penetrates the femoral sheath, where it provides innervation to the femoral triangle (or Scarpa's triangle). The genital branch crosses the inferior epigastric artery (IEA) at its lower end lateral to the junction between the EIA and IEA and enters the inguinal canal through the deep inguinal ring. It travels along with other contents of the inguinal canal along with the spermatic cord in men and the round ligament

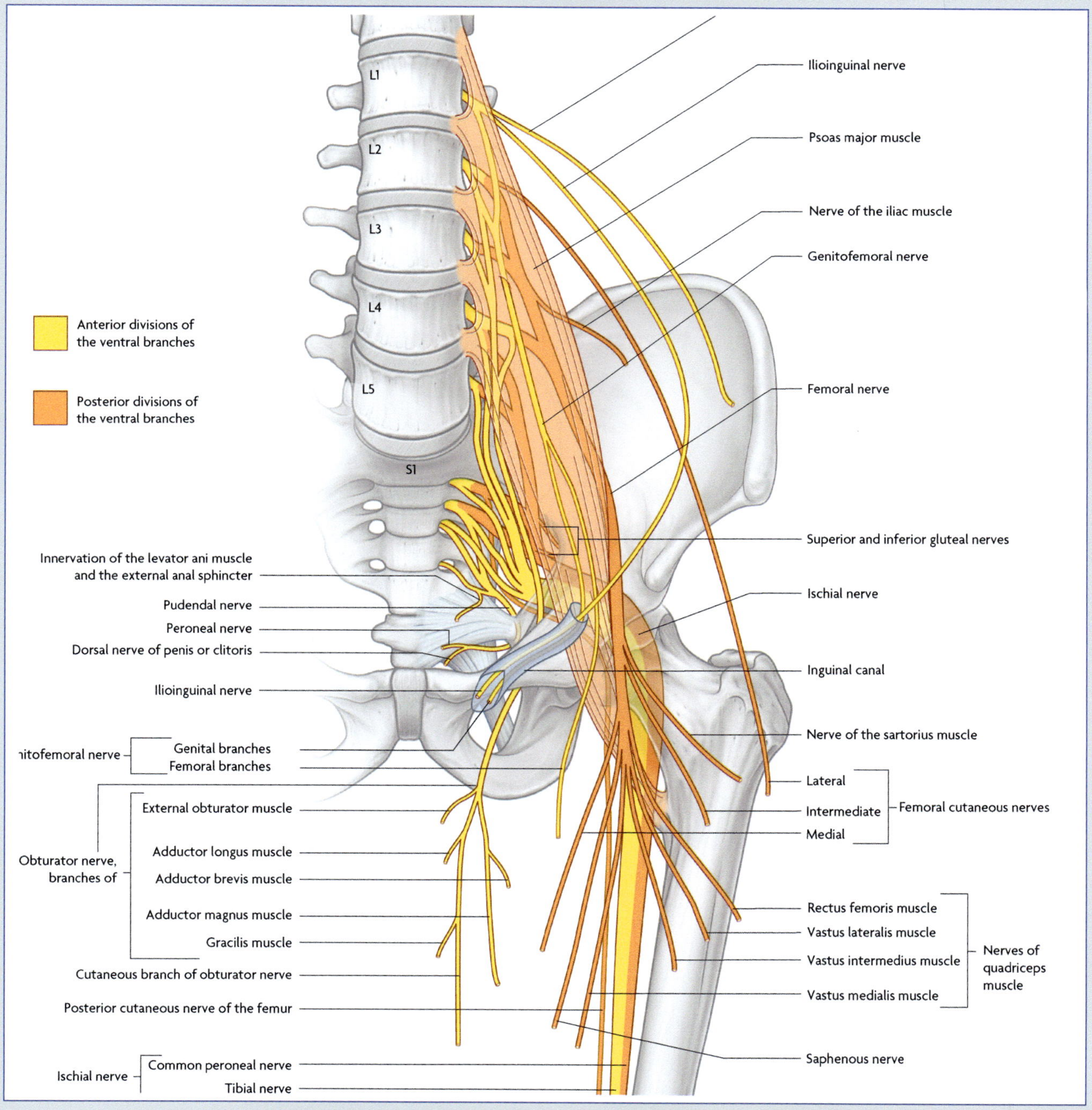

Figure 8.2 Lumbar plexus and related branches.

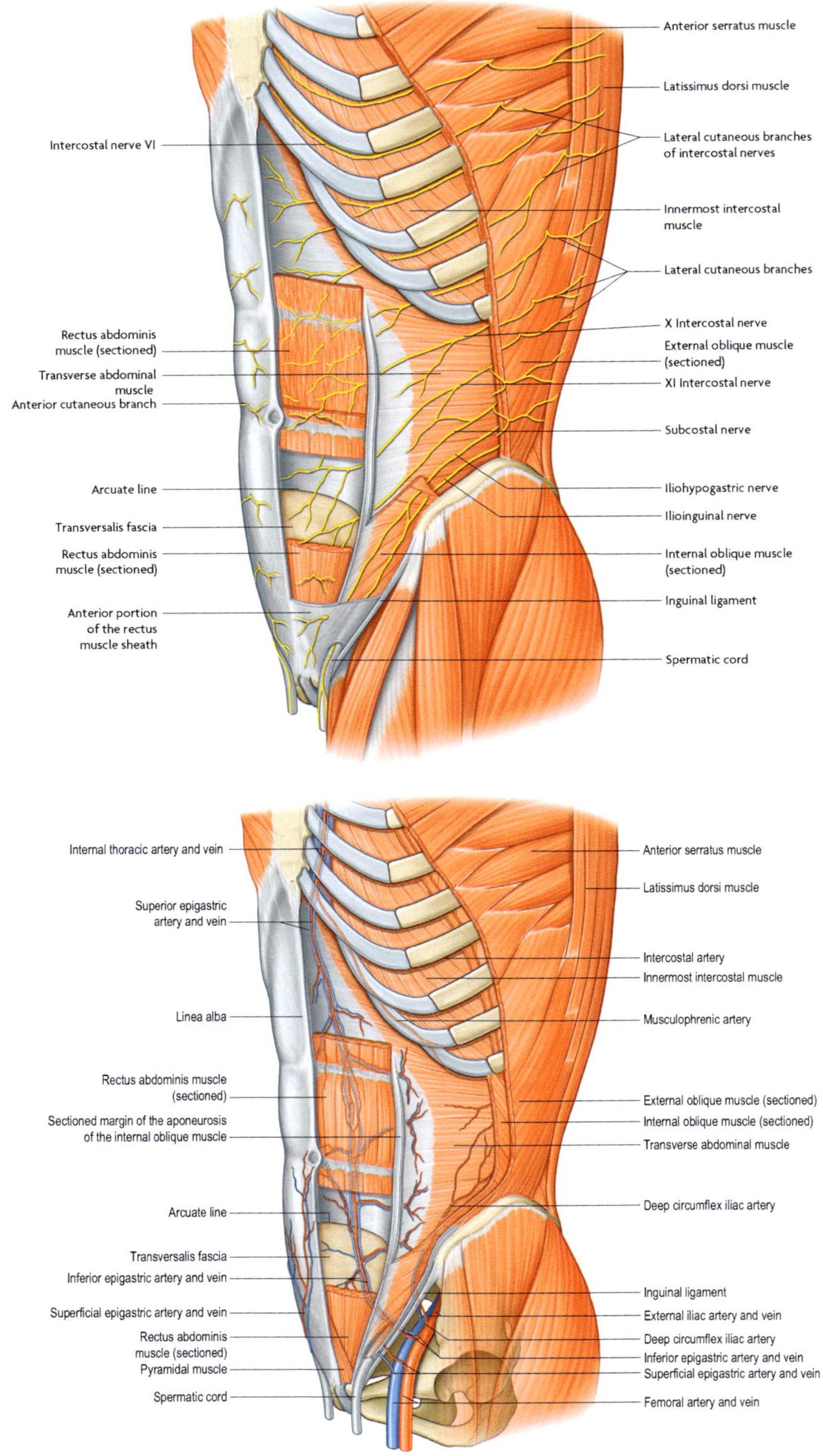

Figure 8.3 Course of the IH and II nerves along the interfascial plane between IOM and TAM.

of the uterus in women. The canal also contains the ilioinguinal nerve and testicular vessels in men or the vessel following the round ligament of the uterus in females. The peculiar characteristic of the border nerves is the presence of a considerable anatomical variability in terms of origin, contribution of spinal nerves, course, and communications among their branches (**Figure 8.4**). Anatomical dissections made on corpses have shown that, although IH and II nerves mainly originate from T12-L1 nerve roots, they can receive a contribution from T11 and L3 spinal nerves in a small number of patients. Moreover, the anastomotic connections among the IH, II, GF, and lateral femoral cutaneous nerves are in common and give rise to a remarkable overlapping of the sensory innervation. Rab et al. delineate four different types of branching patterns in these nerves, and only 20% correspond to their normal distribution. However, the location of IH and II nerves is quite consistently lateral and superior to the anterior superior iliac spine (ASIS) where these nerves are found between the IOM and TAM layers (90%), although the distance from ASIS and the point in which these nerves penetrate TAP can vary widely.

Special anatomical considerations are needed for pediatric patients, in whom the IH and II nerves show characteristics of variability that cannot be superimposed to those of adults running closer to ASIS with peculiar differences based on the different age groups. In view of the existence of a significant anatomical variability at the individual level, the importance of directly visualizing the nerve structures involved through ultrasound-guided imaging techniques is self-evident.

DESCRIPTION OF THE TECHNIQUES

The block of IH and II nerves can be performed with "blind" or ultrasound- guided technique. If blocks are performed on awake patients, the authors suggest to provide adequate sedo-analgesia through the association of benzodiazepine at low doses and opioids (midazolam 0,02 mg/kg^{-1}, sufentanil 0,1-0,15 mcg/kg^{-1} or fentanyl

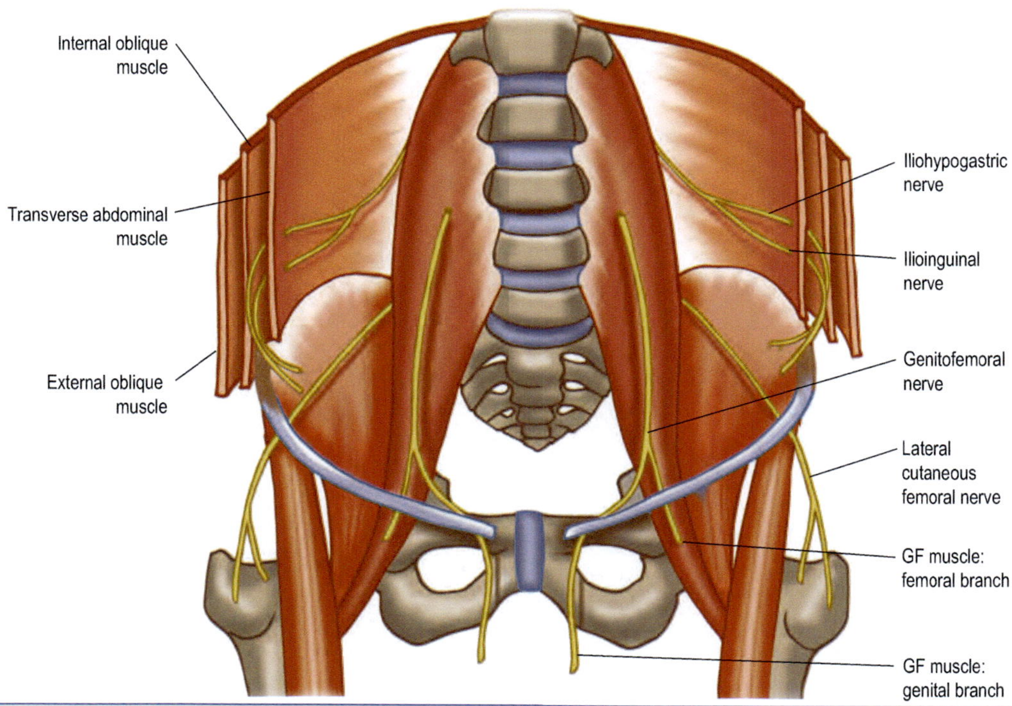

Figure 8.4 Muscle ratios, courses, and communications of IH, II, and GF nerves. Note the anatomical variability characteristic of "border nerves".

1-2 mcg/kg^{-1}); it is preferable to perform the block under general anesthesia in pediatric patients. As previously discussed, the high rate of individual anatomical variability of the target nerves explains the possible onset of iatrogenic complications and the high percentages of block failure (10-40%) linked to blind techniques based only on anatomical landmarks. The introduction of ultrasounds in the daily clinical practice has allowed to overcome the limit due to the wide anatomical variability of these nerve, thus improving the efficacy and safety related to the execution of the block of the border nerves. The advantages of the ultrasound guidance include the identification of the anatomical structures involved, the constant visualization of the needle trajectory, and the possibility of documenting the correct diffusion of local anesthetic (LA), thus allowing to reduce the necessary quantities to achieve a successful block, with a lower incidence of complications compared to the standard techniques. Currently, the use of ultrasounds for blocking the IH and II nerves is highly recommended (Grade A recommendations, level of evidence Ib-IIb), both in adult and in pediatric population. As the IH and II nerves are relatively superficial and usually located within 4 cm from the skin, the use of a high-frequency linear probe (5-15 MHz) would suffice to get a correct ultrasound visualization; in obese patients, it might be useful to increase the scanning depth with a medium-frequency linear probe. ASIS palpation provides an initial anatomical landmark to positioning of the transducer. After accurate skin disinfection with 2% chlorhexidine or iodopovidone and with the patient in supine position, the sterile sheath-covered probe is positioned cranially and medially to ASIS, perpendicularly to the inguinal ligament, and along the imaginary line that connects ASIS with the navel (**Figure 8.5**). At this level the bone prominence of ASIS appears as a hyperechogenic structure with posterior shadow cone, with the subcutaneous adipose tissue and three muscle layers of the abdominal wall (EOM, IOM, and TAM) adjacent to it. Immediately below TAM, it is possible to identify the transversalis fascia, situated just above the peritoneum, easily recognizable due to the peristaltic movements of the bowel.

Once the three muscle layers of the abdominal wall have been identified, the IH and II nerves can be visualized as two hyperechogenic ovular structures, within 1 cm from one another, along the fascial plane between IOM and TAM (**Figure 8.6**). The II nerve is normally located near the landmark of the iliac crest bone (about 4-8 cm), while the IH nerve runs more medially at about 5-15 cm from ASIS.

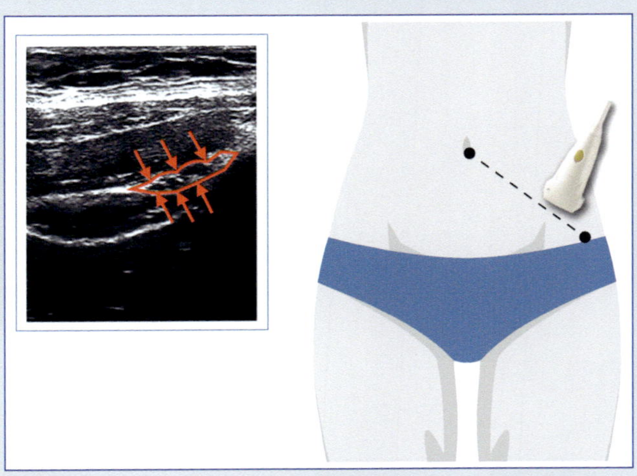

Figure 8.5 Position of the probe for the identification of the IH and II nerves and the muscular structures involved.

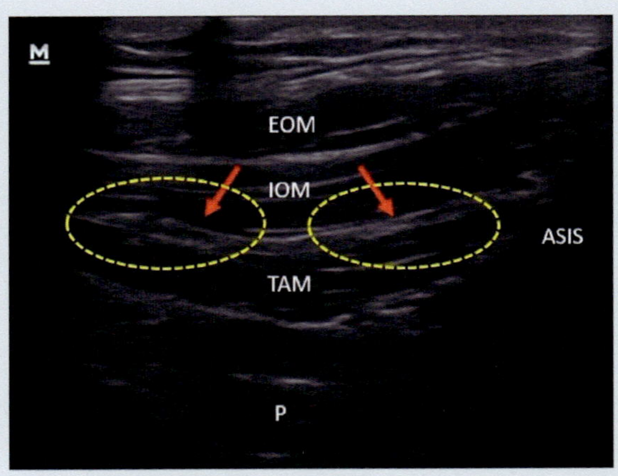

Figure 8.6 Sonoanatomy of IH and II nerves. It is possible to note the nerves (red arrow) that run in TAP and that look like hypoechoic oval structures with the characterizing hyperechoic appearance. ASIS: anterior superior iliac spine; EOM: external oblique muscle; IOM: internal oblique muscles; P: peritoneal cavity; TAM: transverse abdominal muscle.

The block target is to distribute the anesthetic solution around the previously mentioned nerves, while they pass between IOM and TAM. The diffusion of LA involves the characteristic opening of the interfascial plane between the two muscles, which represents a marker of block success (**Figure 8.7**, **Flow chart 8.1 online**).

Both with landmark and ultrasound-guided approach, confirmation of the nervous target can be obtained with an electroneurostimulator (ENS) which, with a voltage higher than 2 mA, may produce paresthesia in the inguinal area. The block can be performed with both an "in-plane" and an "out-plane" approach. A 22 G 50-90 mm needle (SonoPlex stim Pajunk®) is inserted through the subcutaneous tissue, preferably with an "in-plane" approach, from medial to lateral direction, 1-2 cm medially in relation to the probe, constantly following the trajectory up to the plane between IOM and TAM crossed by the nerves. The sensation of a "pop" will signal to the operator the entry into the target fascial plane; at this point, an anesthetic solution is injected after suction test and hydrolocation through the injection of 2-3 ml of saline solution, to make sure that the needle tip is correctly positioned. The confirmation of the correct LA distribution is given by the "real-time" visualization of the biconvex lens-shaped image that progressively separates IOM and TAM. However, although this ultrasound sign can simulate a correct technical execution, it does not completely rule out the possibility of a perifascial injection. Therefore, the authors suggest always confirming the correct execution of the fascial blocks by verifying the "double V" sign. If the injection is correctly performed, the LA diffusion inside the target fascial plane will determine the "opening" of the plane itself and the separation of the two fasciae, which will be bilaterally visible through the characteristic ultrasound "double V" sign (**Video 8.1**).

The "out of plane" technique may be a reasonable choice for obese patients; as in these circumstances the needle tip cannot be always visible during the procedure, the intermittent administration of 0.5-1 ml refracted boluses of normal saline is recommended to correctly localize the needle tip inside the target plane before LA injection. The "out of plane" may be the preferable technique in some cases as it is easier and causes less patient discomfort due to needle depth and trajectory. If the operator finds difficulties in identifying the structures concerned, it is recommended to use, as an anatomical landmark, the deep circumflex iliac artery, which runs in the same plane together with the two nerves (**Figure 8.8**), while its pulsatility can be easily identified by color Doppler function (**Figure 8.9**).

Sometimes, it is possible to visualize a third nerve structure that runs medially to the target nerves within the interfascial plane between IOM and TAM, in other words, the subcostal nerve (12th intercostal nerve); the accidental block of this nerve, which can be mixed up with the IH and II nerves, can cause an aberrant distribution of the anesthetic level. As the IH and II nerves run close in-

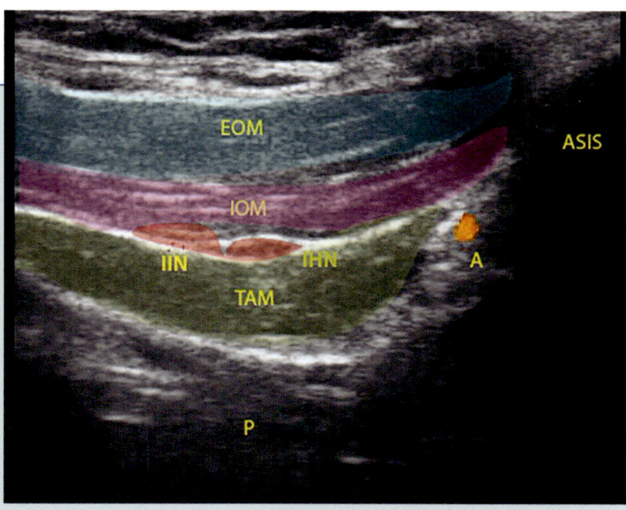

Figure 8.7 Target of iliohypogastric/Ilioinguinal nerve block. A: deep circumflex iliac artery; ASIS: anterior superior iliac spine; EOM: external oblique muscle; IHN: iliohypogastric nerve; IIN: ilioinguinal nerve; IOM: internal oblique muscle; P: peritoneum; TAM: transverse abdominal muscle. Note the distribution of LA around the target nerves, with the "opening" of the fascial plane between IOM and TAM.

Video 8.1 US-guided Ilioinguinal and Iliohypogastric nerve block. Note "double V sign".

side the target fascial plane (sometimes, as a common trunk) and frequently overlap in the sensory innervation, a selective block of the single nerves can be difficult to perform even in expert hands, especially in patients with scarring due to previous surgical interventions; in these circumstances, it is recommended to simply inject the anesthetic solution inside the fascial plane between IOM and TAM, avoiding to separate the two nerves.

As to the block of the GF nerve, numerous approaches have been described in the literature, both with landmark and ultrasound-guided technique. There are different methods to scan and identify the genital branch of the GF nerve although no validated standardized technique has been described yet.

The landmark technique proposed for blocking the femoral branch of the GF nerve requires the patient in supine position with a pillow under the knees to extend the hip joint. This technique relies on palpating the pubic tubercle and injecting LA lateral to it. Another approach requires direct injection into the inguinal canal while performing surgery. Unfortunately, using blind technique the needle is likely to enter the spermatic cord or even the peritoneum, resulting in trauma of the structures inside the spermatic cord or bowel.

The ultrasound-guided block of the genital branch of the GF nerve (described by Peng) requires the use of a high-frequency linear probe (6-13 MHz) and the visualization of the inguinal canal. With the patient in supine position, the probe is positioned perpendicularly to the inguinal ligament and laterally to the pubic tubercle. If the inguinal canal turns out to be difficult to visualize, the femoral artery can be used as anatomical landmark (**Figure 8.10**). Moving the probe in cephalic direction, the operator identifies a transition point in which the iliac artery splits

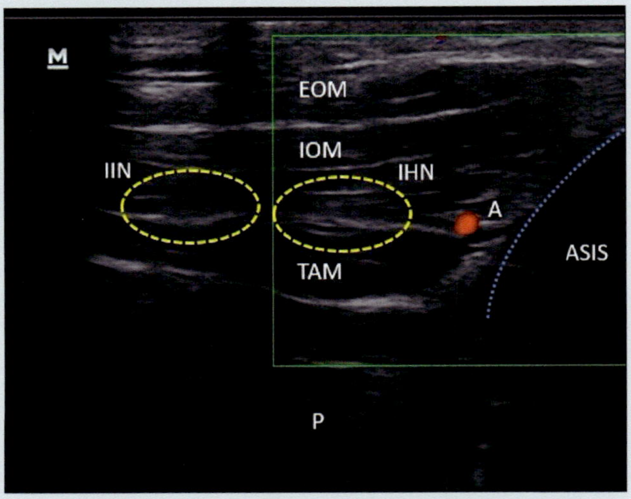

Figure 8.8 Course of the circumflex iliac artery. A: deep circumflex iliac artery; ASIS: anterior superior iliac spine; EOM: external oblique muscle; IHN: iliohypogastric nerve; IIN: ilioinguinal nerve (IIN); IOM: internal oblique muscle; P: peritoneum; TAM: transverse abdominal muscle. Note the course of the circumflex iliac artery in the same plane of the target nerve structures.

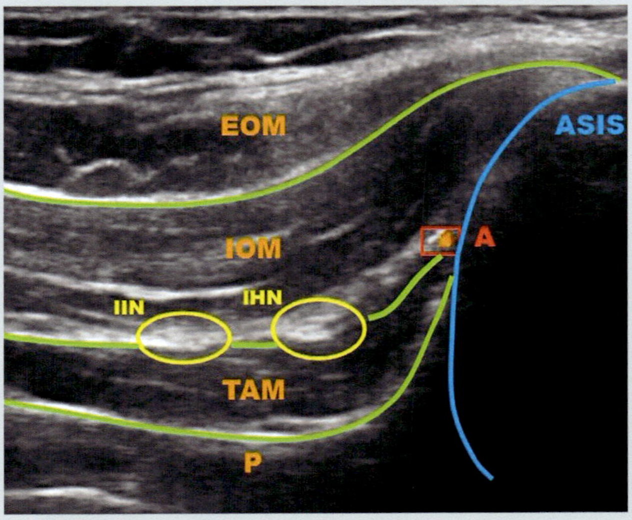

Figure 8.9 Ultrasound visualization of the circumflex iliac artery (A). A: deep circumflex iliac artery; ASIS: anterior superior iliac spine; EOM: external oblique muscle; IHN: iliohypogastric nerve; IIN: ilioinguinal nerve; IOM: internal oblique muscle; P: peritoneum; TAM: transverse abdominal muscle.

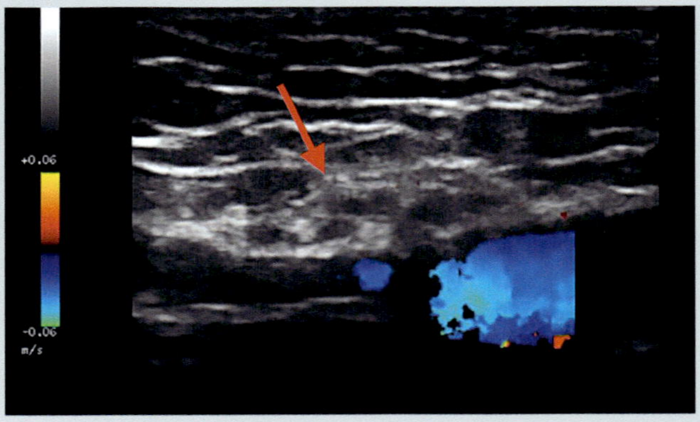

Figure 8.10 Visualization of spermatic cord and femoral artery with color Doppler.

into the femoral artery and EIA, at the level of the external inguinal ring. At this point, the inguinal canal can be identified superficially in relation to the EIA, as a rounded structure that contains the spermatic cord in men and the round ligament of the uterus in women (**Figure 8.11**). The identification of the vascular structures contained inside the inguinal canal can be facilitated by using color-Doppler technique, asking the patient to cough, and performing a Valsalva maneuver to increase blood flow.

Another technique consists of scanning the rectus abdominis muscle at the lower abdomen in transverse plane and identifying the IEA. Moving the probe caudally and parallel to the inguinal ligament, the junction of the IEA with the EIA is identified. The genital branch of the GF nerve entering into the inguinal canal may be identified lateral to EIA.

The ultrasound-guided GF nerve block can be performed with both an "in-plane" and an "out-plane" approach. After the recognition of the target structures inside the inguinal canal, which are not always easy to identify, male patients are administered 4 ml of LA both inside and outside the spermatic cord in the group of the inguinal canal, while female patients are administered 5 ml of LA in the inguinal canal surrounding the round ligament. The authors suggest always carry out suction test and hydrolocation before administering the anesthetic solution, to confirm the correct needle tip localization and to avoid intravascular injection (**Flow chart 8.2 online**).

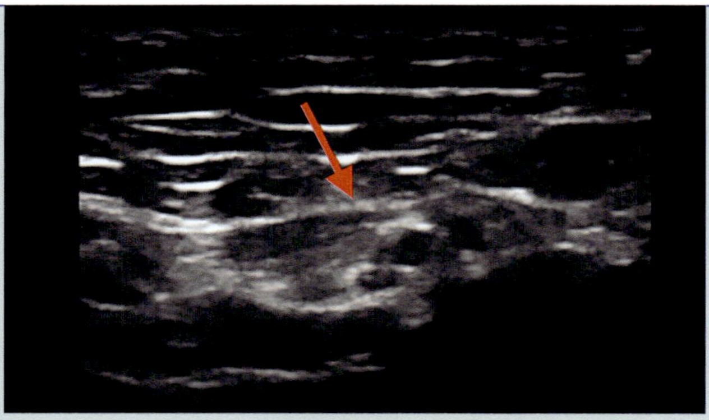

Figure 8.11 Ultrasound visualization of the inguinal canal, superficially to the external iliac artery at the level of the external inguinal ring. Note the inguinal canal that appears as a rounded structure (red arrow).

INDICATIONS AND DOSAGES

The blockade of the border nerves can be used in anesthesiology or for acute and chronic pain treatment, with applications in both adult and pediatric patients. The blocks of the IH and II nerves can provide adequate analgesia in surgeries involving the region between the root of the thigh and the inferior abdominal wall, as an integral part of a multimodal regimen.

The main indications include anesthesia for surgeries that involve the lower abdomen and the inguinal region, such as herniorraphy, orchidopexy, and postoperative analgesia for surgeries in which the Pfannenstiel incision (cesarean section and hysterectomy) is used. It is useful to remember that these blocks cannot be employed as the only anesthetic approach, as they do not provide visceral anesthesia; therefore, the authors always recommend to associate adequate sedo-analgesia or general anesthesia (with the block itself). To avoid general anesthesia in inguinal hernia repairs, some authors think it is useful to associate the TAP block ("double TAP" technique) with the block of the IH and II nerves, or to perform LA infiltration of the hernial sac containing the peritoneum. For inguinal herniorraphy, a possible alternative is to perform blocking of the genital branch of the GF nerve, combined to the block of the IH and II nerves, but it seems to provide benefits only during intraoperative hernial sac traction with no postoperative effect. In the context of the actual pain management, the selective blocks of the IH, II, and GF nerves find applications not just in the treatment of acute and chronic inguinal pain but also in diagnostics, as they help the clinician to make differential diagnoses of chronic pain syndromes which are frequently difficult to identify due to the extreme anatomical variability of these nerves.

As to the doses generally used for blocking the IH and II nerves in adult patients, 10 ml of long-acting LA (0.5% ropivacaine or 0.5% levobupivacaine) for each nerve are usually sufficient to guarantee a successful block. As to the block of the genital branch of the GF nerve, instead, it is recommended to administer in male patients 5 ml of long-acting LA both inside and outside the spermatic cord in the structures of the inguinal canal, and 5 ml of LA in the inguinal canal surrounding the round ligament in female patients. For treatment of chronic pain syndromes, the use of corticosteroids as adjuvants can prolong the analgesic effect.

> **Patients on whom the block should not be performed**
>
> Absolute contraindications:
> - Patient's refusal
> - Known allergy to the ALs used
> - Infection at the level of the injection site or systemic infection
>
> Relative contraindications:
> - Non-collaborating patient/Neurological pathologies
> - Obesity (BMI >35)
> - Previous episodes of coagulopathy (need to assess risk/benefit ratio)
> - Anticoagulant and antiplatelet therapies
> - Scarring at the injection site
> - Difficult visualization of target structures
> - Length of surgery (>120')

COMPLICATIONS AND CONTRAINDICATIONS

The possible complications which can arise when blocking the border nerves are mainly due to the use of blind technique based only on anatomical landmarks. At present, the complications of the IH and II nerve blocks have become rather rare in expert hands thanks to the introduction of ultrasound-guided technique.

The more frequent complications reported in the literature include iatrogenic intravascular injection, bowel perforation, and bleeding with formation of hematomas or ecchymosis (which are more likely to occur in patients affected by coagulation disorders or taking anticoagulant therapy. Other possible adverse events include temporary femoral nerve palsy, urinary retention, and infections. As to the complications related to the GF nerve block, these include infections, ecchymosis, and hematomas. Finally, it is also important to remember the possible occurrence of Local Anesthetic Systemic Toxicity (LAST) often due to reabsorption of the large volumes of LA used, and the block failure resulting from a wrong technical execution. The ultrasound assessment of the LA distribution after performing the block of the IH and II nerves with blind technique has shown that LA is injected around the target nerve structures only in 14% of the cases, with a failure rate block of 45% in terms of lost intra- and postoperative analgesia (**Figure 8.12**). Ultrasound guidance provides an excellent imaging technique through a direct visualization of the anatomical structures involved, improving the success rate and reducing complication risks compared to the standard techniques. Ultrasound-guided nerve block has been validated in a cadaver study with 95% accuracy in localizing target nerves.

The absolute contraindications related to these LRA techniques are extremely limited and basically include patient's refusal, documented allergy to the LA, and infective processes localized to the injection site and/or with a systemic diffusion.

Relative contraindications, instead, include high BMI and the presence of surgical scars involving the anatomical area of the block which can negatively affect the correct identification of the target structures.

> **Complications**
> - Bowel perforation
> - Hematomas or ecchymoses
> - Local or systemic infections
> - Temporary femoral nerve palsy
> - Urinary retention
> - Accidental intravascular injection
> - Local anesthetic systemic toxicity (LAST)
> - Block failure

APPLICATIONS IN THE PEDIATRIC SETTING

The indication of the IH and II nerve blocks in pediatric patients includes the intra- and postoperative analgesia for inguinal canal surgery: inguinal hernia, hydrocele (the first-choice technique in these cases), and cryptorchidism. In pediatric patients, it is import-

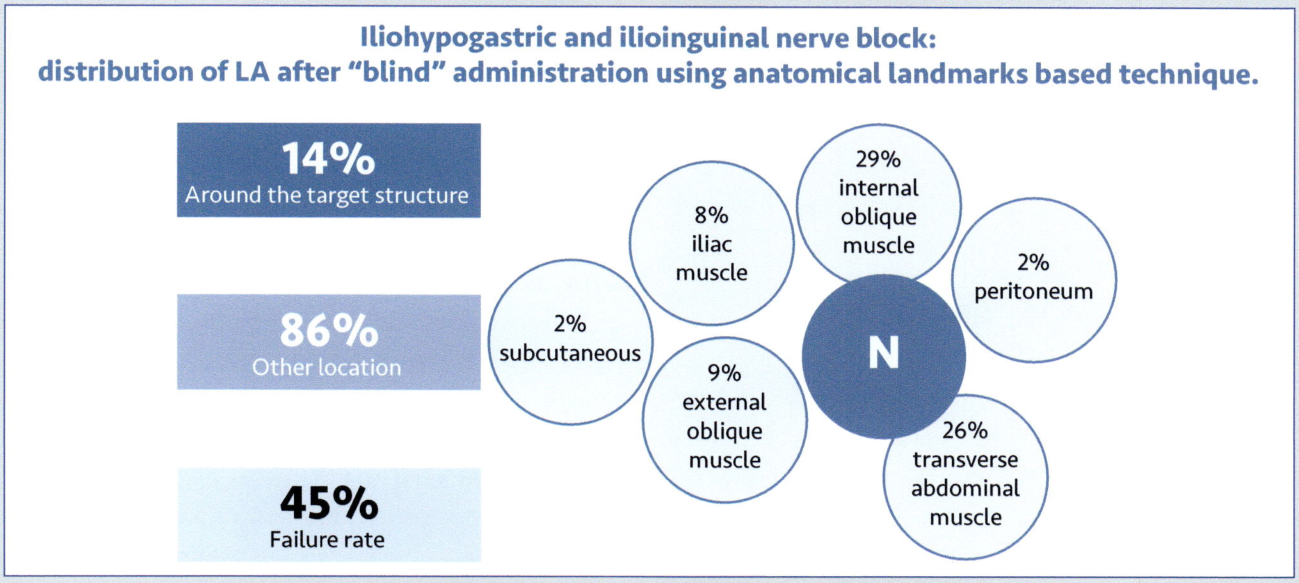

Figure 8.12 Iliohypogastric and ilioinguinal nerve block: distribution of LA after "blind" administration using anatomical landmarks.

ant to perform the block always after the induction of a light general anesthesia or a deep sedation. As this is a wall block, in the first two cases it has a similar efficacy to caudal anesthesia; in the case of cryptorchidism, it surely has a lower efficacy, because the testicle is an organ with a complex visceral innervation related to the mid-thoracic metamers, and the scrotum has a variable innervation partially dependent on the II nerve. During inguinal canal surgery, surgical manipulations of the deep structures (testicle, peritoneum, omentum) are not covered by this block and, therefore, an in-depth of both anesthetic or sedation plan related (to the peripheral block) might be needed. When this can be predicted (for example, newborns with incarcerated hernia), caudal anesthesia can guarantee a better performance. A comparison between the TAP block and the blocks of the IH and II nerves, in the inguinal canal surgery, has instead rewarded the latter, especially for the extent of the postoperative analgesia. The ultrasound-guided IH and II nerve blocks in pediatric patients can be performed with the "in-plane" technique and with a direction that is both medial and lateral (more comfortable in infants). In pediatric patients, these nerves are superficial: therefore, the needle must be inserted as close as possible to the ultrasound probe and must run nearly parallel to it. The LA injection around the two nerves should cause the separation within the fascia of IOM and TAM, similarly to the TAP block.

To date, there are no precise evidence-based recommendations related to the LA doses and concentrations or the adjuvants to be used in pediatric patients undergoing LRA. Therefore, it is necessary to take into consideration the fact that pediatric patients have a little known pharmacokinetics of the LA used and their plasma absorption LA is higher, with resulting increased risk of LAST. Generally, 0.1-0.3 ml/kg of LA (but also 0.075 ml/kg, according to some authors) is enough to block the two nerves, and this allows to perform the block bilaterally, remaining at the same time far from toxic dosages (0.25-0.375% levobupivacaine or 0.25-0.375% ropivacaine can be used, reserving higher concentrations for older children). If the block is correctly performed, the onset time is short (5 minutes). The most recent recommendations from the European Society of Regional Anaesthesia and Pain Therapy (ESRA) and the American Society of Regional Anesthesia and Pain Medicine (ASRA) suggest that ultrasound-guided fascial plane blocks in pediatric patients can be performed in the clinical practice with a high rate of success and safety by using the recommended doses of bupivacaine or ropivacaine that go from 0.25 to 0.75 mg/kg (Evidence B1). However, when an ultrasound-guided bilateral block is performed in pediatric patients, a volume of 0.15 ml/kg for each side is adequate to achieve effective analgesia.

INDICATION OF CHRONIC PAIN

Most of the patients affected by chronic pain have a previous history of surgery. The incidence of debilitating chronic inguinal pain following abdominal surgery varies from 0.5% to 6%. As they have a relatively superficial course, the border nerves are at risk of iatrogenic lesions during lower abdominal surgery such as open appendectomy, inguinal herniorrhaphy, cesarean section or hysterectomy (low Pfannenstiel incision) or after trocar insertion during laparoscopic or robotic surgeries. The resulting nervous injury can facilitate the onset of a chronic painful symptomatology in the anatomical site involved.

In a small percentage of patients the onset of chronic pain may be related to previous trauma, which can manifest itself with two characteristic patterns. The early presentation is self-explanatory, while the late one may be due to reduced mobility of the nerves, which are used to glide between muscle and fascia planes with movement. With scarring, the mobility decreases which contributes to microtrauma of the nerves.

Although the exact etiology of this pain has not been still fully understood, it is possible that it might have an important neuropathic component (allodynia, hyperalgesia). The patients frequently report a burning pain, described as an intense and continuous burning, associated with a sensation similar to paresthesias at the level of the inguinal region and with irradiation to the hemiscrotum, upper leg, and back.

Specifically, the involvement of the IH or II nerves causes pain in the lower abdominal wall which sometimes radiates to the genital area. The diagnosis remains primarily clinical because there is no pathognomonic imaging, laboratory and electrophysiology investigation for inguinal neuralgia. So, it is important for the clinician to differentiate this from the visceral pain that is deep seated and poorly localized. Sensory change with objective signs is sometimes present. Other physical signs include a discrete tender spot, abnormal pain sensitivity (allodynia and hyperalgesia), and Tinel's sign.

GF neuralgia is a common cause of abdominopelvic pain. It may be caused by blunt trauma, compression along the course of the nerve, lower abdominal, groin, or pelvic surgery and injury to nerve following hernia repair especially laparoscopic surgery (12-43%) or spontaneous. GF neuralgia can be a debilitating condition and is difficult to treat due to anatomical variability and difficulty identifying the nerve reliably. Diagnosis is mainly clinical based on the history and the dermatomal distribution of pain, which is mainly neuropathic in nature. There is overlap between the dermatomal supply of the II and GF nerves, thus it should be considered when GF nerve pathology is suspected. When the GF nerve is involved, the patients usually report burning, paresthesia, or numbness in the lower abdomen radiating to medial thigh with extension to the labia majora in women and the anterior surface of the scrotum or testicle in men; the cremasteric reflex might be absent. The pain is frequently episodic and is exacerbated by deambulation or seated position, with important psychological and quality of life repercussions. Patients tend to hold a "novice skier's" position to relieve the strain on the nerves. Spinal extension tends to exacerbate the pain. Physical examination reveals cutaneous neuropathic sensory changes and Tinel's sign may be present on tapping along the inguinal ligament.

The first pharmacological option choice includes the use of drugs active on neuropathic pain (gabapentin, pregabalin), tricyclic antidepressants, and opiates. However, the considerable individual anatomical variability of the sensory innervation and patients' reported symptoms make diagnostic classification difficult and refractory to standard therapies. Unfortunately, as suggested by the recent literature, the persistence of the painful symptoms over time can trigger a cascade of neuronal biochemical changes (central sensitization) capable of leading to the development of a "pain memory" and promoting its chronicization.

In the light of this evidence, an interventional approach is frequently needed in the treatment of these conditions. A selective block of the nerves involved can be useful not just in the treatment of the algic symptomatology, but especially for diagnostic purposes, because it can guide the clinician in the comprehension of the chronic inguinal pain etiology. This block serve both diagnostic and therapeutic roles. In particular, the blocks of the IH, II, and GF nerves play a key role as diagnostic tool to distinguish between neuropathies and radiculopathies and, in the case of success, they can be therapeutically used in chronic inguinal pain management.

In these cases, the patient usually undergoes a diagnostic block with LA/steroids and, in a subsequent phase and if a temporary benefit is reported, approaches prolonging this benefit (such as radiofrequency and ablative techniques) can be taken into consideration. If the patient responds well to the analgesic injection with effects lasting for a few weeks, it is worthwhile to repeat the injections. Because of the potential systemic effects of steroids, it is prudent to avoid frequent repeated injections. The alternative options are pulsed radiofrequency, surgical nerve exploration and release (triple neurectomy), or implantation of peripheral nerve stimulator.

In the related literature, several case reports have documented the clinical efficacy of both ultrasound-guided blocks of the IH, II, and GF nerves and pulsed radiofrequency in the treatment of the severe chronic forms of inguinodynia and orchialgia, and this is for both diagnostic and therapeutic purposes. Further studies and clinical trials are needed to consolidate the scientific evidence supporting the efficacy and safety of these LRA techniques, both from an anesthesiological and a "modern" management of acute and chronic pain point of view.

RECOMMENDED READING

- Abrahams M, Derby R, Horn JL. Update on ultrasound for truncal blocks: a review of the evidence. Reg Anesth Pain Med. 2016; 41:275-88.
- Alfieri S, Amid PK, Campanelli G, et al. International guidelines for prevention and management of postoperative chronic pain following inguinal hernia surgery. Hernia. 2011;15(3):239-49.
- Bischoff J, Koscielniak-Nielsen Z, Kehlet H, Werner M. Ultrasound-guided ilioinguinal/iliohypogastric nerve blocks for persistent inguinal postherniorrhaphy pain. Anesth Analg. 2012;114 (6):1323-9.
- Campos NA, Chiles JH, Plunkett AR. Ultrasound-guided cryoablation of genitofemoral nerve for chronic inguinal pain. Pain Physician. 2009;12(6):997-1000.
- Eichenberger U, Greher M, Kirchmair L, Curatolo M, Moriggl B. Ultrasound-guided blocks of the ilioinguinal and iliohypogastric nerve: accuracy of a selective new technique confirmed by anatomical dissection. Br J Anaesth. 2006;97(2):238-43.
- Fusco P, Marinangeli F. Blocchi nervosi ecoguidati del tronco e della parete addominale. Edra Milano, 2016.
- Hadzic A. Hadzic's Textbook of Regional Anesthesia and Acute Pain Management, Second Edition. Mc Graw Hill. Copyright 2017.
- Jankovic D, Peng P. Regional Nerve Blocks in Anesthesia and Pain Therapy. Traditional and Ultrasound-Guided Techniques. Fourth Edition. Springer International Publishing Switzerland, 2015.
- Peng PW. Ilioinguinal, iliohypogastric and genitofemoral nerve. In: Peng PW, editor. Ultrasound for pain medicine intervention: a practical guide, vol 2. Pelvic pain. Philip Peng educational series. 1st ed. iBook, California, CA: Apple Inc.; 2013. p. 16-23.
- Peng PW, Tumber PS. Ultrasound-guided interventional procedures for patients with chronic pelvic pain - a description of techniques and review of literature. Pain Physician. 2008;11(2):215-24.
- Reinpold W, Schroeder AD, Schroeder M, Berger C, Rohr M, Wehrenberg U. Retroperitoneal anatomy of the iliohypogastric, ilioinguinal, genitofemoral, and lateral femoral cutaneous nerve: consequences for prevention and treatment of chronic inguinodynia. Hernia. 2015;19:539-48.
- Sasaoka N, Kawaguchi M, Yoshitani K, Kato H, Suzuki A, Furuya H. Evaluation of Genitofemoral Nerve Block, in Addition to Ilioinguinal and Iliohypogastric Nerve Block, during Inguinal Hernia Repair in Children. British Journal of Anaesthesia. 2005; Vol. 94, No. 2:243-6.
- Shanthanna H. Successful treatment of genitofemoral neuralgia using ultrasound-guided injection: a case report and short review of literature. Case Rep Anesthesiol. 2014;2014:371703.
- Steffel L, Kim TE, Howard SK, et al. Comparative Effectiveness of Two Ultrasound-Guided Regional Block Techniques for Surgical Anesthesia in Open Unilateral Inguinal Hernia Repair. J Ultrasound Med.2016 Jan;35(1):177-82.
- Suresh S, Ecoffey C, Bosenberg A, Lonnqvist P, de Oliveira Jr GS, de Leon Casasola O, de Andrés J, Ivani G. The European Society of Regional Anaesthesia and Pain Therapy/American Society of Regional Anesthesia and Pain Medicine Recommendations on Local Anesthetics and Adjuvants Dosage in Pediatric Regional Anesthesia. Reg Anesth Pain Med. 2018;43:211-6.
- Terkawi AS, Romdhane K. Ultrasound-guided pulsed radiofrequency ablation of the genital branch of the genitofemoral nerve for treatment of intractable orchalgia. Saudi J Anaesth. 2014;8(2):294-8.
- Thomassen I, van Suijlekom JA, van de Gaag A, Ponten JE, Nienhuijs SW. Ultrasound-guided ilioinguinal/iliohypogastric nerve blocks for chronic pain after inguinal hernia repair. Hernia J Hernias Abdom Wall Surg. 2013;17(3):329-32.
- Van Schoor AN, Boon JM, Bosemberg AT, et al. Anatomical considerations of the pediatric ilioinguinal/iliohypogastric nerve block. Paediatr Anaesth. 2005;15(5):371-7.

- Weintraud M, Lundblad M, Kettner SC, et al. Ultrasound versus landmark-based technique for ilioinguinal-iliohypogastric nerve blockade in children: the implications on plasma levels of ropivacaine. Anesth Analg. 2009;108(5):1488-92.
- Weintraud M, Marhofer P, Bösenberg A, et al. Ilioinguinal/il- iohypogastric blocks in children: where do we administer the local anesthetic without direct visualization? Anesth Analg. 2008;106(1):89-93.
- Abiy S, Ayalew N, Eshete A et al. Comparison of bilateral ilioinguinal-iliohypogastric nerve block versus transversus abdominis nerve block for postoperative pain management for parturient undergoing elective cesarean section in Dilla University Referral Hospital, Ethiopia. A randomized controlled trial. Int J Surg Open. 2020;26:22-29
- Coppens S, Gidts J, Huynen P, Van de Velle M, Joshi GP on behalf of the PROSPECT Working Group collaboration. Pain management after open inguinal hernia repair. An updated systematic review and procedure-specific postoperative pain management (PROSPECT/ESRA) recommendations. Acta Anaesthesiologica Belgica.2020;71:45-56
- Kacmaz M, Bolat H. Comparison of spinal anaesthesia versus ilioinguinal-iliohypogastric nerve block applied with tumescent anaesthesia for single side inguinal hernia. Hernia. 2020;24:1049-1056. Doi: 10.1007/s10029-020-02163-0
- Kunihisa Hotta. Regional anesthesia in the time of COVID-19: a minireview. J Anesth.2021 Jun;35(3):341-344. doi: 10.1007/s00540-020-02834-3. Epub 2020 Jul 25
- Torrano V, Cappelleri G, Russo G, Fusco PF, Behr A, Monzani R, Tritapepe L. SIAARTI BPC per gli anestesisti. Raccomandazioni per l'utilizzo dell'anestesia locoregionale (ALR) nel paziente chirurgico Covid-19. 07/05/2020. https://www.siaarti.it/news

CLINICAL CASE 1 – THE ASSOCIATION OF ULTRASOUND (US)-GUIDED ILIOINGUINAL (II)/ILIOHYPOGASTRIC (IH) NERVE BLOCKS AND GENITOFEMORAL (GF) NERVE BLOCK AS ANESTHETIC TECHNIQUE FOR INGUINAL HERNIORRAPHY

Clinical history and anamnesis We reported the use of US-guided II/IH and GF nerve block in a 70-year-old man, ASA 3, who was scheduled for elective inguinal hernia repair. His medical history included moderate aortic stenosis and severe pulmonary fibrosis.

Materials and methods Written informed consent was obtained. After sedo-analgesia with sufentanyl 5 μg and midazolam 2 mg, patient received US-guided II/IH nerve blocks as sole anesthetic technique. GF nerve block was also associated for reducing pain and attenuating hemodynamic responses at the sac traction.

Technique description For II/IH nerve block, a linear probe was placed in oblique fashion at the line joining the umbilicus and the ASIS (**Figure 8.13**). In asepsis a 22 G 90 mm echogenic needle (SonoPlex stim Pajunk®) was inserterd from medial to lateral direction and Levobupivacaine 0.5% 20 ml was injected to open the fascial plane between transverse abdominis and internal oblique muscles, adjacent to the deep circumflex iliac artery (**Figure 8.14**). Then, the probe was placed parallel and 1.25 cm above the inguinal ligament, at the level of the internal inguinal ring. After Color doppler assessment, genital branch of GF nerve block was performed by injecting Levobupivacaine 0.5% 5 ml was injected medially to external iliac artery inside the inguinal canal. Intraoperative sedation with easy arousability was ensured using intravenously propofol infusion (3 mg/kg/h). Oxygen (4 l/min) was supplemented by Venturi mask and end tidal CO_2 was monitored. A reliable anesthesia of the inguinal area maintaining hemodynamic stability was obtained. Scheduled postoperative analgesia was acetaminophen 1 g every 8 h, with rescue dose of ketorolac 30 mg. Patient reported a good quality postoperative analgesia (NRS <3) and no complications were recorded.

Conclusions Inguinal herniorraphy is one of the most frequent operations performed and the high incidence of chronic postsurgical pain often affects the quality of life of patients. The inguinal area receives highly variable sensory innervation from II and IH nerves with a contribution of the genital branch of GF nerve which may be also involved in nociceptive afferent inputs during inguinal hernia repair. Our experience suggested this anesthetic technique, as part of a multimodal analgesic regimen, could represent a viable alternative to general and neuraxial anesthesia for inguinal hernia repair in day surgery, avoiding hypotension due to sympathetic block that may be dangerous in high risk patient with low cardiac reserve.

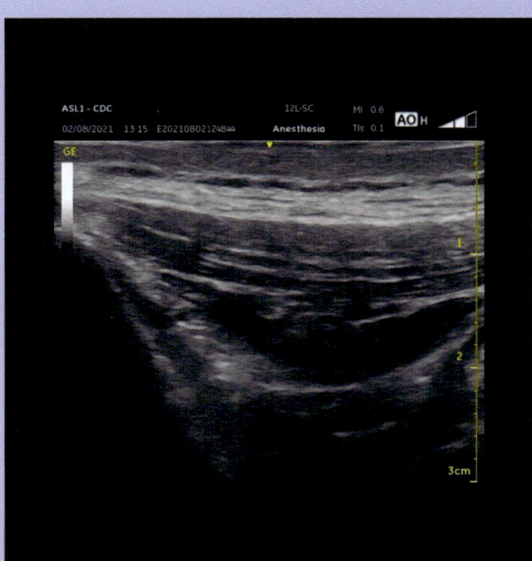

Figure 8.13 Essential sonoanatomy for II/IH nerve blocks.

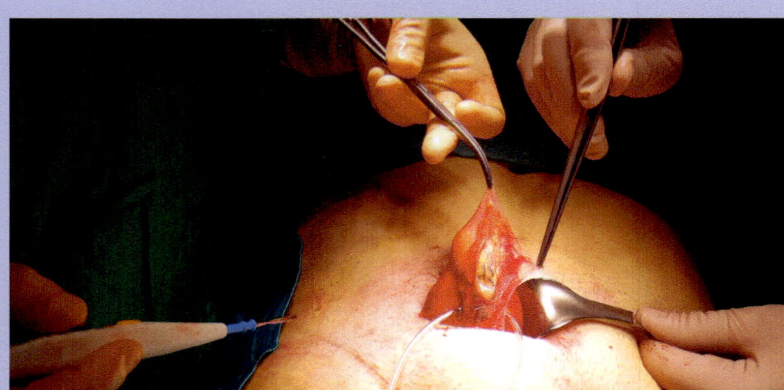

Figure 8.14 Surgeons performing inguinal hernia repair.

CLINICAL CASE 2 – ULTRASOUND (US)-GUIDED ILIOINGUINAL (II)/ ILIOHYPOGASTRIC (IH) NERVE BLOCK ASSOCIATED TO AWAKE SEDATION FOR ANESTHESIA IN INGUINAL HERNIOPLASTY

Clinical history and anamnesis We reported the use of US-guided II/IH in a 60-year-old patient, ASA 2, who presented to the emergency room for a pain in the right groin with no-reducible swelling. From the objective examination and instrumental examinations, it is a strangulate inguinal hernia with indication for surgery. This a male suffering from permanent atrial fibrillation being treated with clopidogrel 75 mg/die. The patient had lunch 2 hours earlier.

Materials and methods Written informed consent was obtained. US-guided II/IH nerve block with sedo-analgesia was proposed to the patient because he had a contraindication to subarachnoid anesthesia due to the intake of clopidogrel, the patient had a full stomach.

Technique description The puncture area and ultrasound probe (linear transducer 5-15 MHz) were prepared in a sterile manner. The inguinal region was scanned with the probe indicator resting on the ASIS in the direction of the umbilicus and II and IH nerves were visualized between the internal oblique and transversal muscles, immediately adjacent. The puncture was performed with a 22 G 90 mm echogenic needle (SonoPlex stim Pajunk®) using "in plane approach" and administering 10 ml of 0,75% ropivacaine with sufficient spread (**Figure 8.15 A**, **B**). Sedation was performed only with Fentanyl 0.05 μg and midazolam 0.03 mg/kg IV. Surgery was completed in 35 min, the patient never complained of pain. Acetaminophen 1 gr IV was administered at the end of surgery and then every 8 hours. Postoperative pain was assessed using the NRS pain scale at time o and at 2, 6, 12 and 24 hours after surgery. Ketorolac 30 mg, prescribed as rescue analgesic, was never required. Pain never exceed 1 on the NRS pain scale. No postoperative nausea and vomiting or femoral nerve block were recorded. The patient was discharged from the hospital after 36 h.

Conclusions US-guided II/IH nerve block could be considered a valid LRA technique for inguinal hernioplasty, especially in high risk patients. This approach provides excellent postoperative pain control reducing additional analgesic consumption with shorter recovery time after surgery.

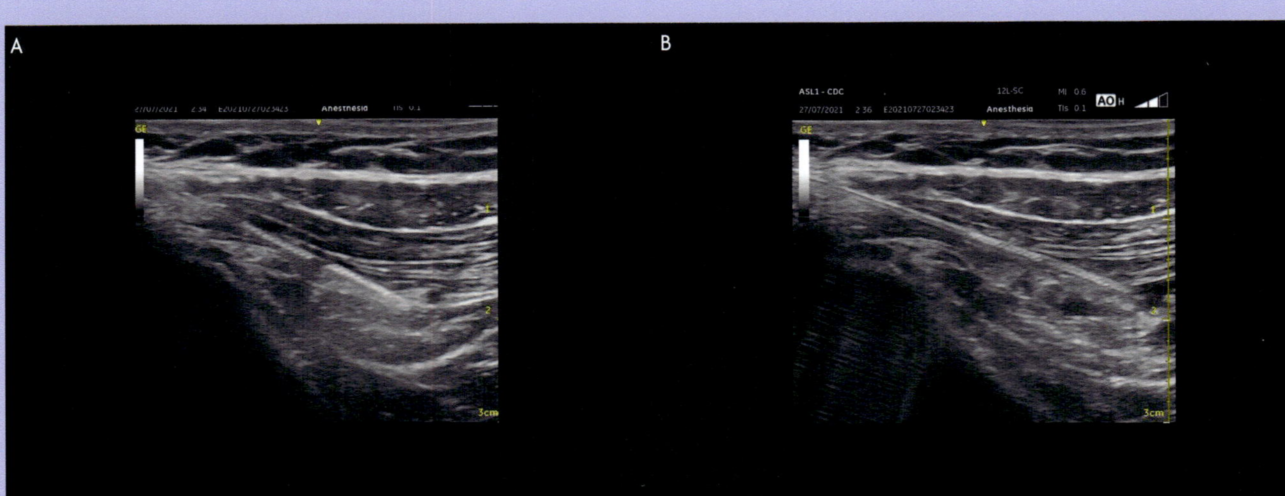

Figure 8.15 A US-guided II/IH nerve block. **B** Ultrasound visualization of the spread of the anesthetic injected in the target fascial plane.

Rectus sheath block

Gianluca Russo, Vito Torrano, Giuseppe Gazzerro, Gilda Tornatore

The rectus sheath block, or blockade of the posterior fascia of the rectus muscle, provides a good analgesia in the median region of the abdominal wall, from the terminal branches of T7 to T11, and it is a useful technique for surgery requiring the incision on the midline (**Figure 9.1**).

This technique was first described by Schleich in 1899 and used to ensure a good myoresolution of the anterior abdominal wall in major surgery.

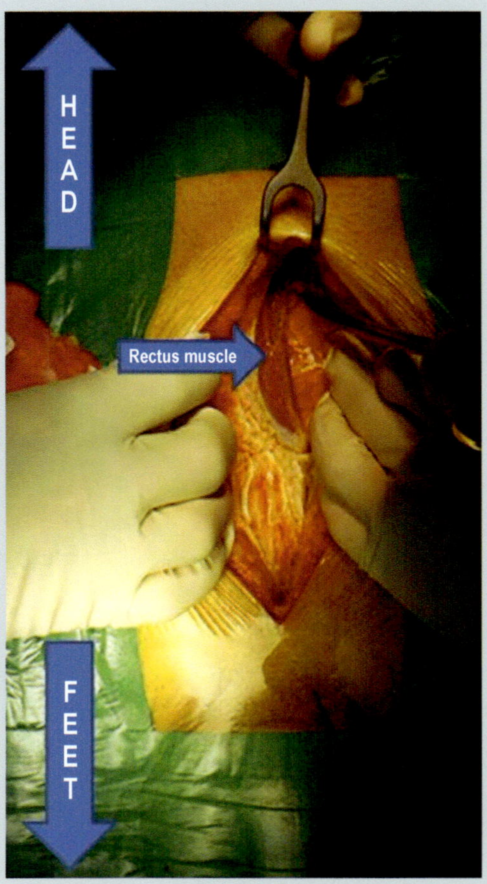

Figure 9.1 Median laparotomy incision: the right rectus abdominis muscle fascia is visible.

In 1996, Ferguson introduced the use of the blockade of the rectus abdominis muscle fascia for perioperative analgesia for umbilical hernioplasty in pediatric patients. Since then, this anesthesiological technique has started to be increasingly widespread and used to provide analgesia in different types of surgical procedures, such as umbilical hernioplasties, epigastric hernioplasties, pylorus myotomies, laparoscopic surgery and other small surgical incisions of the midline.

Traditionally, the rectus sheath block is a blind technique relying on the loss of resistance perceived as the needle tip passes through the rectus abdominis fascia and the muscle plane.

Local anesthetic injection into the posterior sheath of the rectus abdominis muscle ensures a specific and predictable somatic anesthesia of the anterior wall of the abdomen, adequate for umbilical surgery or for procedures in the surface area around the umbilicus. Suprapubic surgical incisions, conversely, require the addition of ilioinguinal or transversus abdominis plane blockade.

For major surgery involving the peritoneum and the viscera, multimodal pain management or the use of peridural analgesia should be considered.

The transversus abdominis plane (TAP block) is a validated technique used for anterolateral abdominal wall analgesia. The TAP block is performed laterally on the abdomen and the local anesthetic is injected between the internal oblique muscle and the transverse muscle. The spread of the sensory block of the TAP block differs from that of the rectus sheath block; in fact, the blockade of the rectus abdominis muscle provides a sensory block of the entire central region of the abdomen (**Figure 9.2**), whereas the TAP block ensures a wider sensory blockade with a lower cranial extension. Compared to the TAP block, the single shot blockade

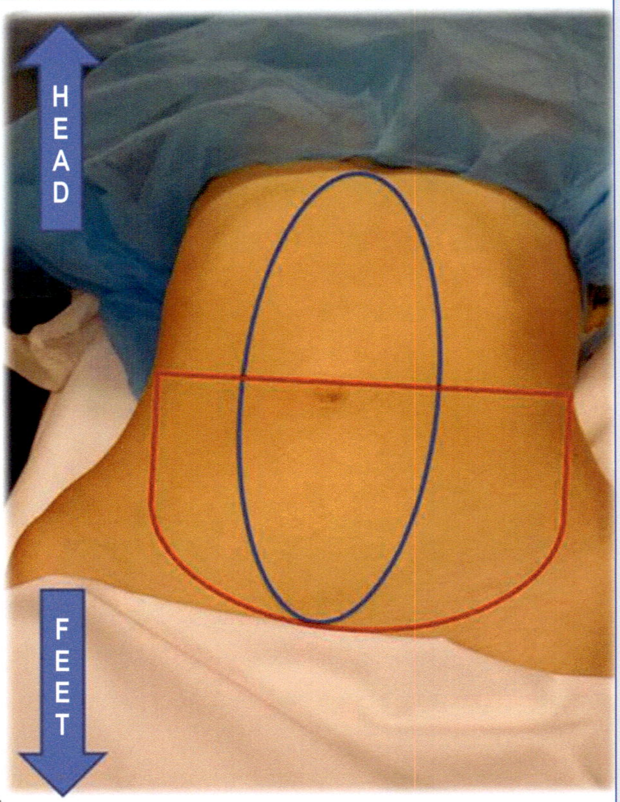

Figure 9.2 Comparison between the sensory block obtained with the bilateral rectus sheath block (blue area) and the sensory block obtained with the bilateral block of the transversus abdominis plane (red area).

of the posterior fascia of the rectus muscle ensures a better, but shorter in duration, analgesic coverage. In order to extend the block duration, two catheters should be placed, one on each side, to obtain a continuous or scheduled bolus infusion of local anesthetic in the post-operative period. On the other hand, a single injection of anesthetic into the transversus abdominis plane shows to be effective in achieving a reduction in pain intensity and opiate consumption for several days in the postoperative period, and it is therefore preferable if a single injection of local anesthetic is performed. Therefore, the rectus muscle fascia block should only be used for postoperative analgesia of median laparotomy if the procedure includes the placing of two catheters required for continuous infusion of local anesthetic in the posterior rectus sheath.

Positioning a peripheral nerve catheter may have several benefits over the placement of an epidural-catheter. First of all, the block of the rectus sheath is not associated with the sympathetic block typically caused by neuraxial blocks, thus avoiding the hemodynamic modifications commonly seen with this type of blocks.

In addition, unlike in neuroaxial blocks, the blockade of the rectus muscle fascia is a better option in patients with coagulopathies or receiving any antiaggregation or anticoagulation. The continuous block of the rectus sheath also permits an early mobilization. In fact, while ensuring a good postoperative analgesia, it preserves the mobility and strength of the lower limbs, allowing a rapid mobilization in the immediate postoperative period. This may have many clinical benefits, such as a reduction of the incidence of deep vein thrombosis, pulmonary embolism, atelectasias and pulmonary infections, ultimately leading to a faster recovery.

The placement of a catheter for the continuous block of the rectus sheath can be performed safely during general anesthesia, thus avoiding the anxiety and stress that sometimes accompany the positioning of the epidural catheter while the patient is awake. This could increase the degree of acceptance and satisfaction.

The introduction and spreading of ultrasonography use in locoregional anesthesia in general, and in this technique especially, have allowed anesthesiologists to evaluate in real time the correct positioning of the needle in the desired position and the spread of the local anesthetic. Ultrasonography enables to view and evaluate the anatomical structures related to the block to be performed, the needle during the procedure, and the spread of the local anesthetic.

The benefits of ultrasound-guided anesthesia blocks compared to 'blind' techniques based on tactile perception, even performed by experienced anesthesiologists, have now been recognized by the scientific literature.

Therefore, the ultrasound-guided block of the rectus sheath offers significant benefits, such as providing a clear image of the structures with a non-invasive method, facilitating the correct positioning of the needle tip, and allowing the direct observation of the spread of the local anesthetic within the desired plane. A recent systematic review of the literature on ultrasound-guided blocks recommends the use of the ultrasound guide for the execution of the rectus sheath block in order to increase the success rate. Although we still lack of statistical evidence that the ultrasound-guided block is safer than the blind technique, the visualization of the anatomical structures and of the entire length of the needle should reduce the incidence of punctures of peritoneum, bowel loops or vessels.

ANATOMY AND SONOANATOMY

The abdominal wall consists of three layers: an internal peritoneal layer, an intermediate muscular layer, and an external cutaneous layer. In its lateral portion, three muscles overlap to contribute to its strengthening: the external oblique muscle, the internal oblique muscle, and the transverse abdominal muscle.

Conversely, in the median area, the muscle is unique, solid and it is contained in the rectus sheath: the rectus abdominis muscle. The rectus muscle runs vertically to form the anterior abdominal wall and has the shape of a large tape located on each side of the midline. The belly of the muscle has four transverse tendon inscriptions, that commonly do not affect the entire thickness of the muscle, but are firmly attached to the anterior leaflet of the sheath. The rectus muscle runs vertically to form the anterior abdominal wall and has the shape of a large tape located on each side of the midline. It originates with a large tendon from the pubic symphysis, from the tubercle and from the iliac crest and moving upwards it is fixed in a median position to the xiphoid process and laterally to the cartilagine of the V-VI-VII ribs.

The rectus sheath is formed by the aponeuroses of the oblique external, oblique internal and transverse muscles. An anterior and a posterior wall are distinguished in the sheath, or fascia. The aponeurosis of the external oblique muscle passes in front of the rectus muscle, from the xiphoid process to the pubis, and then reaches the midline where its fascia cross the contralateral fascia at the linea alba, thus contributing to form the anterior wall of the sheath.

The aponeurosis of the internal oblique muscle is divided into two laminae at the lateral edge of the rectus muscle. One passes in front of the muscle and joins the aponeurosis of the external oblique muscle, forming the front wall of the sheath with it; the other one passes behind the muscle, taking part to the constitution of the posterior wall of the sheath.

This bilaminar device of the aponeurosis of the internal oblique muscle is observed only in the upper three fifths of the rectus muscle; in its lower part, the entire aponeurosisis in front of the muscle. The aponeurosis of the transverse muscle passes, in the upper three-fifths, behind the rectus muscle and joins the posterior lamina of the aponeurosis of the internal oblique muscle, forming the posterior wall of the sheath; in the lower two-fifths of the muscle, it passes, instead, in front of the rectus muscle and joins the aponeurosis of the internal and external oblique muscles, as a part of the anterior wall of the sheath.

Hence, at the boundary between the upper three-fifths and the lower two-fifths of the muscle, the posterior sheath of the rectus muscle changes its constitution: above this level, it consists of the posterior layer of the aponeurosis of the internal oblique muscle and by the aponeurosis of the transverse muscle, while below it consists of the sole transversalis fascia, since the previous formations pass to the front side of the muscle (**Figure 9.3**). The arcuate or semicircular line of Douglas demarcates the lower limit of the posterior layer of the rectus sheath.

The rectus abdominis muscle is mainly supplied by the superior and inferior epigastric arteries. The superior epigastric artery is a terminal branch of the internal thoracic artery, while the inferior epigastric arterie, is a branch of the external iliac artery. The superior epigastric artery penetrates the thickness of the rectus abdominis muscle and anastomoses with the inferior epigastric artery at the level of the Douglas line arcuate.

The innervation of the anterolateral wall of the abdomen originates from the anterior cutaneous branches of the spinal nerves T7 to L1. The nerve terminations

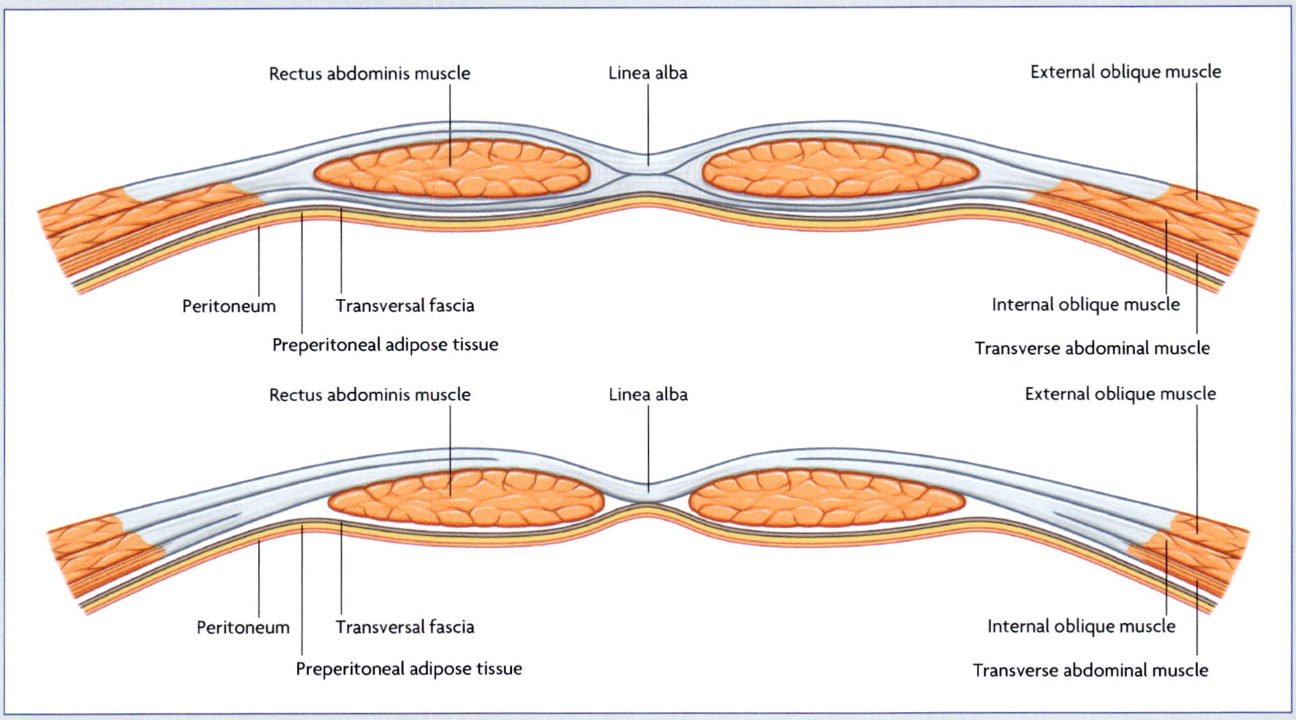

Figure 9.3 Formation of the rectus muscle fascia above and below the arcuate line.

of the anterior branches include the intercostal nerves (T7-T11), the subcostal nerve (T12), and the ilioinguinal and iliohypogastric nerves (L1).

The intercostal nerves T7 to T11 come out of the intercostal space and branch out into the neurovascular plane, between the internal oblique muscle and the transverse abdominal muscle.

The subcostal nerve (T12) and the ilioinguinal and iliohypogastric nerves also branch out into the plane between the internal oblique muscle and the transverse abdominis muscle, and provide innervation of these muscles. Nerves T7-T12 continue anteriorly from the transverse muscle plane to pierce the rectus muscle fascia and end as cutaneous nerves. The intercostal nerves originating from spinal nerves T7-T11 generally run, in their course toward the abdominal wall, which they innervate, between the posterior wall of the rectus muscle and the posterior rectus sheath.

Nerves T7-T11 provide the sensory innervation of the rectus muscles and the overlying cutaneous region. Nerve T7 provides the sensory innervation of the epigastric region, while nerve T10 innervates the periumbilical region.

Ultrasonography allows for an easy recognition of the muscular anatomical structures of the anterior wall of the abdomen. With a high-frequency (6-13 MHz) linear probe, it is possible to scan the anterior abdominal wall from the xiphoid apophysis to the pubic symphysis transversally or longitudinally. The rectus muscles will appear as hypoechoic structures (**Figure 9.4**) surrounded by the hyperechoic image of the anterior and posterior sheath above the arcuate line, while posteriorly only the hyperechoic transversalis fascia may be viewed under the arcuate line. Therefore, it is important to identify the rectus abdominis muscle and the double hyperechoic line under the muscle itself (a double line consisting of the posterior wall of the rectus muscle sheath and the transversalis fascia) (**Figure 9.5**). Moving laterally with the probe, the hypoechoic muscle structures of the external oblique muscle, internal oblique

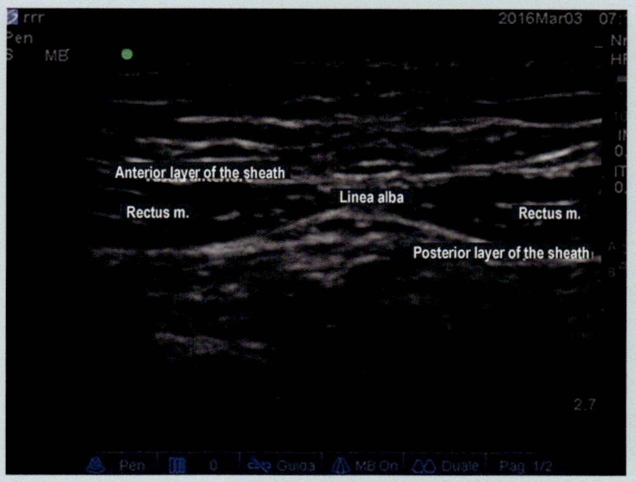

Figure 9.4 Rectus abdominis muscles wrapped in their sheath. The anterior and posterior layers of the sheath converge medially to form the linea alba.

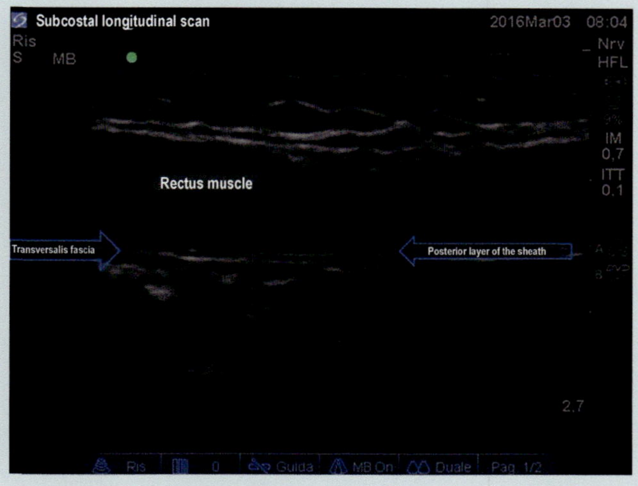

Figure 9.5 Identification of the double hyperechoic line under the rectus muscle, which consists of the posterior layer of the sheath of the rectus muscle and the transversalis fascia.

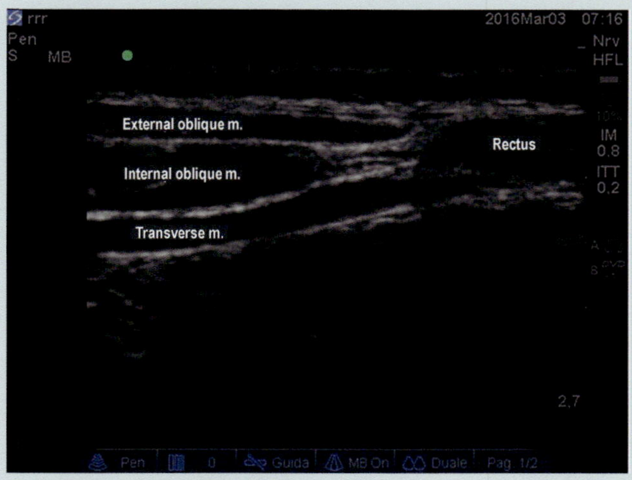

Figure 9.6 Aponeurosis of the external oblique, internal oblique and transverse abdominal muscles, which forms the fascia of the rectus abdominis muscles along the medial line.

muscle and transverse abdominal muscle, with their related hyperechoic muscle fascia, may be recognized. Ultrasonography also shows how the aponeurosis of the external oblique, internal oblique and transverse abdominis muscles medially form the fascia that wraps the rectus abdominis muscles (**Figure 9.6**).

TARGET OF THE BLOCK

Two blind techniques have been described in the past. Both methods aimed to block the terminal branches of the intercostal nerves (7th-11th) within the rectus muscle fascia, but in different manners.

The method described by Courreges consists in injecting one quarter of the LA volume (0.5 ml kg 1) in the subcutaneous tissue and the second quarter after perceiving the passage of the rectus muscle sheath. This double injection was considered to be absolutely necessary by the Author because, in 30% of patients, the cutaneous terminal branches of intercostal nerves T7 to T11 branch out in the subcutaneous tissue before entering the rectus muscle sheath.

Subsequently, Mori and Yap proved that all intercostal nerves, from T7 to T11, penetrate into the rectus muscle sheath at its lateral edge and branch out for at least 5 cm before entering the muscle (only occasionally they enter the rectus muscle immediately after penetrating the lateral margin of its sheath). Ferguson also relied on tactile perception to identify the correct position of the needle as it passed through the tissues (through a "scratching sensations" or "palpable gives") and described a technique consisting of injecting local anesthetic beyond the rectus muscle into the virtual space between the posterior face of the rectus abdominis muscle and its posterior fascia.

However, this technique has not been used in clinical practice, mostly due to doubts regarding the needle tip positioning accuracy, especially relative to the underlying peritoneal structures. The introduction of ultrasonography in the clinical practice of locoregional anesthesia, allowed anesthesiologists to better position the needle tip in the posterior fascia of the rectus muscle and spread the local anesthetic.

The display, upon LA injection, of a hypoechoic, biconvex liquid bag that progressively separates the two planes described, confirms the correct positioning of the needle tip, which can be obtained with an in-plane or an out-of-plane technique.

Unlike the front sheath of the rectus muscle, which has different tendinous insertions, these are not present in the posterior one; this allows the local anesthetic to spread into cephalic and caudal directions within the ipsilateral compartment from a single injection site, thus blocking the anterior branches of thoracic nerves from T7-T11, which provide sensory innervation to the rectus abdominis muscle and the overlying skin.

In conclusion, this anesthesia technique does not allow the nerve structures to be directly viewed, but the local anesthetic is injected under ultrasound guidance into the fascial plane and spreads along that plane around the intercostal nerve terminations. Injections made into the muscle belly cause the blockade to fail.

DESCRIPTION OF THE ULTRASOUND-GUIDED TECHNIQUE

The following equipment is required to perform the block:

- Ultrasound system equipped with a high-frequency linear probe (6-13 MHz);
- Probe cover, not necessarily sterile, for single-shot block;
- Standard cart for locoregional anesthesia;
- Antiseptic agent for skin and glove disinfection, not necessarily sterile, for single-shot block;
- 50 mm, 20-21 G (Sonotap®) TAP block needle;
- 20-40 ml of local anesthetic (levobupivacaine 0.25% or ropivacaine 0.375%).

The block can be performed with the patient awake, seated or anesthetized. Usually, it is performed after induction and intubation, but before surgical incision. The block may also be performed after the end of surgery, before awakening, if the procedure involved the rectus muscle (e.g., to create a stoma or for a paramedian incision). The block may also be used as a "rescue" block performed on awake patients immediately after surgery when pain is not adequately controlled. Patients usually report minimal procedure-related pain.

However, an intravenous cannula must always be correctly positioned before performing the technique. Furthermore, continuous monitoring of vital signs should also be performed during the whole procedure and the necessary medications and devices to deal with any emergency situation due to possible complications, e.g. toxicity of the local anesthetic, must always be available.

The usual methods for ensuring asepsis, especially in procedures performed to position perinervous or perifascial catheters, include dressing with sterile gloves and sterile drapes, as well as the using a face mask and a head cover. The sterile probe cover and the sterile gel are also mandatory during catheter placement for a continuous blockade.

The rectus abdominis muscle fascia may be displayed with the ultrasound probe in a transversal direction laterally to the umbilical region or longitudinally above the umbilical level, always with the patient supine. A linear probe (6-13 MHz) can be used to perform the block, with a depth setting of approximately 2-6 cm depending on the patient size. A 50 mm footprint probe is ideal for abdominal wall blocks, as it allows the operator a better view compared to smaller probes.

The Sonotap® 50 mm, diameter 20-21 G needle is inserted using an in-plane technique, with an angle of less than 45°, lateromedially to the probe positioned transversally in the umbilical region, paying attention to view the entire length of the needle and its tip during the procedure (**Figure 9.7**).

A bolus dose of 10 ml of levobupivacaine 0.25% (or ropivacaine 0.375%) is injected under ultrasound guidance to view its correct positioning and spreading. The ultrasound display allows for the identification of the rectus abdominis muscles and of the double hyperechoic line under the muscle itself (a double line consisting of the posterior sheath of the rectus muscle and the transversalis fascia). Under direct visualization, the needle tip must be advanced to the desired position, behind the rectus muscle and above the underlying muscle sheath (**Figure 9.8**, **Video 9.1**, **9.2**).

The injection of the local anesthetic will hydro-dissect the rectus muscle from the posterior wall of its sheath (**Figure 9.9**).

The block may also be performed with a Tuohy 18 G needle, with a catheter inserted into the space between the posterior face of the rectus muscle and its sheath. For catheter insertion, the use of an in-plane technique is preferred, with the probe positioned longitudinally below the costal margin (**Figures 9.10**, **9.11**). Usually, the catheter is inserted at least 8 cm into the space created between the posterior face of the rectus muscle and its sheath.

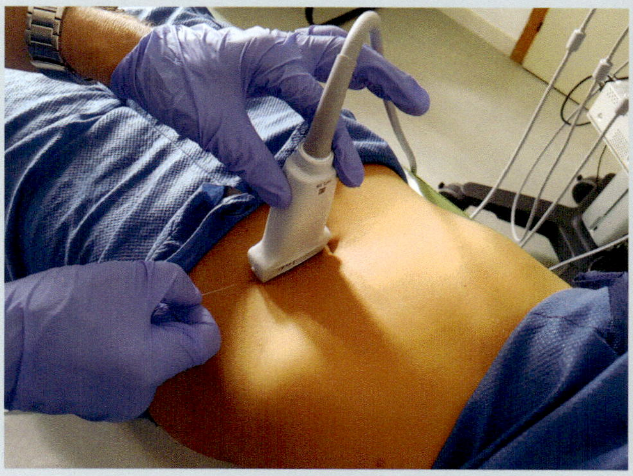

Figure 9.7 In-plane technique with lateromedial needle tip entry and high-frequency linear probe in the paraumbilical transverse position.

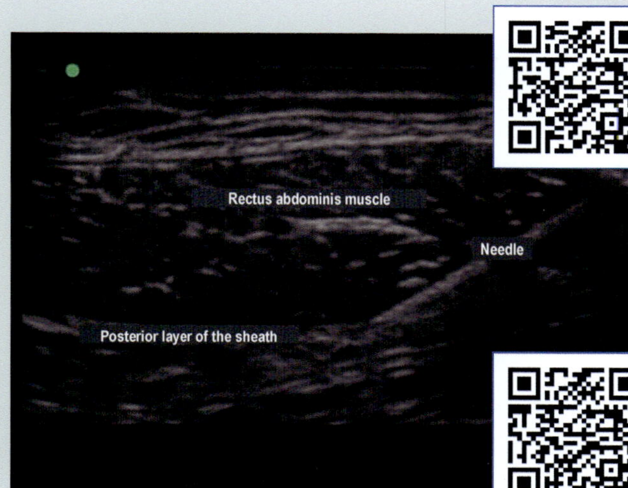

Figure 9.8 The in-plane technique and the lateromedial approach allow to view the needle tip reaching the desired target: the posterior layer of the sheath of the rectus muscle.

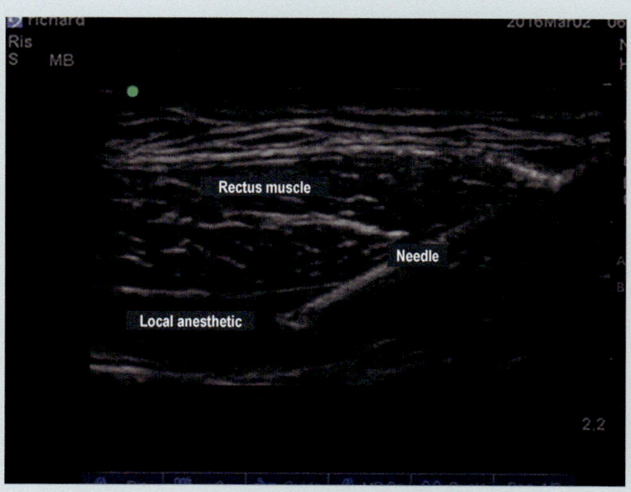

Figure 9.9 The local anesthetic injection separates the rectus muscle from the posterior sheath wall.

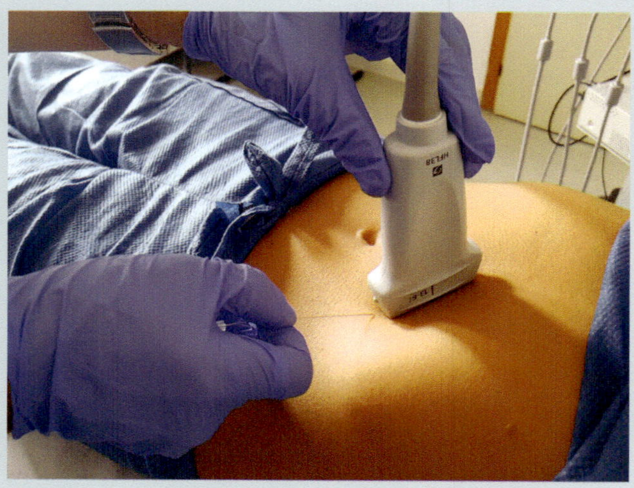

Figure 9.10 In-plane technique with lateromedial direction of the needle tip and high-frequency linear probe in subcostal longitudinal position.

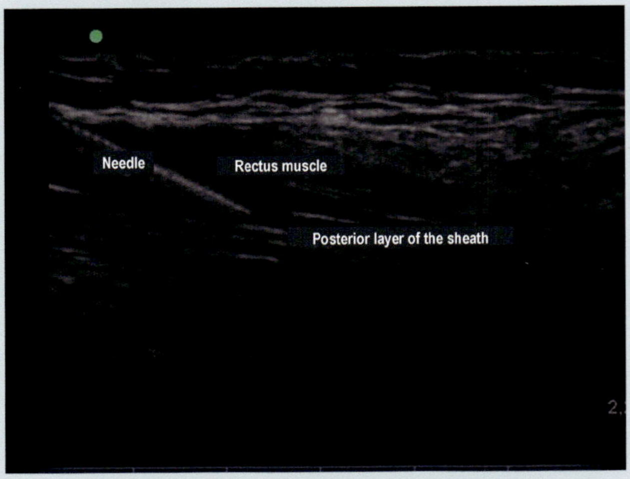

Figure 9.11 In-plane technique and lateromedial needle approach.

Depending on the insertion angle and patient constitution, the catheter depth to the skin may vary between 12 and 15 cm.

With the insertion point just below the costal margin, this measure should ensure that the catheter tip is approximately at umbilical level. The catheter should be fixed in a high and lateral position, in order to not interfere with the surgical field. For median laparotomy incisions, this technique must be repeated on each side to ensure a good complete and bilateral analgesia.

The lateromedial catheter positioning technique performed by using the cannula on the needle (Ecatheter®) was described by Tsui in 2014, but this technique may obviously be used with the probe inserted subcostally and longitudinally, with a cranio-caudal, in-plane insertion of the cannula-needle and subsequently of the catheter. The benefit of this technique is that it can be performed by a single operator, maintaining the entire procedure visualization. A 10 ml bolus of levobupivacaine 0.25% (or ropivacaine 0.375%) can be injected into each of the catheters to ensure the sensory blockade for approximately 6-8 hours. This bolus should therefore be repeated manually or by electronic infusion pumps every 6-8 hours.

CONTINUOUS BLOCK OF THE RECTUS MUSCLE SHEATH

For midline or paramedian incisions extending above the umbilicus, the continuous block of the rectus muscle fascia is recommended.

Surgical incisions along the midline require the placement of a bilateral catheter, while paramedian incisions require the placement of only one catheter in the posterior fascia of the rectus muscle in the same side of the incision.

The surgical insertion of the catheter into the posterior sheath of the rectus muscle was described by Cornish in 2007. Surgically-positioned catheters present the advantage of being positioned under the direct visualization of the rectus abdominis muscle.

The disadvantages of positioning the catheter through the abdominal cavity include the potential contamination and loss of the natural sterility of the rectus muscle compartment (when the passage of the Tuohy needle connects the posterior sheath of the rectus muscle with the peritoneum). In addition, the hole created may cause a leak of local anesthetic into the abdominal cavity, resulting in a loss of effectiveness of the block.

Ultrasound-guided placement across the anterior abdominal wall allows the posterior sheath to remain intact, thus avoiding any leaks of local anesthetic and maintaining the sterility of the rectus abdominis compartment. Positioning the catheters before the surgical incision helps optimizing intraoperative analgesia and minimizing the sympathetic response to the surgical procedure.

For Pfannenstiel incisions or transverse incisions under the umbilicus, the blockade of the transversus abdominis plane (TAP block) is preferable.

For Kocher, incisions or transverse incisions above the umbilicus, the blockade of the transverse subcostal muscle plane also showed good results for postoperative analgesia. If the transverse incision is supra-umbilical and includes the coverage area of both blocks, the two techniques can be performed simultaneously, but with a particular attention not to exceed the maximum dose of local anesthetic (**Flow chart 9.1 online**).

LOCAL ANESTHETIC INDICATIONS AND DOSAGES

The block is performed by injecting 10 ml of a local long-acting anesthetic agent per side.

In clinical practice, antalgic doses such as levobupivacaine 0.25% or ropivacaine 0.375% are preferably used, since the block is associated with deep sedation or general anesthesia depending on the procedure and on clinical needs. Using these concentrations, volumes can also be increased up to 20 ml per side if the visualization of the anesthetic spread is not satisfactory to the operator.

In laparotomy midline incisions, the block must be performed bilaterally, therefore a particular care should be paid not to exceed the maximum doses (**Table 9.1**).

Cases where the block is NOT recommended

Contraindications:

- patient's refusal
- allergy to the LA
- infection at the injection site

COMPLICATIONS AND CONTRAINDICATIONS

Every locoregional anesthesia technique carries the risk of causing infections, bleeding or damage to anatomical structures.

Doctors should be aware that the upper and lower epigastric vessels pass in the posterior sheath of the rectus muscle, so there is a potential risk of placing the needle tip or the catheter in these vessels.

The intravascular injection of local anesthetic could occur, resulting in a risk of systemic toxicity from local anesthetic agents.

An accidental puncture of the epigastric vessels may form a hematoma (bruise).

If the procedure is not carried out correctly, with an adequate ultrasound visualization of the anatomical structures and needle tip, it is always possible to prick the posterior sheath of the rectus abdominis muscle, the peritoneum and the underlying bowel loops.

However, a correct use of ultrasound guidance will considerably reduce this risk.

The superficial positioning of the catheters in the posterior sheath of the rectus muscle and the distance from nerve and vascular structures make this technique safe. In fact, even in case of infections or hematomas, the complications would still be less serious than those in the peridural space. At present, however, no complications due to the ultrasound-guided positioning of the catheter in the rectus muscle fascia have been reported in the literature.

Complications

- Vascular puncture (if performed by inexperienced operators)
- Hematoma (accidental puncture of epigastric vessels)
- Puncture of the posterior sheath of the rectus abdominis muscle, peritoneum and of underlying bowel loops
- Increased risk of LAST (linked to high volumes of LA used or to failure to comply with maximum recommended doses)

TABLE 9.1 RECOMMENDED DOSAGES FOR THE EXECUTION OF THE RECTUS ABDOMINIS MUSCLE FASCIA BLOCK

	Local anesthetic volume	Concentration and local anesthetic recommended	Maximum allowed dose of local anesthetic
Adult	0.2-0.4 ml/kg per side (10-20 ml per side)	Ropivacaine 0.375% Levobupivacaine 0.25%	1 mg/kg per side

BLOCKADE OF THE SHEATH OF THE RECTUS ABDOMINIS MUSCLE FASCIA IN PEDIATRIC PATIENTS

Anatomy and sonoanatomy are superimposable in adults and children.

The aim of the technique is to anesthetize the terminal branches of the intercostal nerves which innervate the periumbilical abdominal wall when crossing the rectus abdominis muscle fascia.

The ultrasound-guided technique in children involves the use of the following materials: a high-frequency linear probe (7-12 MHz), a sterile probe cover, sterile gel, a short bevel needle (4-10 cm, 22 G), sterile drapes, and an antiseptic solution to set up a sterile field.

The probe must be placed transversally and laterally to the umbilicus to identify: the hypoechoic rectus muscle that separates the subcutaneous tissue from the peritoneum, its superficial and deep fascia, and its (hyperechoic) lateral margin, from which the aponeuroses of the internal oblique and transversal abdominal muscle originate. With the patient in supine position, the approach will be in-plane and lateral-to-medial.

To avoid lower epigastric vessel perforation, a more lateral needle insertion point should be chosen, so that the needle crosses the external oblique and internal oblique muscles, thus entering in the lateral portion of the rectus muscle deep fascia. With this procedure, the needle will not directly enter the belly of the muscle, which prevents lower epigastric vessel damage.

Intermittent injections of saline during the advancement of the needle are recommended to confirm the position of the needle tip. The target of the block is to inject the local anesthetic between the rectus muscle and its deep fascia; the spread of the anesthetic solution between the two structures mentioned above can be observed during the injection. A dose of 0.1-0.2 ml/kg of levobupivacaine 0.25% or ropivacaine 0.2% per side will suffice.

Complications are rare and mild: puncture of a bowel loop and vascular puncture with formation of a hematoma in the abdominal wall.

The use of low volumes of local anesthetic makes the risk of systemic toxicity virtually irrelevant. This technique has virtually no contraindications.

BLOCKADE OF THE RECTUS ABDOMINIS MUSCLE AND CHRONIC PAIN

Rectus abdominis sheath block finds its main indication in the management of chronic abdominal pain over postoperative analgesia, with a diagnostic and therapeutic value that has been demonstrated especially in abdominal cutaneous nerve entrapment syndromes (ACNES), in iatrogenic neural damage, in myofascial painful syndromes. Finally, as demonstrated by a work by Skinner et al. of 2007, promising results were obtained using corticosteroids as adjuvants: the combined injection of a local anesthetic agent and a steroid agent seems to result in a double action consisting in the temporary interruption of the nerve conduction and in the reduction of the inflammatory response.

RECOMMENDED READING

- Abrahams MS, Horn JL, Noles LM, Aziz MF. Evidence-based medicine: ultrasound guidance for truncal blocks. Reg Anaesth Pain Med. 2010;35(2 Suppl):S36-42.
- Cornish P, Deacon A. Rectus sheath catheters for continuous analgesia after upper abdominal surgery. ANZ J Surg. 2007;77(1-2):84.
- Courreges P, Poddevin F, Lecoutre D. Para-umbilical block: A new concept for regional anaesthesia in children. Paediatr Anaesth. 1997;7(3):211-4.
- Dolan J, Lucie P, Geary T, Smith M, Kenny G. The rectus sheath block for laparoscopic surgery in adults: A comparison between the loss of resistance and ultrasound guided techniques. Anaesthesia. 2007;62:301-13.
- Ferguson S, Thomas V, Lewis I. The rectus sheath block in paediatric anaesthesia: new indications for an old technique? Paediatr Anaesth. 1996;6(6):463-6.
- Hebbard P. Subcostal transversus abdominis plane block under ultrasound guidance. Anesth Analg. 2008;106(2):674-5.
- Malchow R, Jaeger L, Lam H. Rectus sheath catheters for continuous analgesia after laparotomy - without postoperative opioid use. Pain Med. 2011;12(7):1124-9.
- McDonnell JG, O'Donnell B, Curley G, et al. The analgesic efficacy of transversus abdominis plane block after abdominal surgery: a prospective randomized controlled trial. Anesth Analg. 2007; 104(1):193-7.
- Mori H, Akita K, Hata Y. Anatomical study of innervated transverse rectus abdominis musculocutaneous and deep inferior epigastric perforator flaps. Surg Radiol Anat. 2007;29(2):149-54.

- O'Donnell BD, McDonnell JG, McShane AJ. The transversus abdominis plane (TAP) block in open retropubic prostatectomy. Regional Anesthesia and Pain Medicine. 2006;31(1):91.
- Sandeman DJ, Dilley AV. Ultrasound-guided rectus sheath block and catheter placement. ANZ Journal of Surgery. 2008;78(7):621-3.
- Schleich CL. Schmerzlose Operationen. Berlin: Springer; 1899: 240-1.
- Sites BD, Brull R. Ultrasound guidance in peripheral regional anesthesia: philosophy, evidence-based medicine, and techniques. Current Opinion in Anaesthesiology. 2006;19(6):630-9.
- Tsui BC. Ultrasound-guided rectus sheath catheter placement. Anaesthesia. 2014;69:1172-82.
- Webster K, Hubble S. Rectus sheath analgesia in intensive care patients: technique description and case series. Anaesthesia and Intensive Care. 2009;37:855.
- Webster K. The transversus abdominis plane (TAP) block: abdominal plane regional anaesthesia. Update in Anaesthesia. 2008;24(1): 24-9.
- Yap LH, Whiten SC, Forster A, Stevenson JH. The anatomical and neurophysiological basis of the sensate free TRAM and DIEP flaps. Br J Plast Surg. 2002;55(1):35-45.

CLINICAL CASE 1 – SUBXIPHOID CARDIAC DRAINAGE PAIN MANAGEMENT: COULD ULTRASOUND RECTUS SHEATH BLOCK BE THE ANSWER?

Clinical history and anamnesis Pain management after cardiac surgery is very important to enhance the deep breathing, coughing and early ambulation which are critical for respiratory care, early recovery and prognosis. The pain caused by the subxiphoid drainage tube can be from skin incision, rubbing during the tube insertion, continuing irritation between adjacent tissue and the tube, direct injury to the rectus abdominis muscles. Treatment generally involves the use of high doses of strong opioids which results in adverse effects that increase respiratory depression, infection and delay discharge. Based on our experience, the use of locoregional anesthesia techniques can be a valid alternative that can effectively control pain by minimizing these complications. We report ten cases scheduled for elective Coronary Artery Bypass Graft Surgery (CABG) in which Ultrasound Rectus Sheath Block (US-RSB) was performed to manage subxiphoid drainages pain.

Technique description Before admission to Intensive Care Unit (ICU), a strictly aseptic US-RSB was performed in the epigastric region by injection of 10 ml of 0.375% levobupivacaine and dexamethasone 4 mg into the posterior sheath of the rectus abdominal muscles bilaterally. Via an in-plane approach, a 12.5-MHz linear probe and atraumatic 21 G 100 mm needle (SonoPlex stim Pajunk®) was used (**Figure 9.12 A, B**). No complications such as ileal injury, infections and local anesthetic systemic toxicity were recorded. All patients had an extubation time of less than 1 hour after surgery. Only 1 g of acetaminophen every 8 hours was systematically administered without NSAID's or opioids. In the first 24 hours after the procedure, patients reported a good quality analgesia (NRS <3 and an excellent satisfaction rate. All patients reported a good pulmonary capacity: patients had a partial pressure of arterial oxygen to fraction of inspired oxygen ratio of 300 mmHg or more. Oxygen saturation was more than 96%, while partial pressure of arterial oxygen was more than 90 mmHg and partial pressure of arterial carbon dioxide was 35 mmHg, on average.

Materials and methods Written informed consent to the procedure and patient's approval to the publication were obtained.

Conclusions We believe that bilateral ultrasound guided rectus sheath block could be an effective and safe anesthetic technique to manage subxiphoid drainage pain in patients undergoing cardiac surgery, leading to greater comfort for the patient, early pulmonary rehabilitation, without common opioid-related side effects. Further studies are warranted to validate our results.

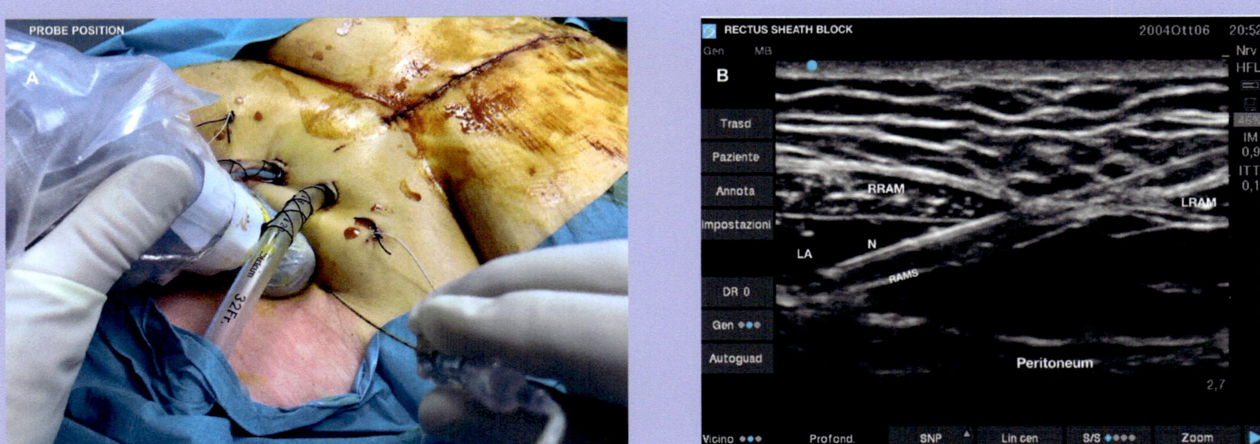

Figure 9.12 A, B Probe position: a linear probe is positioned in the epigastric region below the subxiphoid drainages. Ultrasound rectus sheath block; via an in-plane approach the local anesthetic is injected into the posterior sheath of the rectus abdominal muscles bilaterally. LA: local anesthetic; LRAM: left rectus abdominis muscle; N: needle; RAMS: rectus abdominis muscle sheath; RRAM: right rectus abdominis muscle.

CLINICAL CASE 2 – RECTUS SHEATH BLOCK (RSB) AS A SOLE ANESTHETIC TECHNIQUE FOR UMBILICAL HERNIA REPAIR

Clinical history and anamnesis Rectus sheath block (RSB) has been described both as a sole anesthetic and for preoperative analgesia. The RSB anesthetizes the 9th, 10th and 11th intercostal nerves providing somatic anesthesia to the abdominal wall structures superficial to the peritoneum. We report the case of a 82-year-old, 72 kg male with hypertensive, severe ischemic heart disease, diabetes and chronic obstructive pulmonary disease proposed for an umbilical hernia repair.

Technique description At the first bilaterally, all the structures were identified and color Doppler was used for avoiding vascular structures (inferior and superior epigastric vessels run in the posterior rectus sheath). Then under direct vision with an in-plane real-time technique the needle tip was advanced posterior to the rectus muscle and above the underlying rectus sheath, from lateral to medial, watching the local anesthetic dissects the rectus muscle away from the posterior rectus sheath. 10 ml of 0,5% levobupivacaine and 10 ml of lidocaine 1% were used for each side. Surgery was well tolerated and no haemodynamic instability or any kind of arrhythmia was developed (**Figure 9.13**).

Materials and methods After monitoring pulse oximeter (SpO_2), ECG and non-invasive blood pressure, a bilateral ultrasound guided rectus sheath block was performed with 23-Gauge x 50 mm needle (Sonoplex – Pajunk®).

Conclusions Rectus sheath block (RSB) has been described both as a sole anesthetic and for preoperative analgesia. We showed that RSB can be successfully used for providing both anesthesia and postoperative analgesia for umbilical hernia repair.

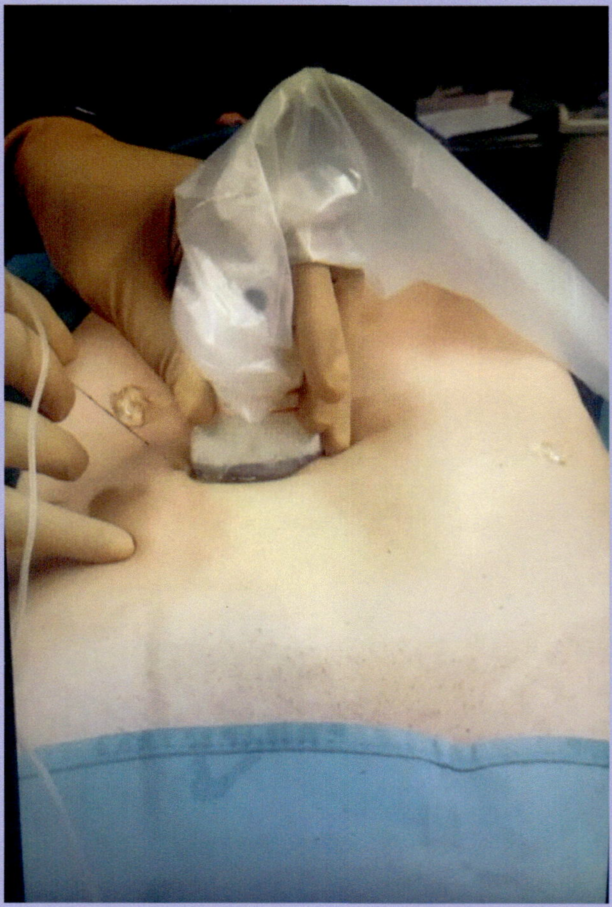

Figure 9.13 In-plane technique with lateromedial needle tip entry and high-frequency linear probe in the paraumbilical transverse position.

CHAPTER
10

Transversalis Fascia Plane (TFP) block

Astrid U. Behr

International literature is not quite yet completely clear on the nomenclature of the various blocks around the quadratus lumborum muscle (QLM). This chapter will be described the approach with the injection site between the transverse abdominal muscle (TAM), the QLM, and the transversalis fascia (TF), with a distribution of the local anesthetic (LA) along the anterior face of the QLM targeting the nerves of T12 and L1

In 2009, Hebbard proposed a variant of the ultrasound-guided Transverse abdominis Plane (TAP) block with a more posterior approach and called it transversalis fascia plane block (TFP Block). The target of the TFP block is the proximal part of nerves T12 and L1, localized between the aponeurosis of TAM and the TF, before their division in anterior and lateral cutaneous branches. This site of injectionis more lateral, and therefore more peripheral than the site of lumbar plexus, but is posterior and more proximal than the TAP, where the lateral and anterior cutaneous branches are already divided. In 2007 Blanco verbally described a similar approach, calling it quadratus lumborum block one (QLB I); later he proposed its evolution with injection site posterior to the QLM, calling it QLB II or posterior QLB.

ANATOMY AND SONOANATOMY

Anatomy

The lumbar plexus is formed by the ventral branches of the first four lumbar nerves (L1-L4) and anastomotic branches coming from the subcostal nerve (T12) and from L5. It is located within the posterior portion of the psoas major muscle (PMM), anteriorly to the transverse processes of the lumbar vertebrae, and in line with the intervertebral foramina. The iliohypogastric (IHGN) and ilioinguinal (IGN) nerves, which originate from L1, are the main target of this block (**Figures 10.1**, **10.2**).

IHGN is a mixed nerve which behaves like an intercostal nerve and arises from the upper part of the lateral border of the PMM, travelling with an oblique direction, to caudal and outward long the anterior (inner) face of the QLM posteriorly to the lower kidney (renal) pole. It glides on the surface of the aponeurosis of the transversus abdominis muscle (TAM), pierces above the level of the iliac crest, thus entering the TAP. Along its course in the TAP, it innervates the TAM and the internal oblique muscle (IOM), and divides into the lateral and anterior sensitive cutaneous branches. The lateral cutaneous branch crosses the IOM and the external oblique muscle (EOM) above the iliac crest, at a slightly posterior level than the lateral cutaneous branch of the subcostal nerve, and innervates the skin of the posterolateral gluteal region. The anterior cutaneous branch runs within the TAP, innervating the respective muscles, and crosses the IOM aponeurosis about 2-4 cm medially and 2 cm caudally to the anterior superioriliac spine.

The anterior cutaneous branch then travels in a medial and caudal direction and, after having sent some branches that pierce the sheath of the rectus abdominis muscle, it crosses the EOM aponeurosis about 3 cm above the superficial inguinal ring to finally distribute into the skin of the pubic region. The IHGN, along its path, communicates with the IGN and subcostal (T12) nerves. The anterior branch of the latter emits a branch for the pyramidal muscle; the lateral cutaneous branch crosses the IOM and EOM, and descends over the iliac crest to provide sensitivity of the anterior part of the gluteal region.

IGN is also a mixed nerve, which is smaller than the IHGN but behaves in the same way. The two nerves run next to each other paired along their way, contracting the same anatomical relationships. IGN emerges from

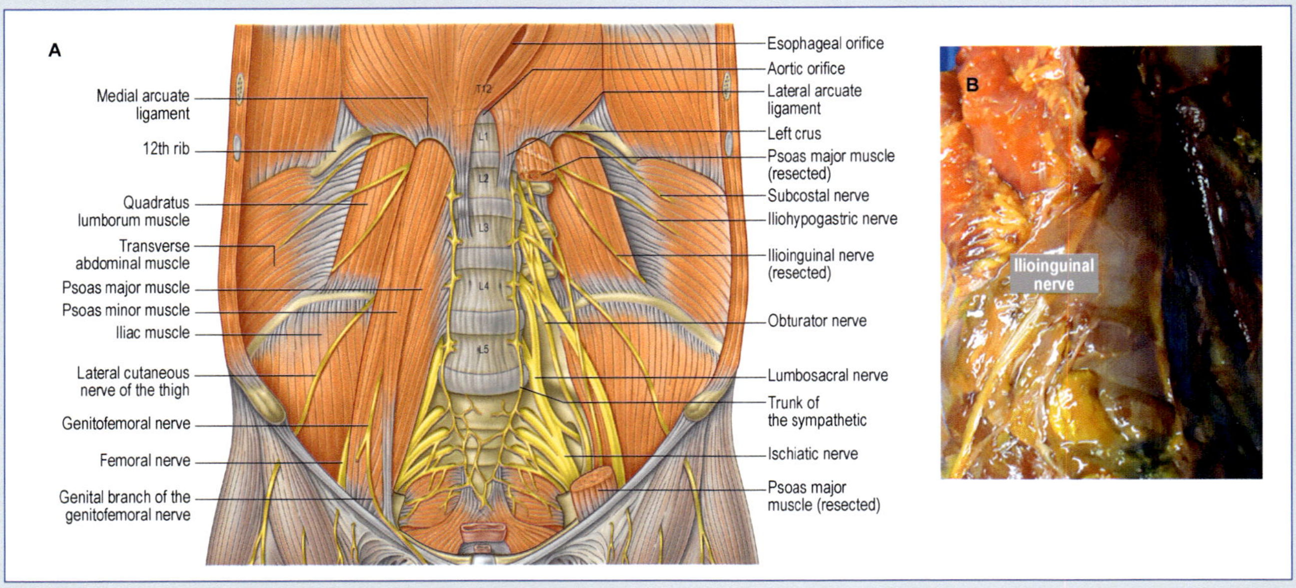

Figure 10.1 A Posterior abdominal wall seen from the inside, with view of the nerves of the lumbar plexus. **B** Detail from dissection on fresh corpse: note the course of the right ilioinguinal nerve (courtesy of Prof. C. Stecco, Department of Human Anatomy, University of Padua).

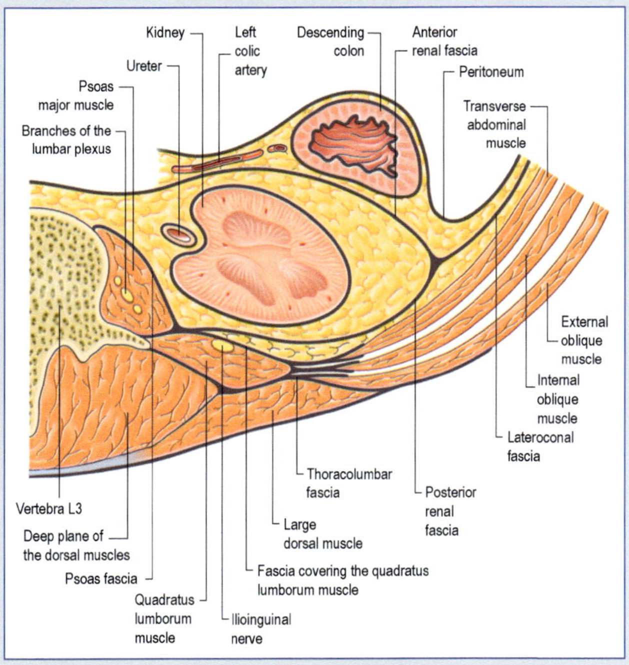

Figure 10.2 Cross-sectional view of the posterior abdominal wall at L3 level: note the nerves of the lumbar plexus contained in the thickness of the psoas major muscle.

the lateral margin of the PMM and together with the IHGN, or at a slightly more caudad level crosses the QLM and the superior part of the iliac muscle obliquely, piercing the TAM near the anterior extremity of the iliac crest. It runs within the TAP in an inferomedial direction, innervates the TAM and IOM, and finally pierces the IOM at a distance of about 2.5 cm medially and 2 cm inferiorly to the anterior superior iliac spine.

A voluminous genital branch which travels in the inguinal canal under the spermatic cord emits near the anterior superior iliac spine and emerges ending in a cutaneous sensitive branch that innervates the skin in the medio-proximal region of the thigh – the skin that covers the mons pubis and the labia majora or the anterior scrotum. In some cases, the IGN may end by joining the IHGN, or be completely absent

These nerves emit their lateral cutaneous branches before entering the TAP or within its very first part and therefore are not always completely approached by LA injection in the TAP. The QLM, which originates from the iliac crest and inserts to the 12th rib and medially to the trasverse process from L1 to L5, together with the TAM, refer to localization of IGN and IHGN, forming the postero-medial border of the fascial plane where we have to inject the LA (**Figure 10.3**).

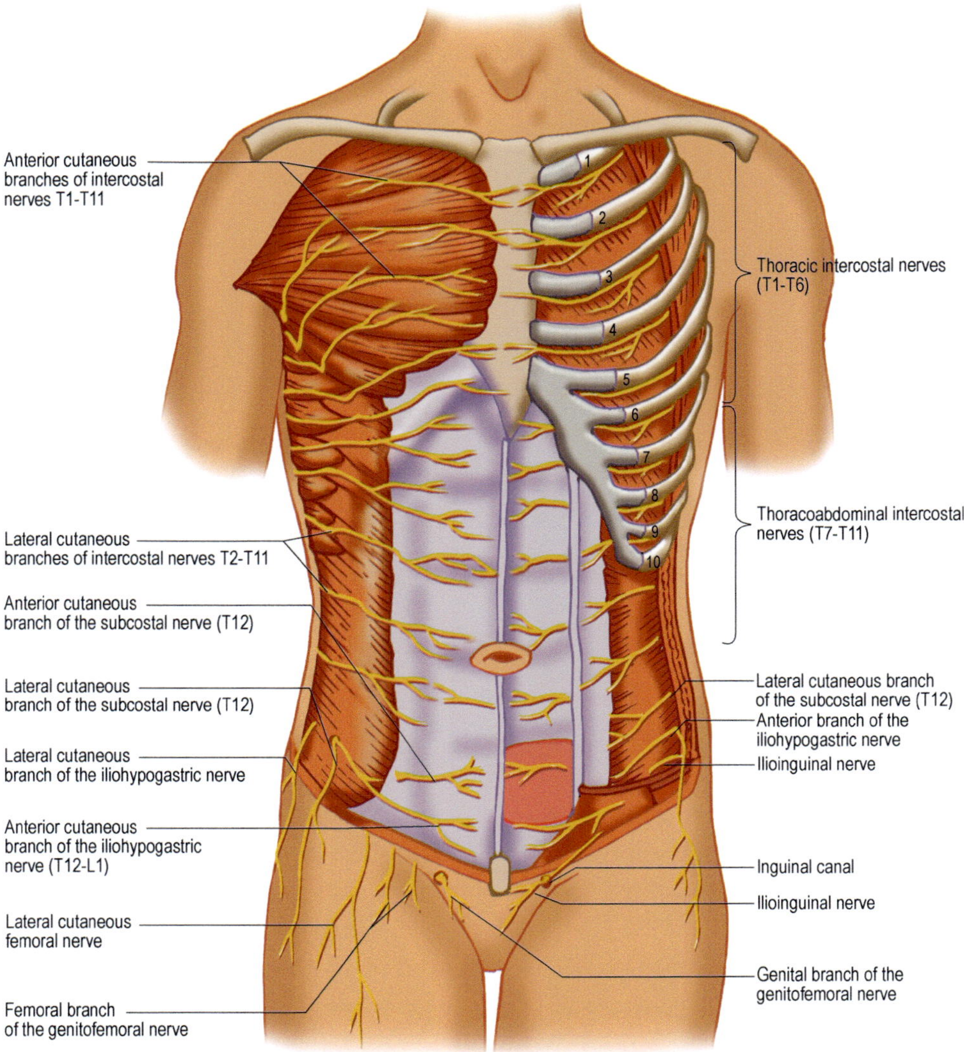

Figure 10.3 View of the nerves of the anterior abdominal wall with perforation points of cutaneous branches.

Sonoanatomy

In a transverse scan with the linear probe between the costal margin and the iliac crest, you can identify under cutis and subcutis the three abdominal muscle layers separated by their hyperechoic fasciae: from external to internal the EOM, then the IOM, the thickest of the three layers, and finally the TAM, the most hypoechoic muscle layer (**Figure 10.4**).

The TF runs immediately under the TAM and is not always clearly distinguishable from the aponeurosis of the muscle. Even deeper to this fascial plane, we find loose connective tissue, described as perinephric or extraperitoneal fat, bordered by the hyperechoic peritoneum with the bowel loops below, recognizable for the peristaltic movement.

Moving the probe posteriorly by following the TAM aponeurosis, medially we can identify the QLM attached to the transverse process of the L4 vertebra. Beneath we can consistently recognize the peritoneum with its hyperechoic aspect and movement bend-

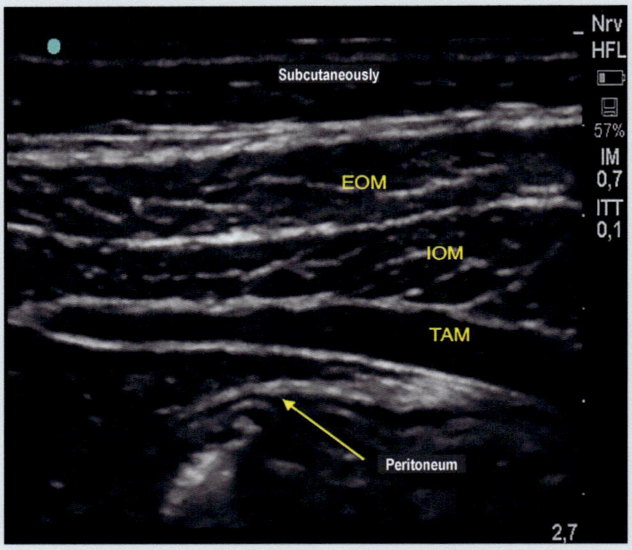

Figure 10.4 Ultrasound image with linear probe positioned in axillary line with depth set at 2.7 cm and marker facing dorsally. EOM: external oblique muscle; IOM: internal oblique muscle; TAM: transverse abdominal muscle.

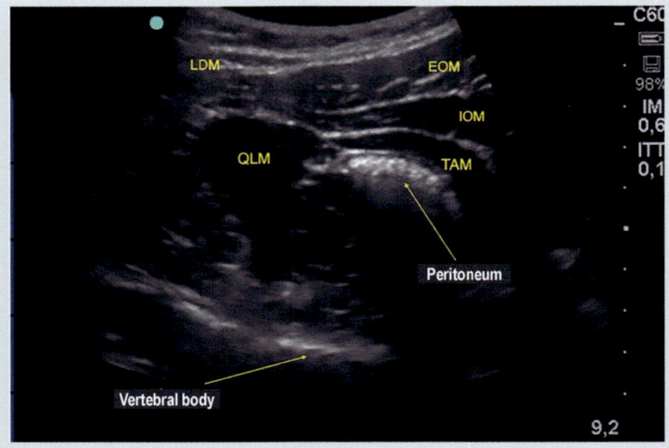

Figure 10.5 Ultrasound image with convex probe in medium axillary line, with depth set at 9.2 cm and marker facing dorsally. The acoustic shadow of the transverse process is absent because it is a projection between the transverse processes of L2-L3. Note the hyper-reflective image of the peritoneum. EOM: external oblique muscle; IOM: internal oblique muscle; LDM: large dorsal muscle; QLM: quadratus lumborum muscle; TAM: transverse abdominal muscle.

ing away from the abdominal muscles in anteroposterior direction, and for the presence because of the loose adipose tissue interposed between the TF and the peritoneum.

This adipose tissue increases near the iliac crest. The most suitable position to appreciate perfect sonoanatomy is at the level of the medial border of TAM, where the muscle comes in contact with the QLM, becomes thinner (tail) and its aponeurosis continues medially with the anterior layer of thoracolumbar fascia (**Figure 10.5**).

DESCRIPTION OF THE ULTRASOUND-GUIDED TECHNIQUE

This approach consists of positioning the needle tip in the plane between the TAM and the TF and the injection of LA anterolaterally with spread to the QLM. The target of this fascial block is the proximal part of the nerves originating from T12 and L1, particularly the IHGN and IGN including the anterior and lateral cutaneous branches in a position between the lumbar plexus and the TAP (**Figure 10.6**).

To better understand the role of the TF in the correct distribution of LA, we performed anatomical dissection in collaboration with the Department of Human Anatomy of the University of Padua. This study allowed us to postulate the hypothesis that despite it being possible to identify a tissue structure compatible with TF from an histological point of view, from an macroscopically and sonographically point of view, the clear distinction of the plane between TF and epimysium of the TAM is not possible (**Figure 10.7**).

Only the advent of US has allowed the execution of this block, but an accurate and correct deposition of LA in the plane between the aponeurosis of the TAM, QLM and TF remains difficult. It seems unlikely that the TF can play a decisive role in compartmentalization of the LA in the course of TFP block due to the difficulty, even with ultrasound, of clearly identifying TF and the delimited small area illustrated in **Figure 10.6**. Normally the needle tip penetrates the posterior fasciae of the TAM and the LA injection ends up in a zone of retroperitoneal or perirenal fat beyond the TAM, defined by Choquet et al. as posterior pararenalretroperitoneal space (PPS).

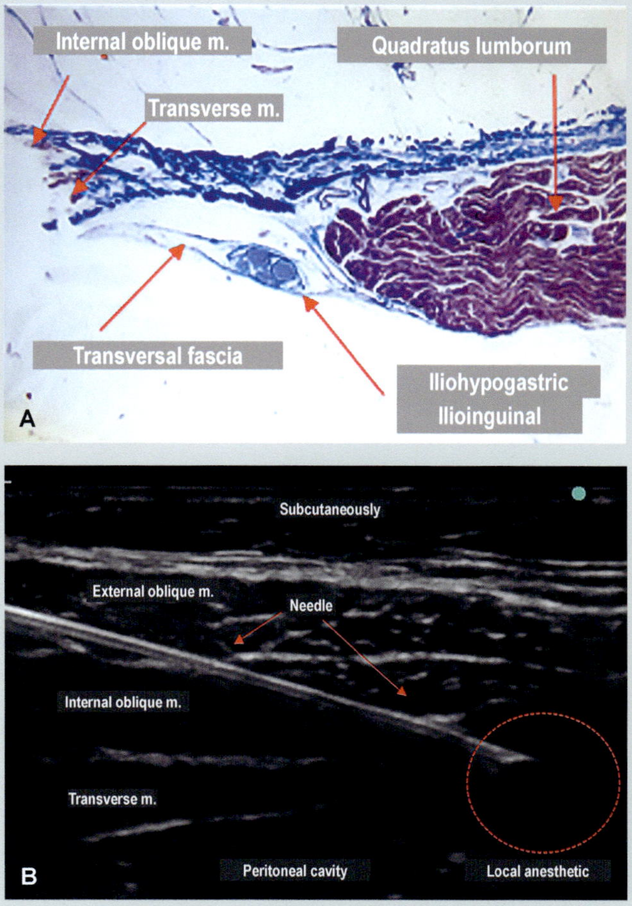

Figure 10.6 A Histological section with H.M. staining showing the transverse fascia (TF) covering the ilioinguinal and iliohypogastric nerves (courtesy of Prof C. Stecco, Department of Human Anatomy, University of Padua). **B** Ultrasound image with linear probe showing the same structures with the needle tip before the QLM: the TF is not detectable.

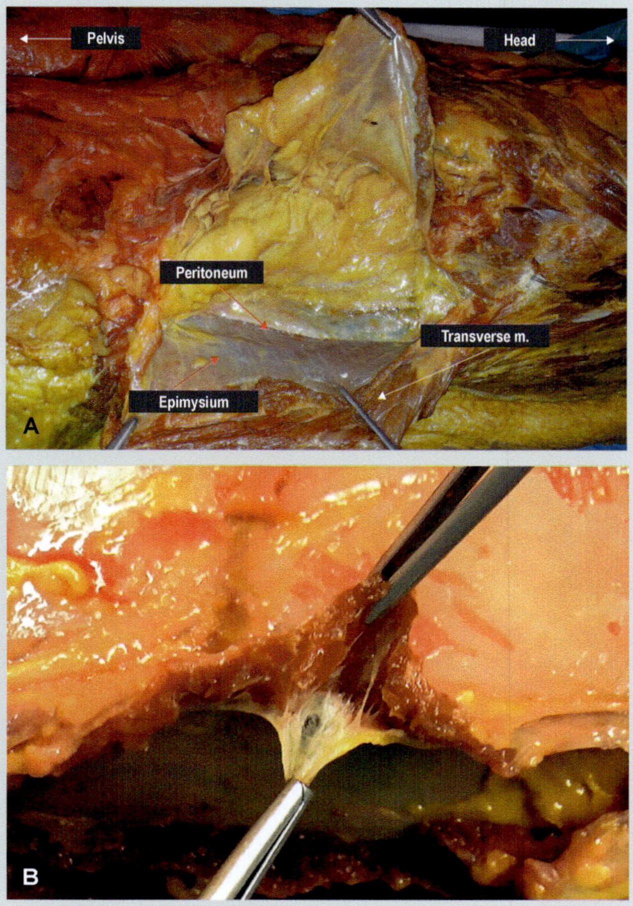

Figure 10.7 A Corpse dissection (courtesy of Prof. C. Stecco, Department of Human Anatomy, University of Padua), lateral abdominal wall: the macroscopic absence of a fascial structure that corresponds to the TF can be noticed. **B** Detail of the dissection: adhesion of the TAM to its fascia (epimysium).

The patient position is supine with a pilet under the buttock, or in lateral decubitus, with the surgical side up. To adopt the most ergonomic position, the operator will place the monitor of the ultrasound machine in front of him, opposite to the selected side.

The ultrasound machine should be equipped with a high-frequency linear probe (6-12 MHz), in obese patients with a low-frequency convex probe (2-6 MHz), with a standard set for nerve blocks including sterile probe cover and gel, ethyl-based disinfectant, sterile towels and gloves, anechogenic needle 21 G x 80-100 mm and two 10 ml syringes with LA. An assistant should be present for aspiration and injection of LA. The block can be performed in the awake patient with adequate analgosedation, otherwise under neuraxial or general anesthesia (**Figure 10.8**).

After accurate skin disinfection, the sterile covered probe is positioned in transverse orientation between the costal margin and the iliac crest on the mid-axillary line. After identification of the three muscle layers (EOM, IOM and TAM) the probe is moved posteriorly following the aponeurosis of the TAM (**Figure 10.9**).

The QLM Is identified medially to the end of TAM along with the underlying hyperechoic and hyperreflective

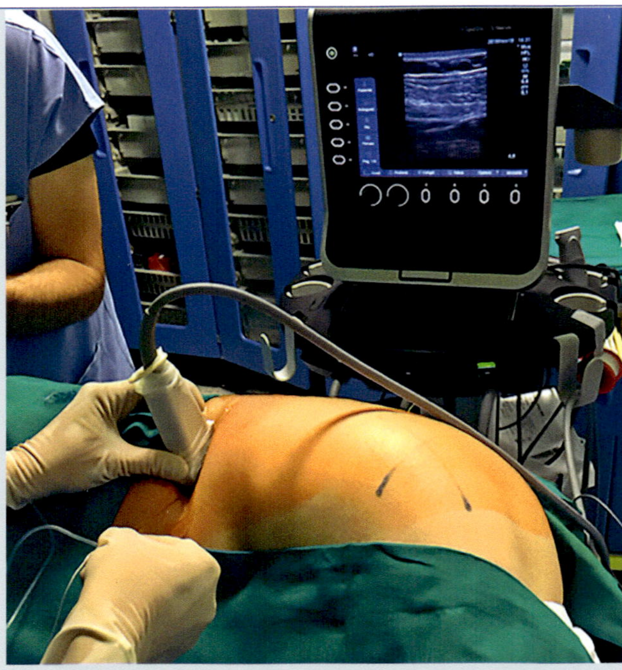

Figure 10.8 Patient in lateral decubitus, with the operator in front and the ultrasound machine in an ergonomic position; the linear probe is in a transversal position on the midaxillary line and the needle direction is anterior towards posterior (lateral towards medial).

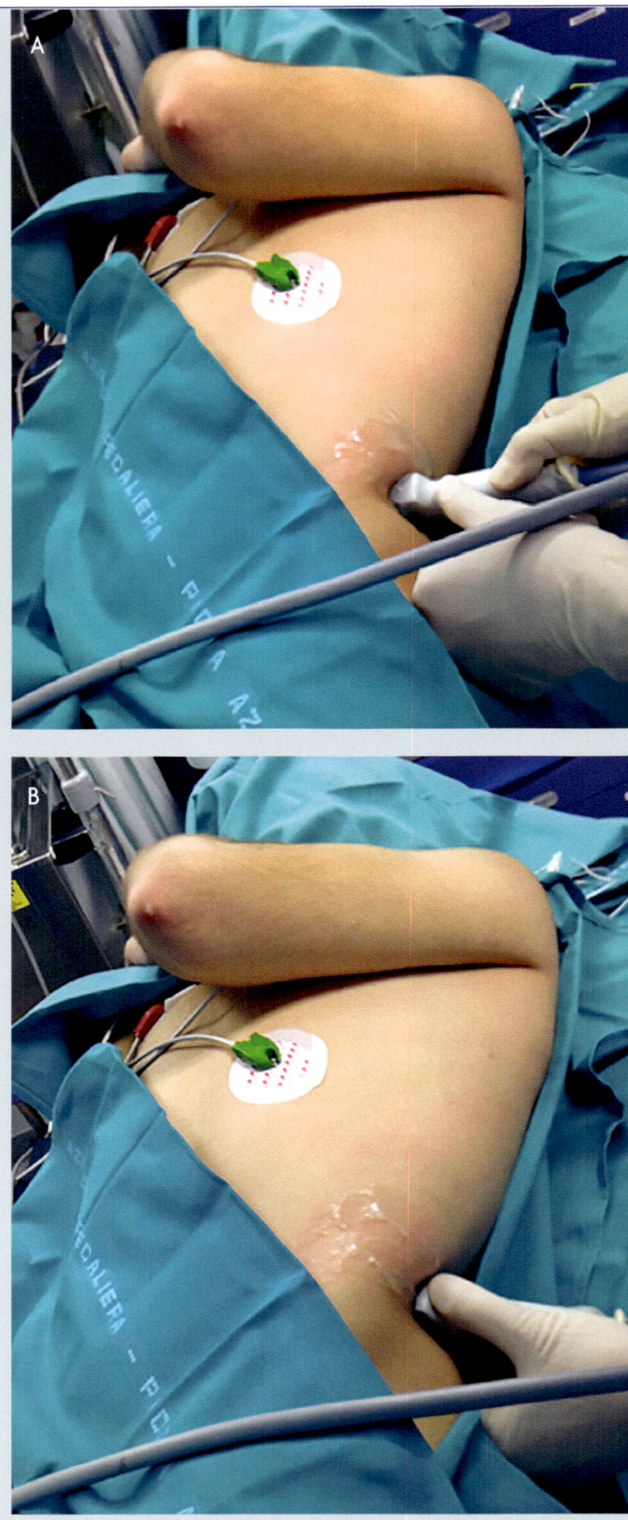

Figure 10.9 Patient in supine decubitus, with a sandbag under the buttock: the linear probe is in a transverse position and is moved towards the back to highlight the tail of the TAM (transverse abdominal muscle) and the QLM (quadratus lumborum muscle).

peritoneum, which bends away from the abdominal muscles in anteroposterior direction. The extraperitoneal and perirenal fat, which increases towards the iliac crest is normally present anterior to TF. Once an optimal sonographic and anatomical image is obtained, the probe will be stabilized and the needle inserted in-plane in an anteroposterior (lateral to medial) direction crossing the subcutaneous tissue, the EOM and IOM and finally reaching the tip of the TAM (**Figures 10.10**, **10.11**).

To improve the angulation and consequently the visibility of the needle, the skin puncture site must be at a distance of about 3-4 cm from the probe, with efforts to further increase this distance in obese patients requiring the use of a longer needle. To reduce risk of intraperitoneal or abdominal organ puncture, we recommend advancing the needle in a anteroposterior (medial) direction, where more adipose tissue is present and to proceed with the hydro-dissection technique, after crossing the 'tail' of the TAM, since the fascia medially is thinner and more difficult to distinguish as a separate plane. The correct needle tip position is confirmed by

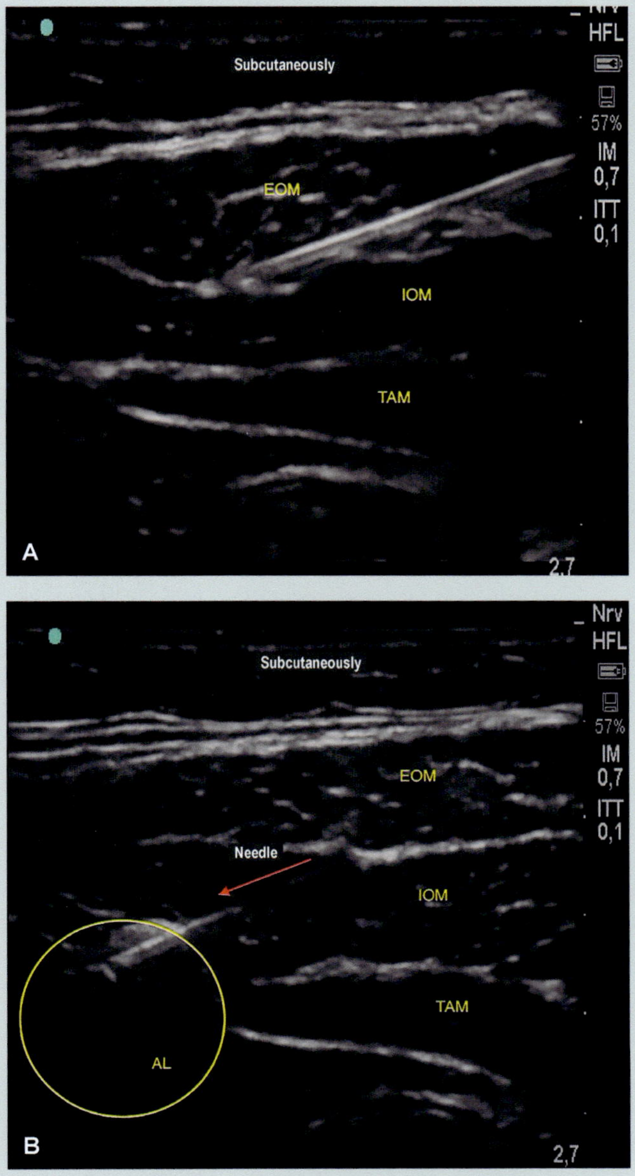

Figure 10.10 A Ultrasound image with linear probe depth set at 2.7 cm and marker oriented posteriorly with needle (21 G X 100 mm) introduced in-plane. **B** Same position with the needle advanced beyond the tail of the TAM (transverse abdominal muscle) and injection of the local anesthetic; the lowering of the peritoneum can be noticed.

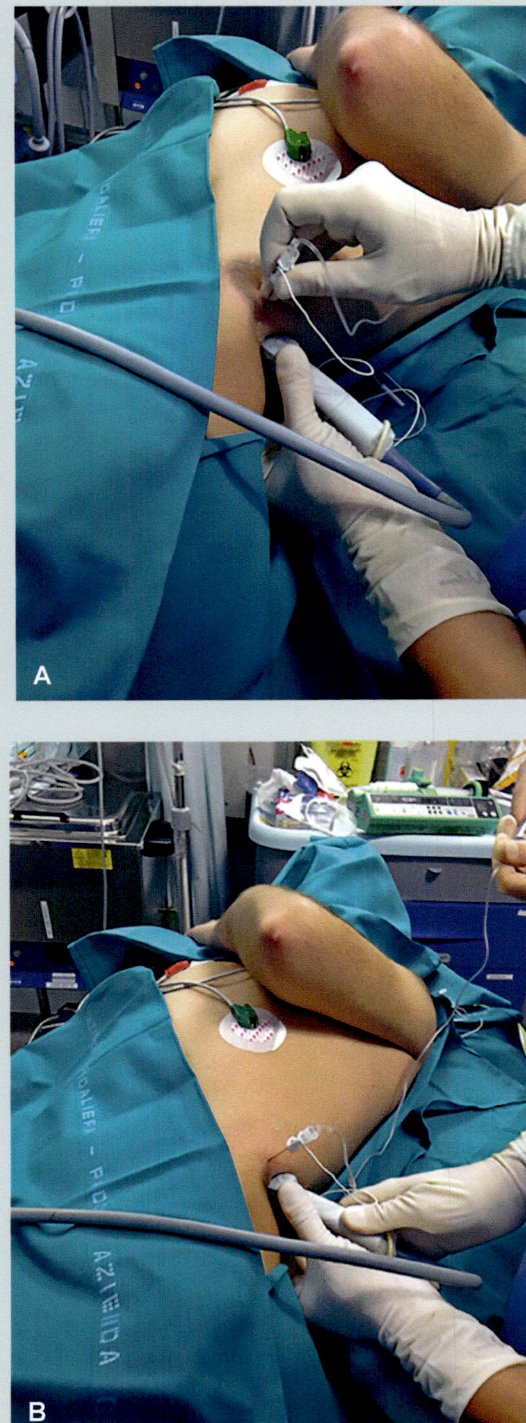

Figure 10.11 A Patient in supine decubitus with a sandbag under the buttock: in-plane insertion of the needle and alignment of the linear probe. **B** Injection of the LA in small volumes, with frequent aspirations between injections.

the medial spread of LA, in front of QLM, observing the splitting of the fascial planes or the breakdown of the retroperitoneal fat. When withdrawing the needle some LA can also be injected in the TAP to extend the block to anterior branches of the nerves superior to T12 (**Flow chart 10.1 online**).

INDICATIONS AND DOSAGES

The TFP block is mainly proposed for the treatment of the somatic component of intra- and postoperative pain, and for prevention of chronic postoperative persistent pain and should whenever possible be included in a multimodal analgesic protocol. The injection of LA in an anatomical site between the lumbar plexus and the TAP, focused on the IGN and IHGN, can provide long-term perioperative analgesia by giving a sensory block of the iliac crest, but also of the great trochanter, the upper lateral part of the thigh, and the lower abdomen. Therefore, this technique can be applied for reconstructive procedures in orthopedic, vertebral and maxillofacial surgery, where bone-harvesting of the iliac crest may result in intense post-operative pain, often greater than the pain in the main surgical territory with a high risk of chronicization. In a randomized study, Parras' et al. compared the efficacy of QLB I to femoral nerve block for postoperative analgesia in patients undergoing endoprosthesis for hip fracture and showed the superiority of QLB in the first 24 hours in terms of reduced pain, time of stay in PACU, and opioid consumption. Clinical evidence is mainly based on case reports with some indication of analgesic technique for the cutaneous analgesia in total hip replacement and revision of hip replacement in orthopedic surgery. In abdominal laparotomic surgery, its application has been proposed for inguinal plastic surgery, for appendicectomy and colorectal surgery, and in vascular surgery for femorofemoral bypass. Some recent randomized studies also demonstrated its efficacy in obstetric surgery as treatment for post-operative pain after Cesarean sections in addition to multimodal analgesia and it was shown to reduce the 24-h opioid consumption and opioid related side effects, while improving patient satisfaction at the same time. Further clinical studies are necessary to investigate efficacy and usefulness of unilateral or bilateral technique, with the possibility of continuous infusion of LA through catheter.

We find variable LA doses in literature, with even higher volumes or concentrations than that recommended for TAP block (**Table 10.1**). The doses should never exceed the maximum levels recommended for the risk of local anesthetic systemic toxicity (LAST) and attention should be paid to reduce concentrations of LA when volumes increase, especially in bilateral application. The precise site of LA injection should be the small area described before between TF and epymisium of TAM, but unfortunately this is difficult to achieve and normally LA spreads anterorlaterally, being dispersed in the retroperitoneal space between perirenal Zuckerkandl's fascia and the QLM. This would certainly explain the need for large volumes of LA (20-30 ml).

TABLE 20.1 DOSAGES AND VOLUMES OF LA TO BE USED IN THE TFP BLOCK

	LA VOLUME	DRUGS	ASSAYS
Adult patient	0.3-0.6 ml/kg per side (15-40 ml per side)	Ropivacaine 0.2%-0.5% Levobupivacaine 0.125%-0.37-5%	2-3 mg/kg
Pediatric patient	0.4 ml/kg per side	Ropivacaine 0.2%-0.5% Levobupivacaine 0.125%-0.375%	2 mg/kg

When TFP block is NOT recommended

Absolute contraindications:
- patient refusal
- true LA allergy
- local infection at injection/procedure site

Relative contraindications:
- surgery at the injection site (catheter)
- disorders of coagulation or platelet aggregation (hematoma)
- day surgery procedures for risk of femoral nerve motor block

COMPLICATIONS AND CONTRAINDICATIONS

The scientific literature does not report descriptions of severe adverse events. Performed by experienced operators ultrasound-guided TFP block is considered a relatively simple and safe technique.

Possible complications are block failure, intraperitoneal injection, bowel lesion, colon and liver puncture, hematomas, or LAST.

There are only few contraindications to the TFP block, which reflect those described for the TAP block, such as a lack of consent to the procedure, anamnesis positive for true LA allergy and infections or other anomalies at the injection site. Relative contraindications are surgery at the injection site and the presence of coagulation or platelet aggregation disorders due to the risk of hematomas. The TFP is a superficial block site, but difficult to compress for hemostas is if needed.

In several cases quadriceps motor block and no hip flexion were reported after performing a TFP block. A motor block due to transient paralysis of the femoral nerve for the spread of LA in both directions, central (lumbar plexus) and distal (femoral nerve), should be considered a consequence more than a complication and for the risk of prolonged discharge times or patient falls a one-day surgery setting may be a relative contraindication for application of TFP block.

Complications

- Intraperitoneal injection
- Bowel lesions – colon and liver puncture
- Hematomas
- Block failure
- LAST
- Lower limb weakness

INDICATIONS IN CHRONIC PAIN

TFP block is indicated in a multimodal analgesia protocol for preventive treatment of chronic postoperative pain after bone graft harvesting from the iliac crest in reconstructive surgery.

RECOMMENDED READING

- Aydin ME, Bedir Z, Yayik AM et al. Subarachnoid block and ultrasound-guided transversalis fascia plane block for caesarean section A randomised, double-blind, placebo-controlled trial. Eur J Anaesthesiol. 2020 Sep;37(9):765-772
- Black ND, Malhas L, Jin R, et al. The analgesic efficacy of the transversalis fascia plane block in iliac crest bone graft harvesting: a randomized controlled trial. Korean J Anesthesiol 2019; 72:336–343
- Blanco R, McDonnell JG. Optimal point of injection: The quadratus lumborum type I and II blocks. Htpp://www.respond2articles.com/ANA/forums/Post/1550.aspx (accessed 26 july 2018)
- Carney J, Finnerty O, Rauf J, et al. Studies on the spread of local anaesthetics solution in transversus abdominis plane blocks. Anaesthesia. 2011; 66:1023-30.
- Chakraborty A1, Goswami J, Patro VA. Ultrasound-guided continuous quadratus lumborum block for postoperative analgesia in a pediatric patient. A&A Case Reports. 2015;4:34-6.
- Chin KJ, Chan V, Hebbard P, et al. Ultrasound-guided transversalis fascia plane block provides analgesia for anterior iliac crest bone graft harvesting. Can J Anesth. 2012;59:122-3.
- Chin KJ. Reply to Dr Choquet et al. Reg Anesth Pain Med 2017; 42:548–549
- Chiono J, Bernard N, Bringuier S, et al. The ultrasound-guided transversus abdominis plane block for anterior iliac crest bone graft postoperative pain relief: a prospective descriptive study. Reg Anesth Pain Med. 2010;35:520-4.
- Choquet O, Capdevila X. Transversalis Fascia Blocks Different Names for the Same Posterior Pararenal Space Block. RAPM. 2017; 42;4:547-8.
- Dakwar E, Vale FL, Uribe JS. Trajectory of the main sensory and motor branches of the lumbar plexus outside the psoas muscle related to the lateral retroperitoneal transpsoas approach. J Neurosurg Spine. 2011;14(2):290-5.
- El-Boghdadly K, Wolmarans M. Standardizing nomenclature in regional anesthesia: an ASRA-ESRA Delphi consensus study of abdominal wall, paraspinal, and chest wall blocks. Reg Anesth Pain Med 2021; 46:571–580. doi:10.1136/rapm-2020-102451
- Elsharkawy H, El-Boghdadly K et al. Quadratus Lumborum Block Anatomical Concepts, Mechanisms, and Techniques. Anesthesiology 2019; 130:322–35.
- Heary RF, Schlenk RP, Sacchieri TA, et al. Persistent iliac crest donor site pain: independent outcome assessment. Neurosurgery. 2002;50:510-7.
- Hebbard PD. Transversalis fascia plane block, a novel ultrasound-guided abdominal wall nerve block. Can J Anesth. 2009; 56:618-20.
- Kadam VR1. Ultrasound guided quadratus lumborum block or posteriortransversus abdominis plane block catheter infusion as a postoperative analgesic technique for abdominal surgery. J Anaesthesiol Clin Pharmacol. 2015;31(1):130-1.
- Kadam VR1. Ultrasound-guided quadratus lumborum block as a postoperative analgesic technique for laparotomy. J Anaesthesiol Clin Pharmacol. 2013;29(4):550-2.
- Kim DH, Kim SJ. Fascial plane blocks: a narrative review of the literature. Reg Anesth Pain Med 2021;46:600–617. doi:10.1136/rapm-2020-101909.
- Klaassen Z, Marshall E, Tubbs RS, et al. Anatomy of the ileoinguinal and iliohypogastric nerves with observations of their spinal nerve contributions. Clinical Anatomy. 2011;23:454-61.
- Krohg A, Ullensvang K, Rosseland L, et al. Analgesic Effect of Ultrasound-Guided Quadratus Lumborum Block After Cesarean Delivery: A Randomized Clinical Trial. Anesth Analg. 2017;8 Febr;126(2):559-65.
- La Colla L, Uskova A, Ben-David B. Single-shot Quadratus Lumborum Block for Postoperative Analgesia After Minimally Invasive Hip Arthroplasty. A New Alternative to Continuous Lumbar Plexus Block? RAPM. 2017; 42;1:125-6.

- Lee S, Goetz T, Gharapetian A. Unanticipated Motor Weakness with Ultrasound Guided Transversalis Fascia Plane Block. A&A case reports. 2015;5:124-5.
- Nielsen T, Moriggl B, Barckman J et al. Cutaneous anaesthesia of hip surgery incisions with iliohypogastric and subcostal nerve blockade: A randomised trial. Acta Anaesthesiol Scand. 2018;1–10.
- Parras T, Blanco R. Randomised trial comparing the transversus abdominis plane block posterior approach or quadratus lumborum block type I with femoral block for postoperative analgesia in femoral neck fracture, both ultrasound-guided. Rev Esp Anestesiol Reanim. 2016; 63;3:141-8.
- Rahn DD, Phelan JN, Roshanravan SM, et al. Anterior abdominal wall nerves and vessel anatomy: clinical implications for gynecologic surgery. Am J Obstet Gynecol. 2010;202:234-5.
- Rebuffat P. Nervi spinali. In: Anatomia funzionale del sistema nervoso. Mazzocchi G, Nussdorfer G. Pubs Libreria Cortina. Padova 1996:344-9.
- Rosario DJ, Jacob S, Luntley J, et al. Mechanism of femoral nerve palsy complicating percutaneous ilioinguinal field block. BJA. 1997;78:314-6.
- Rosenberg PH, Veering BT, Urmey WF. Maximum recommended doses of local anesthetics: a multifactorial concept. Reg Anesth Pain Med. 2004;29:564-75.
- Scimia P, Basso Ricci E, et al. Ultrasound-Guided Transversalis Fascia Plane Block: An Alternative Approach for Anesthesia in Inguinal Herniorrhaphy: A Case Report. AA Pract. 2018 Apr 15;10(8):209-11.
- Serifsoy TE, Tulgar S, Selvi O, et al. Evaluation of ultrasound-guided transversalis fascia plane block for postoperative analgesia in cesarean section: a prospective, randomized, controlled clinical trial. J Clin Anesth 2020; 59:56–60.
- Skandalakis PN, Zoras O, Skandalakis JE, et al. Transversalis, endoabdominal, endothoracic fascia: who's who? Am Surg 2006; 72:16-8.
- Standring S. Parete addominale posteriore e retroperitoneo. In: Anatomia del Gray, 40° edizione eds Trans-edit group Srl Publ Elsevier Masson. Milano 2009:1071-3.
- Tran TM, Ivanusic JJ, Hebbard P, et al. Determination of spread of injectate after ultrasound-guided transversus abdominis plane block: a cadaveric study. Br J Anaesth. 2009;102:123-7.
- Vasques F, Stecco C, Mitri R, De Caro R, Fusco P, Behr AU. Blocking around the transversalis fascia: behind the scene. Minerva Anestesiol. 2018 Mar 27.
- Visoiu M1, Yakovleva N. Continuous postoperative analgesia via quadratus lumborum block - an alternative to transversus abdominis plane block. Paediatr Anaesth. 2013;23(10):959-61.
- Watanabe K, Mitsuda S, Tokumine J, et al. Quadratus lumborum block for femoral–femoral bypass graft placement A case report. Medicine. 2016;95:35.
- Wikner M. Unexpected motor weakness following quadratus lumborum block for gynaecological laparoscopy. Anaesthesia. 2017;72:230-2.

CLINICAL CASE 1 – ULTRASOUND-GUIDED TRANSVERSALIS FASCIA PLANE BLOCK: AN ALTERNATIVE APPROACH FOR ANESTHESIA IN INGUINAL HERNIORRHAPHY

Clinical history and anamnesis We report the use of this technique in a patient undergoing inguinal herniorrhaphy. The patient provided written permission for publication of the report. The patient was a 50-year-old man, American Society of Anesthesiologists physical status III, scheduled to undergo inguinal herniorrhaphy. His medical history included hypertensive cardiomyopathy, a moderate aortic stenosis, and severe pulmonary fibrosis.

Technique description With the patient in a supine position, a high-frequency linear US probe (15 MHz) was placed in a transverse orientation above the iliac crest. The external oblique, internal oblique, and TAMs were identified. The transducer was then moved posteriorly to where the TAM tapers off into its aponeurosis, the thoracolumbar fascia, adjacent to the quadratus lumborum muscle (QLM). Subsequently, a 22-Gauge 80 mm needle (SonoTAP, Pajunk®, Germany) was advanced using an in-plane technique. After having placed the needle tip in the virtual triangular plane located between the posterior edge of the TAM, the QLM, and the underlying transversalis fascia, 20 ml of 0.5% levobupivacaine was injected. We ultrasonically confirmed the downward displacement of the retroperitoneal fat deep into the transversalis fascia and the spread of local anesthetic over the anterior surface of the QLM (**Figure 10.12**).

Materials and methods Intraoperative sedation (score 2 on modified Wilson sedation scale) 8 was provided by intravenous propofol infusion (3 mg/kg/h) and 50 µg fentanyl. Oxygen (4 l/min) was administered by Venturi mask, and end tidal CO_2 was monitored. Reliable surgical analgesia and hemodynamic stability were achieved. Neither blood pressure nor heart rate increased during traction of the hernia sac, and no additional local anesthetic was needed. We assessed the duration of the block by testing the area (homolateral abdominal lower quadrant) for the loss of sensation to pinprick, cold, and touch sensation. By this technique, the duration of the sensory block was about 12 hours. Scheduled postoperative analgesia was provided by intravenous acetaminophen 1 g every eight hours, with intravenous 30 mg ketorolac as rescue medication. Pain intensity was assessed using a numerical rating scale of 0-10. Pain assessment was performed every three hours until hospital discharge. Postoperatively the patient reported a good-quality analgesia. During the first 24 hours after surgery, the numerical rating scale pain score was <3. Only 1g acetaminophen was required. The postoperative period was uneventful.

Conclusions We hypothesized that the US-guided TFPB could provide a reliable block of the nerves T12-L1, which pass in a virtual anatomical triangular plane located between the TAM and the transversalis fascia anterolateral to the QLM, as suggested by Hebbard in his first description. Moreover, our experience suggests that the US-guided TFPB presents a viable alternative to US-guided anterior TAPB and QLB and to general and neuraxial anesthesia. Future prospective studies will be necessary to evaluate the clinical usefulness of US-guided TFPB for inguinal hernia repair and to compare this approach with the other US-guided techniques for IIN, IHN, and GFN blocks and wound infiltration. Further studies will also be needed to investigate if US-guided TFPB may play a role in chronic postsurgical pain prevention after inguinal herniorrhaphy.

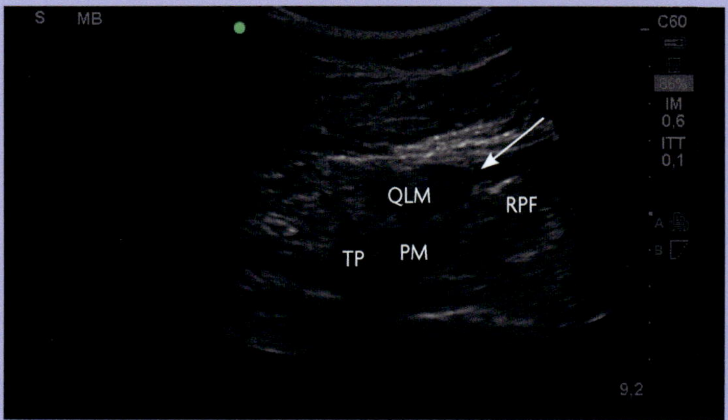

Figure 10.12 Ultrasound-guided transversalis fascia plane block. White arrow indicate the direction of the needle. QLM, quadratus lumborum muscle; RPF, retroperitoneal fat; TP: transverse process.

Quadratus lumborum block (QLB)

Astrid U. Behr, Francesco Vasques

QLB is a recently introduced analgesic block with local anesthetic (LA) injection site adjacent to the quadratus lumborum muscle (QLM). In this new interfascial truncal block distribution of injectate is influenced by fascial anatomy and remains some controversy in understanding of mechanism of action. Different injection site may produce similar spread, but distribution and effect of LA are variable and often unpredictable. Generally FPB will only provide meaningful visceral analgesia if there is LA penetration into the paravertebral space and intervertebral foramina, or via a systhemic LA effect mediated by vascular absorbtion.

The first QLB block, introduced in 2007 by R. Blanco (QLB I), described an approach similar to the transversal fascia plane block (TFP). Observing LA spread by magnetic resonance imaging (MRI), the author noted that an injection posteriorly to QLM, which means into the fascial plane between QLM and latissimus dorsi muscle (LDM), assured not only analgesic action on relevant nerves traveling within the fascial plane but also documented spread in the paravertebral space with the possibility of modulating visceral pain. As a result he abandoned the QLB I technique, preferring the posterior approach then named QLB II.

Borglum et al. instead described a different technique by crossing the QLM from posterior, called the transmuscular approach with site of LA injected anteriorly in the plane between QLM and psoas muscle (PM).

Initially the scientific evidence, mostly based on case reports, suggested that different injection sites around QLM provide various analgesic effects for different mechanisms of action. Maximum distribution of sensory block is reported from dermatomes T7 to L2, in some studies up to the fourth thoracic dermatome. The QL block targets the ilioinguinal (IGN) and iliohypogastric (IHGN) nerves, the ventral rami of T12-L2, and possibly more extensively spreads to as far as T5 and L5 nerve roots. Depending on the approach utilized and other technical factors, analgesia may be provided to the abdominal wall, hip, and possibly other areas. Recent meta-analysis confirms its role as an analgesic block in multimodal postoperative analgesia regimen after abdominal and hip surgery.

ANATOMY AND SONOANATOMY

Anatomy

The QLM is part of the posterior abdominal wall muscles, represents the anatomical reference for QLM blockand can be thought of as an anatomical bridge between the anterolateral musculature of the abdominal wall (EOM, IOM, TAM) and the lumbar paravertebral region (**Figure 11.1**). It recalls the shape of an irregular quadrilateral, caudally larger and cranially narrower and originates inferomedially from the posterior iliac crest and the iliolumbar ligament, while superiorly is attached to the inferior margin of the 12th rib. Medially QLM is in contact to the tips of the transverse process of the first four lumbar vertebras through small tendons, anteromedially it is directly adjacent to the PM, while anteriorly it is separated from colon and kidney by peritoneum and renal fascia. The subcostal nerve (T12), IHGN and IGN travel along the inner surface of QLM, covered by the extension of TF versus medial. Here we find a more or less developed layer of retroperitoneal loose connective tissue: the perinephric fat. Performing the LA injection adjacent to the QLM, the thoracolumbar fascia (TLF) may be the pathway for the spread towards the different nervous structures, the targets of the block. TLF is a multilayer of merged aponeuroses that wrap the posterior abdominal wall muscles and extends from thoracic vertebrae to lumbar vertebrae.

This multifascial structure is composed of three layers,

the anterior, middle and posterior layer of TLF. The first runs anterior to the QLM, the middle layer lies between the QLM and the spinal erector muscles (ESM) and the posterior layer wraps the ESM. The anterior layer continues medially with the epimysium of PM and laterally represents the TF covering the subcostal nerve, the IPN and the IGN. The three abdominal wall muscles (TAM, IOM and EOM) are all bordered by this fascial structure. The QLM extends from the sacral crest and medial third of the external lip of iliac crest to the posterior margin of the humerus bicipital sulcus, always wrapped by the TLF and covered posteriorly by the triangular shaped LDM.

Previously PM has been considered to represent the inferior border of the thoracic paravertebral space at T12 level. Cadaver studies have now demonstrated that it is possible to get dye spread from lumbar paravertebral area to the thoracic paravertebral space. We could speculate that there may be a route of communication through the endothoracic fascia that becomes very thin

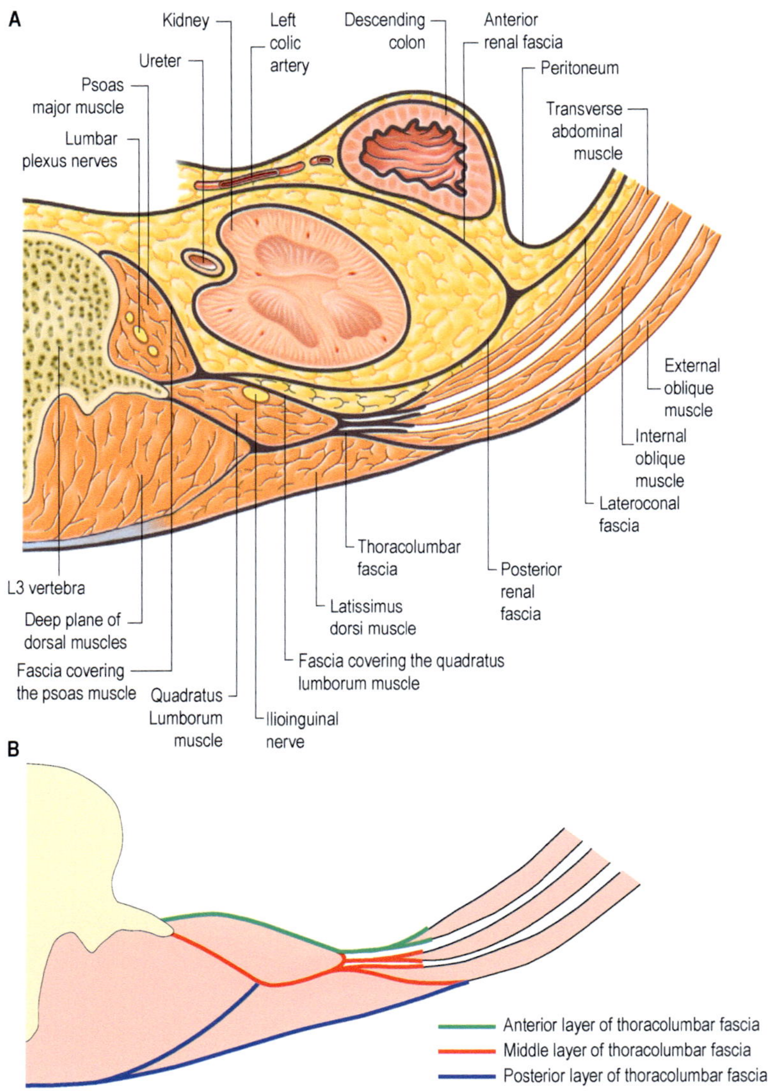

Figure 11.1 A Image of transverse section of abdomen at L3 level, right half. **B** Illustration of three-layer interpretation of thoracolumbar fascia.

at the level of diaphragm and continues and continues caudally with the TF, representing a possible pathway between the area above and below the diaphragm. Karmakar et al. demonstrated in cadaver studies that also the median and lateral arcuate ligament as well as the aortic hiatus might represent a pathway for communication between these different anatomical compartments. The TLF contains mechanoreceptors, nociceptors, and sympathetic fibers. The spread of LA to the paravertebral space and the inhibition of these sympathetic fibers seems to be responsible for the visceral pain coverage provided by this block.

Sonoanatomy

The QLM remains the main reference for correct understanding and performance of QLM block (**Figure 11.2 A, B**). To identify the muscle and surrounding anatomy, generally is preferred the patient in lateral position as it gives more exposure to a complete anatomical view, stability in handling probe and needle and comfort for the patient.

Recommending a curvilinear low-frequency transducer (2-6 MHz) positioned with a transverse scan on the midaxillary line between the iliac crest and the costal margin, the anatomical structures may be correctly identified by the shamrock technique (**Figure 11.2 C**). The acoustic shadow of the transverse process of the lumbar vertebra will represent the stem and ESM, QLM and PM the three leaves of the shamrock (**Figure 11.2 C**). As an alternative the ultrasound image can be recorded the thump up sign where the acoustic shadow of the transverse process represents the thumb and the verte-

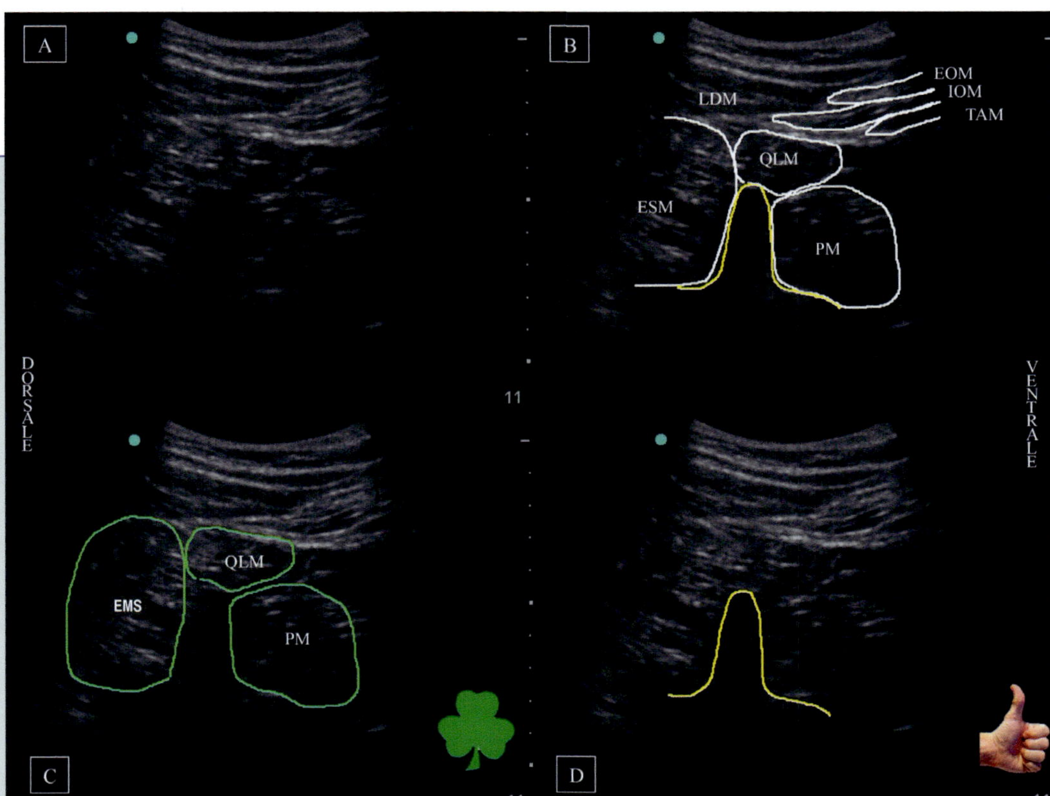

Figure 11.2 A-D Ultrasound image of posterior abdominal wall. A convex array probe is positioned between the costal margin and the iliac crest on the midaxillary line with a transverse orientation. Scan depth 11 cm, probe marker is oriented towards the patient's back. **B-D** The yellow dotted line surrounds the transverse process and the vertebral body. EOM, external oblique muscle; ESM, spinal erector muscle; IOM, internal oblique muscle; LDM, latissimus dorsi muscle; PM, psoas muscle; QLM, quadratus lumborum muscle; TAM, transverse abdominal muscle.

bral body the fist (**Figure 11.2 D**). In this scan the QLM is attached at the top of the thumb and represents with a slightly more hypoechoic aspect than the surrounding muscles and the PM anteromedially, the TAM laterally and the LDM dorsally.
Based on a patient's body habitus and approach chosen injection site, the linear probe may be an alternative. This ensures better resolution, due to a more superficial site of the block and the possibility of clearly identifying the fascial planes, particularly TLF and its relationship with QLM and the other posterior abdominal wall muscles. On the other hand does not permit a complete sonoanatomical view of the previously described scene (**Figure 11.3**).

DESCRIPTION OF TECHNIQUES

QLB is an interfascial plane block between QLM and adjacent posterior abdominal wall muscles, with at least three different possibilities for the injection site. Clinical experience and publications about these blocks are continuously growing with some discussion about nomenclature and clinical indications. Unfortunately, in the available papers, mainly case reports or case series, it is not always clear which approach has been used and until today, despite growing clinical application and evidence, there are no definitive rules or indications about technique, doses, volumes, extent of the block and correct timing. Initially described as primarily somatic blocks, in cadaver studies, the authors observed LA (dye) spread towards the posterior abdominal wall, reaching the thoracic paravertebral space and along the fascial planes a maximum distribution from T4 to L1, with likely somatic and visceral analgesia. We need to specify that dye spread in cadavers occurs differently from in the living and further clinical studies are necessary to understand the correct clinical application of these techniques in abdominal surgery.
Figure 11.4 illustrates in a schematic view the anatomy of the posterior abdominal wall and the different QLB block approaches. LA spread depends partially on the site of injection and technique, resulting in the possibility of reducing LA volumes and doses according to needle position and technique of injection.

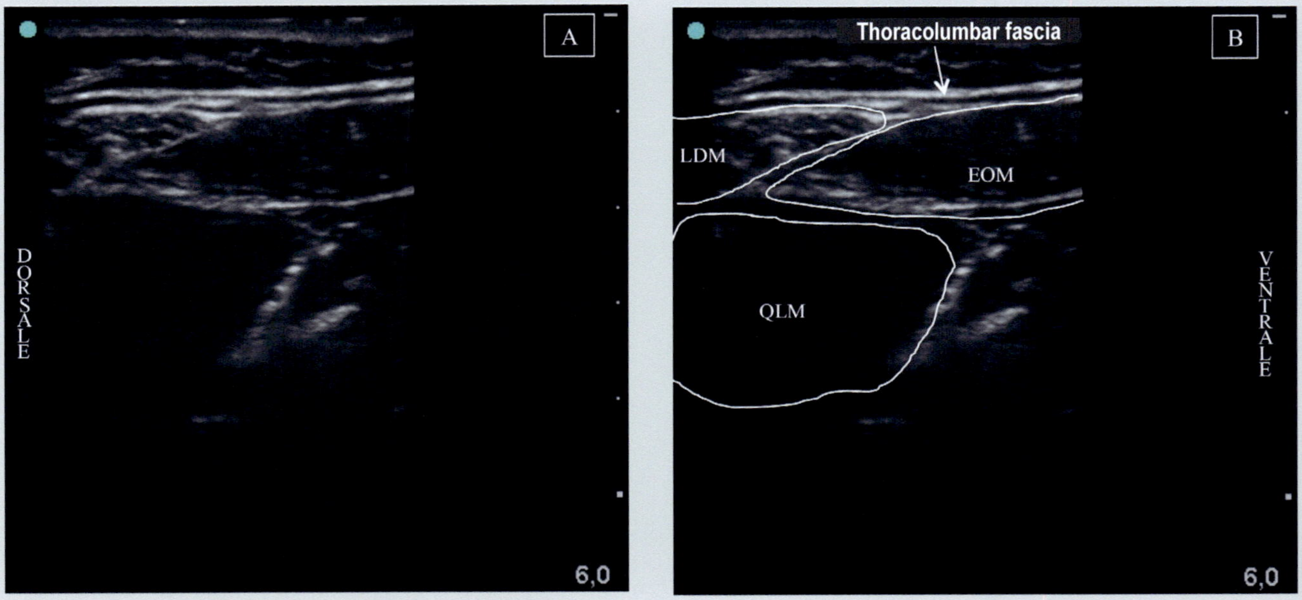

Figure 11.3 A Ultrasound image with linear probe at set depth of 6 cm, probe marker is oriented towards the patient's back. **B** Posterior abdominal wall detail at the cross of latissimus dorsi (LDM), external oblique (EOM) and quadratus lumborum (QLM) muscles. The "hook sign" is visible.

Lateral QLB approach (once QLB I)

Consists of an injection in the fascial plane between the aponeuroses of IOM and TAM at the lateral border of the QLM with an approach very similar to TFP (see Chapter 10). Block technique and LA spread have the same characteristics as that reported by Hebbard (see **Figure 11.4**). The patient is in supine position, linear probe in transverse scan between costal margin and iliac crest and in-plane needle approach from anterior-to-posterior (lateral to medial), needle trajectory crossing the three abdominal muscle layers (EOM, IOM, TAM) and injection lateral to the QLM.

Posterior QLB (once QLB II)

Consists of an injection in the fascial plane between the QLM and ESM, on the posteromedial or posterolateral surface of QLM.

The patient is in supine position with a gel roll under the buttock in slight lateral tilt for more comfortable placing of probe and needle. After accurate skin disinfection, a low frequency probe is positioned between costal margin and iliac crest and moved posteriorly identifying the three layers of the abdominal wall muscles and the posterior border of QLM (**Figure 11.5**).

Proceeding beyond the IOM end, we detect the site where EOM overlaps the QLM (hook sign) and a hyperechoic line, located between QLM and LDM, corresponding to the middle layer of TLF. This area is called lumbar interfascial triangle (LIFT), a triangular space between QLM and LDM, and is the target of the posterior approach. An echogenic needle 21 G x 80-100 mm, will be inserted with an in plane approach from anterior to posterior or from posterior to anterior. Hydrodissection with small bolus of saline help to confirm the ideal position of the needle tip between QLM, ESM and LDM on the posterior surface of the QLM in the middle layer of TLF. MRI studies have shown that injecting in this site allows to get LA spread towards the paravertebral space.

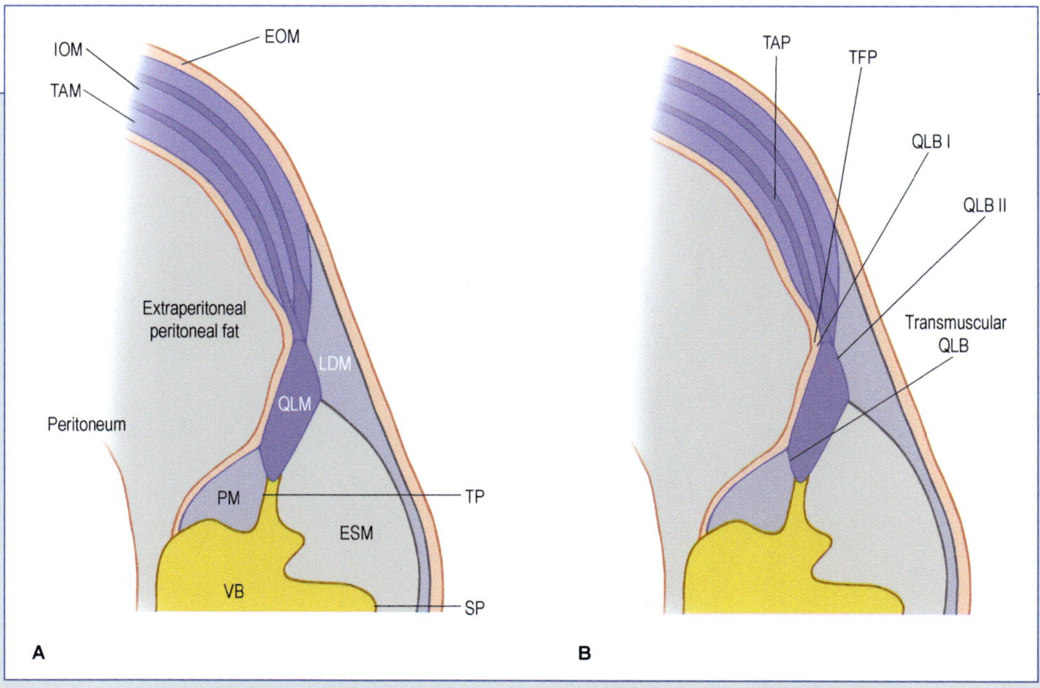

Figure 11.4 **A** Schematic illustration of the right half of posterior abdominal wall. EOM: external oblique muscle; ESM: spinal erector muscle; IOM: internal oblique muscle; LDM: latissimus dorsi muscle; PM: psoas muscle; SP: spinal process; TAM: transverse abdominal muscle; TP: transverse process; VB: vertebral column. **B** The black lines indicate the needle direction and the injection point of local anesthetic in the various indicated nerve blocks. QLB: quadratus lumborum block; TAP: transverse abdominis plane block; TFP: transversalis fascia plane block.

The main advantages of this "evolution" of QLB approach may be the possibility of LA spread towards paravertebral space, a more superficial block site with better ultrasound resolution. The interposition of QLM, separating the peritoneum from injection site contributes for safety by avoiding complications like intraperitoneal or abdominal organ puncture. It is considered an easy and superficial block with an average performance time of less than two minutes in experienced hands of and onset time of circa 30 minutes (**Figure 11.6**, **Video 11.1**).

Anterior QLB (once transmuscular QLB, tQLB or QLB III)

Consists in a transmuscular approach with injection anterior to the QLM in the fascial plane, between QLM and PM. The patient is in sitting position or in lateral decubitus with the side to be blocked up-wards. A convex probe (2-6 MHz) is placed on the midaxillary line between costal margin and iliac crest in a transversal orientation (**Figure 11.7**) and will be moved posteriorly identifying the QLM, lateral to the transverse process of the 4th lumbar vertebra and dorsal to PM.

For better understanding the anatomy for this approach we have to remember the shamrock sign with the transverse process as the stem and PM, QLM and ESM around or the thumb up sign with the QLM attached on lateral margin (tip) of transverse process, (**Figure 11.8**).

According to the approach described by Børglum, an echogenic needle 21 G x 80-100 mm is advanced in-plane from medial or lateral in a postero-anterior direction crossing ESM or LDM and QLM. LA has to be injected in small boluses in the interfascial plane between QLM and PM after repeated negative aspiration test (**Figure 11.8 C**, **D**, **Video 11.2**). This approach, called transmuscular QLB (tQLB) by its author, indicates a consistent spread of LA/dye to the lumbar nerve roots covering femoral nerve, lateral femoral cutaneous nerve, IPN and IGN, can also reach the thoracic paravertebral space (**Flow chart 11.1 online**). MRI studies showed the spread of LA cranially along the QLM reaching beyond the arcuate ligaments to thoracic area.

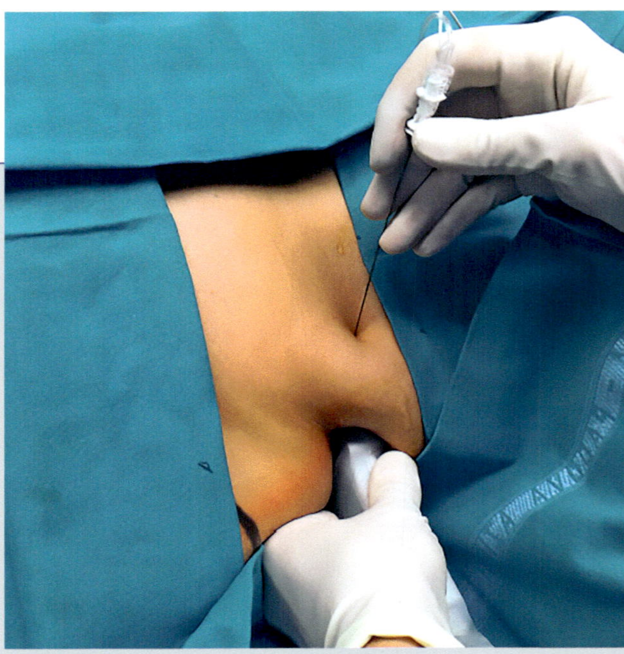

Figure 11.5 Performance of QLB II in supine patient. The convex array probe is placed between the costal margin and the iliac crest on the midaxillary line, orienting the probe marker towards dorsal. The needle is advanced in-plane with an antero-posterior (latero-medial) direction.

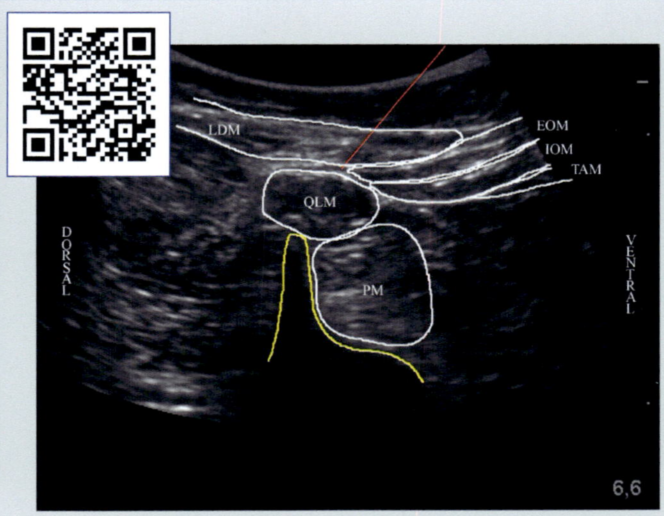

Figure 11.6 Ultrasound image with convex array probe as in **Figure 11.5**. The yellow dotted line shows the transverse process and the vertebral body. The red line shows the needle route and the injection point of local anesthetic in QLB II described by Blanco.

INDICATIONS AND LOCAL ANESTHETIC DOSES

The main indication for this truncal block consists in intra and postoperative pain treatment for abdominal and hip surgery in adult and pediatric patients. The various block techniques have different distribution of LA with not always the same analgesic effects, but there is insufficient evidence to recommend one approach over another for specific surgical types. The ideal outcome for QLB blocks will cover area of analgesia from T7 to L3 with an effect both on somatic and visceral pain. In various reports successful use of QLB (all approaches) has been described for the following surgical procedures: proctosigmoidectomy, hip surgery, above-knee amputation, iliac crest harvest, abdominal hernia repair, breast reconstruction, colostomy closure, radical nephrectomy, lower extremity vascular surgery, total hip arthroplasty, laparotomy and colectomy.

More details for technique and indications with the different approaches are:

- *Lateral QLB*: various RCT demonstrated reduced opioid consumption for 48h after cesarean section and hip surgery. A recent RCT in laparoscopic cholecystectomy reports benefit for postoperative opioid consumption versus continuous iv infusion of lidocaine. The consistent evidence for its analgesic effects for cesarean and abdominal surgery demonstrates also its superiority compared to the TAP block.
- *Posterior QLB*: RCT double blind studies versus placebo or versus TAP block documented an opioid sparing effect after cesarean section. Similar studies in laparoscopic gynecologic surgery confirm this block as helpful in reducing postoperative pain. It has also been studied for its analgesic affects in laparoscopic cholecystectomy and in hip and vertebral surgery. There are some case reports with bilateral catheter and continuous infusion of ropivacaine in abdominal surgery. Chronic neuropathic disorders, such as abdominal wall allodynia after multiple surgery, seems to benefit

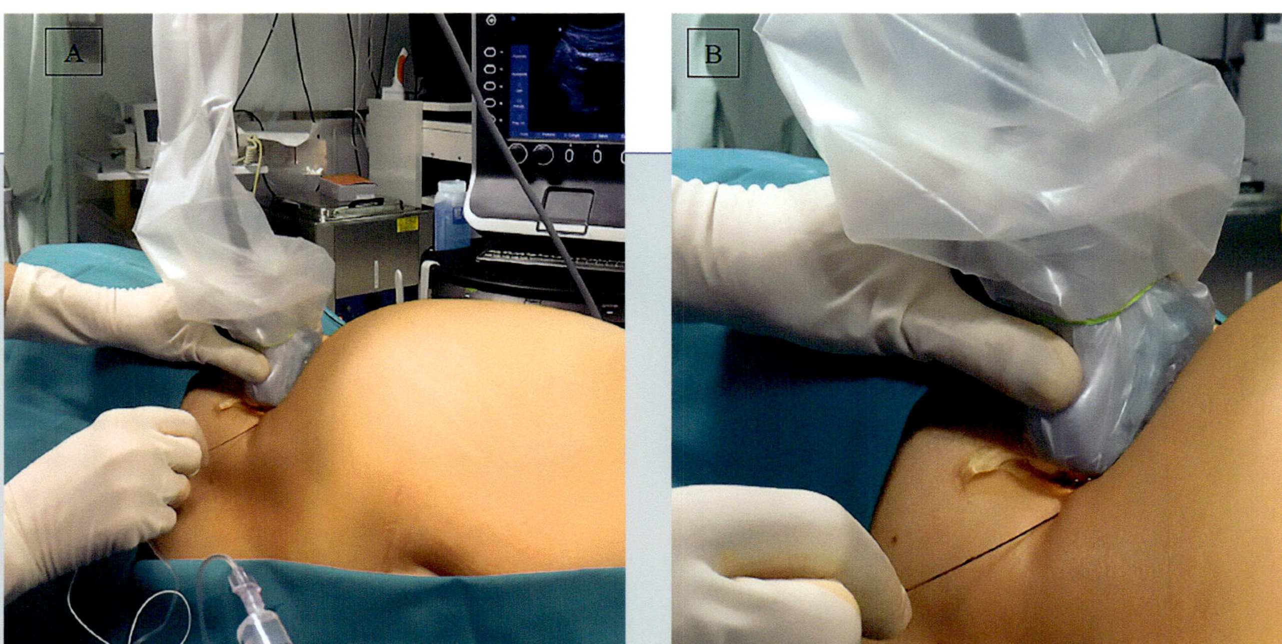

Figure 11.7 A Patient in lateral position for performing a tQLB described by Børglum. For the most ergonomic position, the operator is at the patient's back with the ultrasound machine in front, An assistant injects small boluses of local anesthetic with intermittent aspiration. **B** Detail of in-plane probe-needle alignment. The site of puncture is at an appropriate distance from the probe, to optimize needle visibility and maneuverability.

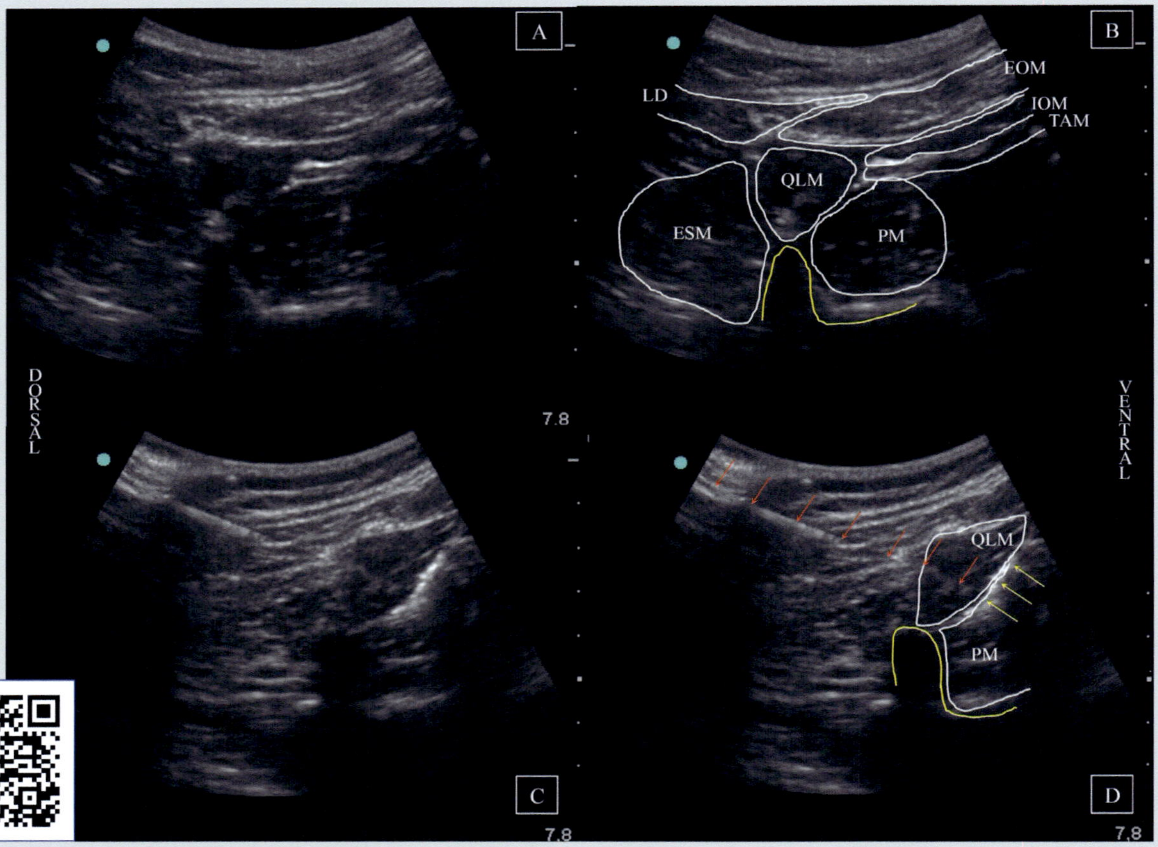

Figure 11.8 A Ultrasound image of posterior abdominal wall during transmuscular QLB by Børglum. A convex array probe is positioned between the costal margin and the iliac crest on the midaxillary line with a transverse orientation. Scan depth 8 cm, the probe marker is oriented toward dorsal. **B** LDM, latissimu dorsi muscle; QLM, quadratus lumborum muscle; EOM, external oblique muscle; IOM, internal oblique muscle; TAM, transverse abdominal muscle; PM, psoas muscle; ESM, erector spine muscle. The yellow dotted line surrounds the transverse process and the vertebral body. **C** Needle in-plane trajectory through the abdominal wall muscles and local anesthetic spread in the plane between QLM and PM. **D** Same image. Red arrows indicate the needle trajectory crossing the abdominal wall; yellow arrows indicate the anterior layer of thoracolumbar fascia; the yellow dotted line surrounds the transverse process. PM, psoas muscle; QLM, quadratus lumborum muscle.

from bilateral continuous infusion of LA by catheter.

- *Anterior QLB*: there is a large degree of heterogeneity in studies for tQLB, but the initial indications in abdominal surgery are confirmed by various studies. Apart from an evidence-based application for caesarean section, less pain and a postoperative opioid sparing effect are demonstrated in 2 RCT with QLB versus placebo for percutaneous nephrolithotomy and QLB versus TAP block in laparoscopic bariatric surgery. There are further indications for prosthetic hip surgery and for prevention of persistent postsurgical pain after iliac crest harvest. Unilateral and bilateral catheter positioning and infusion with LA and intermittent bolus for several days were described in cases of nephrectomy and hip surgery.

Cadaver studies showed variable results. Dam and Moriggl's experience confirms dye spread towards subcostal nerve, IHGN and IGN and thoracic spread mainly posteriorly to the arcuate ligaments (T9-T12), Carline's research, claims that dye was never detected inside the lumbar plexus, PM or in the lumbar sympathetic trunk. A recent systematic review and meta-analysis to determine the role of ultrasound-guided quadratus lumborum block for postoperative analgesia, included data from 27 studies with 1557 patients. The main findings were that QLB reduces postoperative opioid consumption, prolongs the time to the first rescue opioid analgesic and diminishes the incidence of PONV after abdominal, obstetric, gynecologic, urologic and hip surgery in adult patients.

Unfortunately, there is a scarcity of studies that compare different QLB techniques and only one study compares QLB versus epidural analgesia, where the results clearly favoured the epidural block, indicating superiority of the central block as a regional analgesic technique. These issues will be clarified only in future when ongoing clinical trials are completed and new RC studies designed.

Who cannot have a block

Absolute contraindications:

- patient refusal
- true LA allergy
- local infection at injection/procedure site

Relative contraindications:

- surgery near the injection site (catheter)
- disorders of coagulation or platelet aggregation (hematoma)

COMPLICATIONS AND CONTRAINDICATIONS

All complications described for the TAP block may be present but reported complications and adverse effects related to QLB are minimal. There may be some considerations related to safety to prefer one technique over the other. If the anatomical site of posterior QLB is more superficial, in particular with the QLM inserted between the peritoneum and the needle tip, peritoneal injection or abdominal organ puncture are more difficult to achieve (intestinal lesion, renal hematoma).

The QLB procedures are generally performed at a significant distance from sensitive structures and do not appear to have serious complications like neuraxial and paravertebral blockade, such as epidural hematoma, epidural abscess, and pneumothorax. In addition, interfascial plane blocks may be associated with less risk of serious bleeding complications in the presence of anticoagulation or antiplatelet therapy relative to neuraxial and paravertebral. The risks of bleeding complications are not yet known and there is actually no stratification of the risk. The posterior and lateral approach are using a fascial plane through where pass the abdominal branches of lumbar arteries, but is considered a compressible area. The anterior approach has to be considered a deep block site with risk of retroperitoneal spread of hematoma and where hemostatic compression will be difficult to apply. Nonetheless, there remains potential for clinically significant hematoma and the procedure must be avoided in patients with blood coagulation and platelet aggregation disorders. The important vascularization of fascial planes means also more risk of absorption of LA and LAST (local anesthetic systemic toxicity). Reported symptoms of LAST after QLB were arrhythmias in two cases, tinnitus in three and a metallic taste in nine patients.

There are no reported cases of infectious complications from QLB and little has been published regarding the frequency of reported side effects. The incidence of limb weakness after anterior and posterior QLB is low, but can contribute to delay mobilization and discharge in few patients.

Complications

- Intraperitoneal injection
- Abdominal organ puncture
- Renal or retroperitoneal hematoma
- LAST
- Block failure
- Limb weakness

CHRONIC PAIN INDICATION

The QLB seems to also have indication in chronic pain treatment and for the prevention of chronic postsurgical pain (**Table 11.1**).

TABLE 11.1 DOSES AND VOLUMES OF LA IN QLB

	VOLUME OF AT	MEDICATIONS	DOSES
Adult patient	0.3-0.6 ml/kg per side (15-25 ml per side)	Ropivacaine 0.2%-0.5% Levobupivacaine 0.125%-0.37-5%	2-3 mg/kg

RECOMMENDED READING

- Abrahams M, Derby R, Horn J. Update on ultrasound for truncal blocks: a review of the evidence. Reg Anesth Pain Med. 2016; 41, 2: 275-88.
- Adhikary SD, El-Boghdadly K, Nasralah Z, et al. A radiologic and anatomic assessment of injectated spread following transmuscular quadratus lumborum block in cadavers. Anaesthesia. 2017;72: 73-9.
- Baidya DK, Maitra S, Arora MK, et al. Quadratus lumborum block: an effective method of perioperative analgesia in children undergoing pyeloplasty. J Clin Anesth. 2015;27:694.
- Behr AU, Vasquez F. The Thumb-up: a different view of the Shamrock lumbar plexus block. Minerva Anestesiol. 2018 May 28.
- Blanco R, Ansari T, Girgis E. Quadratus lumborum block for postoperative pain after caesarean section. Eur J Anaesthesiol. 2015; 32:1-7.
- Blanco R, Ansari T, Riad W, Shetty N. Quadratus lumborum block versus transversus abdominis plane block for postoperative pain after cesarean delivery. Regional Anesthesia and Pain Medicine. 2016;41(6):757-62.
- Blanco R, McDonnell JG. Optimal point of injection: The quadratus lumborum type I and II blocks. Htpp://www.respond2articles.com/ANA/forums/Post/1550.aspx (accessed 10 july 2018).
- Børglum J, Christensen AF, Hoegberg LCG, et al. Bilateral-dual transversus abdominis (BD-TAP) block or thoracic paravertebral block (TPVB)? Distribution patterns, dermatomal anaesthesia and LA pharmacokinetics. Reg Anesth Pain Med. 2012;37(7):E136-9.
- Børglum J, Moriggl B, Jensen K, et al. Ultrasound-guided transmuscular quadratus lumborum blockade. Br J Anaesth. 2013.
- Carline L, McLeod GA, Lamb C. A cadaver study comparing spread of dye and nerve involvement after three different quadratus lumborum blocks. BJA. 2016;117(3):387-94.
- Carney J, Finnerty O, Rauf J, et al. Studies on the spread of local anaesthetics solution in transversus abdominis plane blocks. Anaesthesia. 2011;66:1023-30.
- Carvalho R, Segura E, do Cèu Loureiro M, et al. Quadratus lumborum block in chronic pain after abdominal hernia repair: Case report. Rev Bras Anestesiol. 2017 Jan - Feb;67(1):107-9.
- Dam M, Moriggl B, Hansen CK, Hoerman R, et al. The Pathway of Injectate Spread With the Transmuscular Quadratus Lumborum Block: A Cadaver Study. Anesth Analg. 2017.
- El-Boghdadly K, Elsharkawy H, Short A. Quadratus Lumborum Block Nomenclature and Anatomical Considerations Reg Anesth Pain Med. 2016;41(4):548-9.
- El-Boghdadly K, Wolmarans M. Standardizing nomenclature in regional anesthesia: an ASRA-ESRA Delphi consensus study of abdominal wall, paraspinal, and chest wall blocks. Reg Anesth Pain Med 2021;46:571–580. doi:10.1136/rapm-2020-102451 (eventualmente togliere articolo di El-Boghdadly del 2016)
- Elsharkawy H, El.Boghdadly K, Kolli S, et al. Injectade spread following anterior subcostal and posterior approach to the quadratus lumborum block. Eur J Anaesthesiol. 2017;34:587-95.
- Elsharkawy H, El-Boghdadly K et al. Quadratus Lumborum Block Anatomical Concepts, Mechanisms, and Techniques. Anesthesiology 2019; 130:322–35. (eventualmente togliere articolo di Elsharkawy del 2017).
- Hansen CK, Dam M, Bendtsen TF, Børglum J. Ultrasound-guided quadratus lumborum blocks: definition of the clinical relevant endpoint of injection and the safest approach. A Case Rep. 2016;6:39.
- Hebbard PD. Transversalis fascia plane block, a novel ultrasound-guided abdominal wall nerve block. Can J Anesth. 2009; 56: 618-20.
- Hockett M, Hembrador S, Lee A. Quadratus Lumborum Block for Postoperative Pain in Total Hip Arthroplasty: A Case Report. A & A case reports 2016;7(6):129-31.
- Ishio J. Komasawa N, Kido H, et al. Evaluation of ultrasound-guided posterior quadratus lumborum block for postoperative analgesia after laparoscopic gynecologic surgery. J Clin Anesth. 2017; 41, 1-4.
- Kang W, Lu D, Yang X, et al. Postoperative analgesic effects of various quadratus lumborum block approaches following cesarean section: a randomized controlled trial. J Pain Res 2019; 12:2305–2312.
- Karmakar MK, Gin T, Ho AMH. Ipsilateral thoracolumbar anaesthesia and paravertebral spread after low thoracic paravertebral injection. BJA. 2001; 87(2):312-6.
- Kim DH, Kim SJ. Fascial plane blocks: a narrative review of the literature. Reg Anesth Pain Med 2021;46:600–617. doi:10.1136/rapm-2020-101909.
- Korgvee A, Junttila E, KoskinenH et al. Ultrasound-guided quadratus lumborum block for postoperative analgesia A systematic review and meta-analysis. Eur J Anaesthesiol 2021; 38:115–129.
- Lönnquist PA, Hildingsson U. The caudal boundary of the thoracic paravertebral space. A study in human cadavers. Anaesthesia. 1992;47:1051-2.
- Murouchi T, Iwasaki S, Yamakage M. Quadratus lumborum block: analgesic effects and chronological ropivacaine concentrations after laparoscopic surgery," Reg Anesth Pain Med. 2016;41(2):146-50.
- Parras T, Blanco R. Randomised trial comparing the transversus abdominis plane block posterior approach or quadratus lumborum block type I with femoral block for postoperative analgesia in femoral neck fracture, both ultrasound-guided. Rev Esp Anestesiol Reanim. 2016;63(3):141-8.
- Rebuffat P. Nervi spinali. In: Anatomia funzionale del sistema nervoso. Mazzocchi G, Nussdorfer G Pubs Libreria Cortina, Padova 1996:344-9.
- Rosenberg PH, Veering BT, Urmey WF. Maximum recommended doses of local anesthetics: a multifactorial concept. Reg Anesth Pain Med. 2004;29:564-75.
- Rozen WM, Tran TM, Ashton MW, et al. Refining the course of the thoracolumbar nerves: a new understanding of the innervation of the anterior abdominal wall. Clin Anat. 2008;21:325-33.
- Saito T, Den S, Tanuma K, et al. Anatomical basis for paraver-

tebral anesthetic block: fluid communication between the thoracic and lumbar paravertebral regions. Surg Radiol Anat. 1999;21:359-63.
- Sato M. An antero-lateral approach to ultrasound-guided lumbar plexus block in supine position combined with quadratus lumborum block using single-needle insertion for pediatric hip surgery. Ped Anesth. 2017;27:1064-5.
- Sauter AR, Ullensvang K, Bendtsen TF, et al. The 'Shamrock Method' - a new and promising technique for ultrasound guided lumbar plexus blocks. Br J Anaesth 2013: e-letter, Published 26 February 2013, http://bja.oxfordjournals.org/fo.
- Schuenke MD, Vieming A, Van Hoof T. A description of the lumbar interfascial triangle and its relation with the lateral raphe: Anatomical constituents of load transfer through the lateral margin of the thoracolumbar fascia. J Anat. 2012;221:568-76.
- Shaaban M, Sakr Esa W, Maheshwari K, et al. Bilateral Continuous Quadratus Lumborum Block for Acute Postoperative Abdominal Pain as a Rescue After Opioid-Induced Respiratory Depression. A&A Case Rep. 2015;5:107-11.
- Sondekoppam RV, Ip V, Johnston DF, et al. Ultrasound-guided lateral-medial transmuscular quadratus lumborum block for analgesia following anterior iliac crest bone graft harvesting: a clinical and anatomical study. Can J Anesth 2018;65(2):178-87.
- Sondekoppam RV. Continuous quadratus lumborum block analgesia for total hip arthroplasty revision. J of Clin Anest. 2016;35;235-7.
- Standring S. Parete addominale posteriore e retroperitoneo. In: Anatomia del Gray, 40° edizione eds Trans-edit group Srl Publ Elsevier Masson, Milano 2009: 1061- 3.
- Tamura T, Yokota S et al. Local anesthetic spread into the paravertebral space with two types of quadratus lumborum blocks: a crossover volunteer study. Journal of Anesthesia (2019) 33:26–32.
- Ueshima H, Otake H, Lin J. Ultrasound-Guided Quadratus Lumborum Block: An Updated Review of Anatomy and Techniques. Biomed Res Int. 2017;2017:2752876.
- Ueshima H, Otake H. Clinical experiences of unilateral anterior sub-costal quadratus lumborum block for a nephrectomy. J Clin Anesth 2018;44:120.
- Ueshima H, Otake H. Lumbar vertebra surgery performed with a bilateral posterior quadratus lumborum block. J of Clin Anesth. 2017;41:61.
- Ueshima H, Otake H. The Ultrasound guided continuous transmuscular quadratus lumborum block in an effective analgesia for total hip arthroplasty. J Clin Anesth. 2016;1:35.
- Vasques F, Behr AU, Weinberg G, et al. A Review of Local Anesthetic Systemic Toxicity 2015;40(6):698-705.
- Vasques F, Stecco C, Mitri R, De Caro R, Fusco P, Behr AU. Blocking around the transversalis fascia: behind the scene. Minerva Anestesiol. 2018 Mar 27.

CLINICAL CASE 1 – COULD THE ULTRASOUND-GUIDED QUADRATUS LUMBORUM BLOCK TYPE 2 BE A VIABLE ALTERNATIVE TO EPIDURAL ANALGESIA FOR POSTOPERATIVE PAIN RELIEF IN LAPAROSCOPIC ABDOMINAL SURGERY?

Clinical history and anamnesis Although epidural analgesia is commonly considered the gold standard for post-operative pain management in abdominal surgery, there is increasing evidence in literature that less invasive, alternative regional techniques, such as the ultrasound-guided quadratus lumborum block type 2 (US-QLB 2) could be as effective as epidural analgesia, in particular after laparoscopic surgical procedures.
A 52-year-old patient, ASA 2, underwent laparoscopic right hemi-colectomy. Written informed consent was obtained.

Technique description After induction of general anesthesia, we performed the US-QLB 2 by injecting 20 ml of 0,375% levobupivacaine for each side, in the fascial plane between quadratus lumborum and latissimus dorsi muscles. Before the end of surgery, 1 g of acetaminophen and Ketorolac 30 mg were intravenously administered (**Figures 11.9**, **11.10**).

Materials and methods Intraoperative hemodynamic stability was obtained. In the first 24 hours after surgery, patient reported a prolonged pain relief. Only 3 g of acetaminophen and ketorolac 90 mg were administered, with no opioids needed. No discomfort or complications were recorded postoperatively.

Conclusions This case report suggested that US-QLB 2 could provide long-lasting analgesia and improve visceral pain control, likely due to extension of local anesthetic into the paravertebral space. The spread to the thoracic paravertebral space is believed to result from the embryonic origin of the QL and PM muscles in the thoracic cage and the continuation of the transversalis fascia with the endothoracic fascia at the level of the arcuate ligaments at the diaphragm. Further studies are needed to confirm if this technique may be considered a safe and effective alternative to epidural analgesia in laparoscopic surgery.

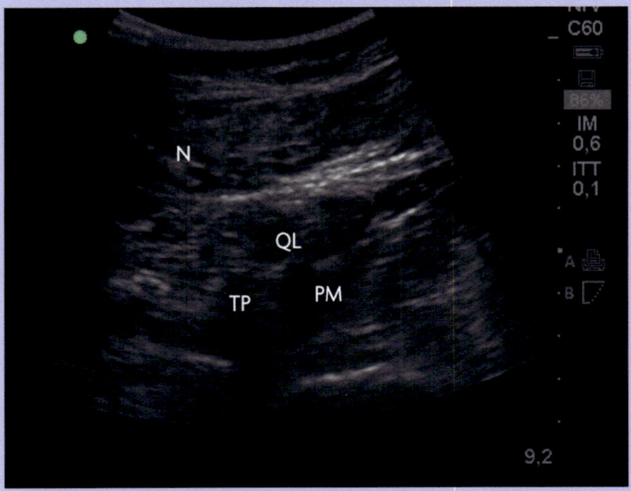

Figure 11.9 Needle directed towards the QL. TP: transvers process, N: needle, QL: quadratus lomborum, PM: psoas muscle.

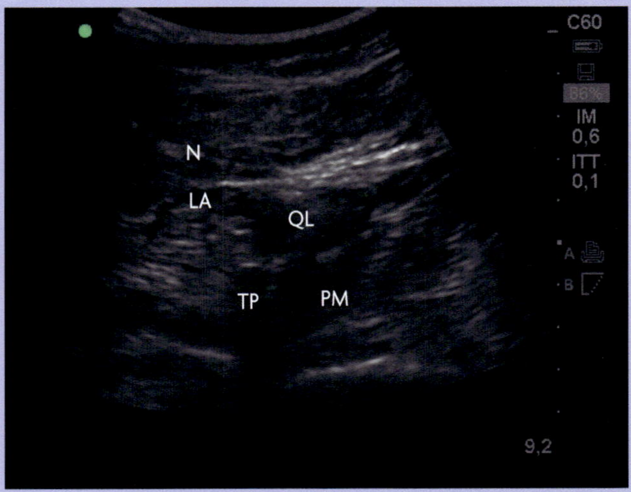

Figure 11.10 Spread of LA below the thoracolumbar fascia. TP: transvers process, N: needle, QL: quadratus lomborum, PM: psoas muscle, LA: local anesthetic.

CHAPTER 12

Ultrasound-guided trunk and abdominal wall blocks in children

Vittorio Lucchetta, Giuseppe Paladini, Nicola Zadra

In the last twenty years locoregional anesthesia (LRA) has been widely used also in Pediatrics, thanks to its excellent profiles of efficacy and safety.

The recent discovery of potential toxic effects of general anesthetic drugs on the developing brain of many mammals, bearing the risk of long-term cognitive impairment, has raised the concern of similar neurotoxic effects on children.

Acknowledged literature and international organizations such as the FDA (Food and Drug Administration) suggest to adopt all possible strategies to reduce children exposure to general anesthesia in their first years. Based on this, LRA is considered to have an added value in Pediatrics, as this is the anesthetic technique which better allows to reduce the total dose of general anesthetics during surgery.

Recent epidemiological studies have shown how LRA in children is associated with a low complication morbidity (total 0.42%) and that their extent is mostly moderate, but especially that the peripheral blocks are likely to cause complications six times less than the central blocks. As in the adult population, pediatric thoracic and abdominal surgeries – once managed with neuraxial anesthesia – have become a field for peripheral blocks, which will be described in this chapter:

- thoracic paravertebral block;
- transversus abdominis plane (TAP) block;
- ilioinguinal and iliohypogastric nerve block;
- rectus sheath block;
- erector spinae plane block.

All these blocks can play an important role in a multimodal management of intraoperative and postoperative pain in pediatric surgery.

Anatomy and sonoanatomy of every single block are the same that are described in detail for adults, so we suggest you to refer to those chapters for further description.

In children, we often work on a superficial level and on small areas, so a small high-frequency probe (7-12 MHz) allows to perform most peripheral blocks, as are described in this chapter (**Figure 12.1**).

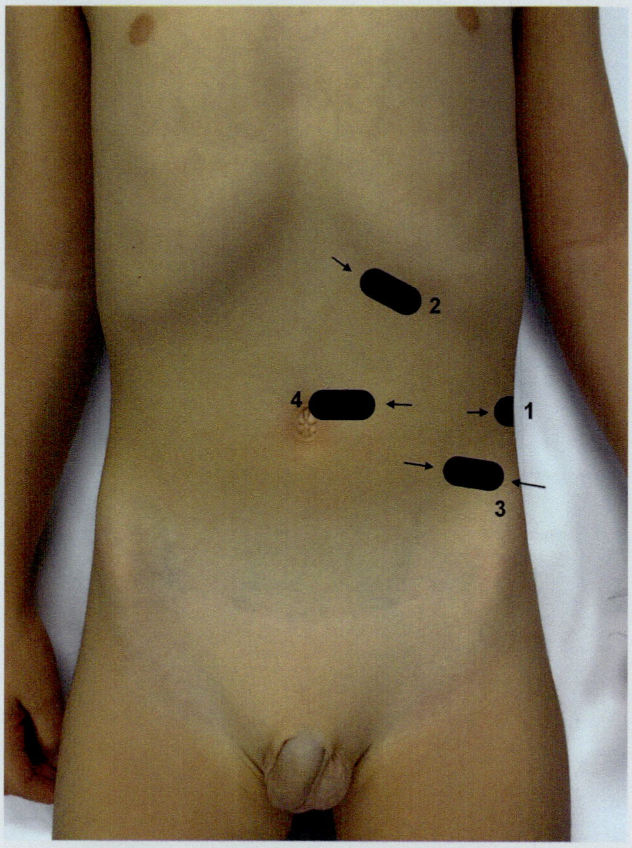

Figure 12.1 Landmarks for US transducer and needle positioning for the abdominal wall blocks. 1: TAP block; 2: subcostal TAP block; 3: iliohypogastric and ilioinguinal nerve block; 4: rectus sheath block.

The peripheral block technique can be used in children as well as in adults, while the local and the general anesthesia management are different, as children always require a deep sedation or general anesthesia combined with the block. Performing an anesthetic block on a deeply sedated patient or under general anesthesia has pros and cons. Among the former, the procedure can be performed on an immobile and unconscious patient; if a child is under general anesthesia, there is complete control of his vitals and we benefit from the protective role of general anesthetic drugs on the central nervous system (CNS) from any toxic effect. Among the cons, the anesthesiologist can gather less direct clinical information in case of technical errors or possible complications; this means that the block technique must be meticulous, and the injection of local anesthetics must be performed according to precise rules, as there are no neurological warnings of acute intoxication, caused by local anesthetics, and the test dose, which is commonly administered to adults, is meaningless in a sedated child. The anesthetic injection must be slow and fractionated, interrupted by frequent aspiration tests and combined with a close exam of ECG tracing, with special care for the T wave, which may appear higher in an acute intoxication from local anesthetics, especially if adrenaline is added. The ultrasound-guided injection by in-plane technique is even safer, allowing direct visualization of the needle tip and the surrounding structures.

THORACIC PARAVERTEBRAL BLOCK

Anatomy and sonoanatomy

The paravertebral space is a wedge-shaped space, whose posterior boundary is formed by the posterior costotransverse ligament and the internal intercostal membrane, the anterior boundary is the parietal pleura, and the base is formed by the vertebral discs and bodies and the intervertebral foramina. As anatomy and sonoanatomy in children do not differ from adults, please refer to Chapter 2.

Block target

Paravertebral analgesia is obtained by injecting local anesthetic along the vertebral column close to the spinal nerves. The anesthetic spread along the column, in front of the transverse processes, produces a multilevel anesthetic block. The anesthetic can spread also laterally along the intercostal spaces and medially in the epidural space, so in some cases the thoracic paravertebral block (PVB) appears as an epidural block, with a bilateral spread. The mechanism of action of the PVB is mutimodal, but it primarily bears an anesthetic effect on the homolateral spinal nerves and the sympathetic chain.

Description of the technique

The use of thoracic paravertebral block was described in children for the first time by P.A. Lonnqvist in 1992, 87 years after the technique had been introduced in adults. For the traditional approach, as in the adult, the needle must be inserted dorsally, 1.5-3 cm laterally to the cranial border of the spinous process; the needle is advanced until it touches the transverse process of the underlying vertebra, then redirected cranially, in order to proceed beyond the process. This technique was based on a loss of resistance (using air or saline) as the needle crossed the costotransverse ligament. Either a short-bevel or a Tuohy needle can be used. This "blind" technique can enjoy the use of a nerve stimulator to elicit the contraction of the abdominal muscles, once the needle has reached its target.

The introduction of thoracoscopy offered the chance for an interesting approach to the thoracic PVB, guided by direct visualization. This technique is particularly useful when a continuous block is needed, as it is possible to visually control the insertion of the needle and the advancement of the catheter under the parietal pleura, thanks to the thoracoscopic guide used by surgeons for the operation (**Figure 12.2**); likewise, this technique can be performed under thoracotomy.

The addition of ultrasound guidance to the LRA techniques opened new frontiers, allowing to monitor in real time both the placement of the needle in the paravertebral space and the spread of the local anesthetic, increasing the safety and efficacy of the method. The ultrasound-guided PVB technique is the same in adults as in children. In children the block is always performed after the general anesthesia or sedation

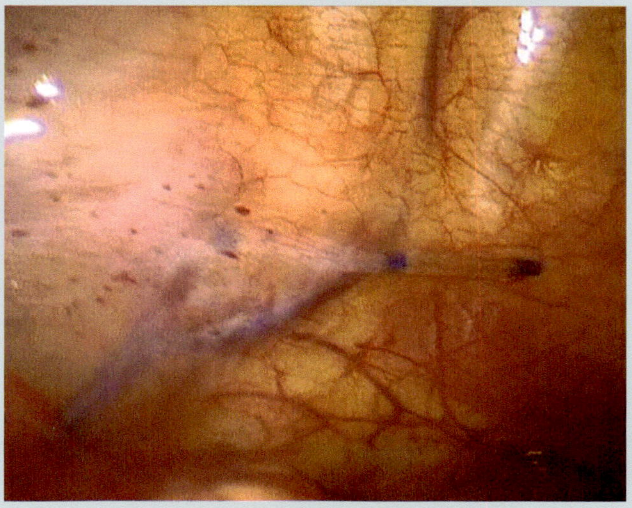

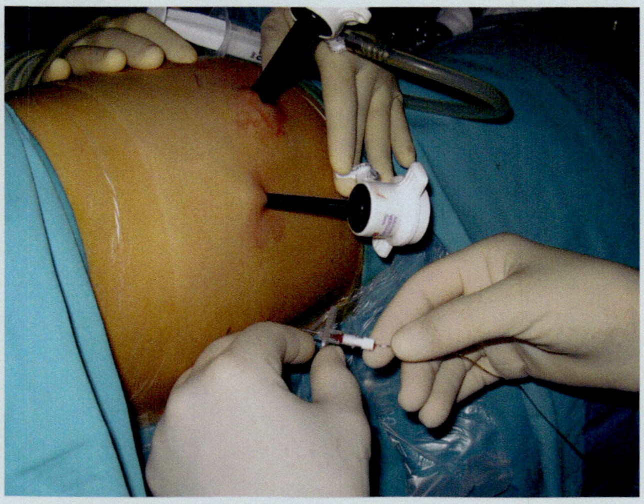

Figure 12.2 A thoracic paravertebral catheter positioned under thoracoscopic guidance.

and patients are placed in lateral decubitus position, with the affected side upwards; a prone position can be used to perform a bilateral block.

To perform an ultrasound-guided block, the following material is necessary: a high frequency linear probe (7-12 MHz), a sterile probe cover, sterile gel, a short bevel needle or Tuohy needle (better if with extension), sterile drapes and an antiseptic solution to create a sterile field.

The ultrasound transducer is positioned in order to obtain a transverse scan of the column, visualizing the spinous process, which will appear as an upside down hyperechogenic V, with a shadow cone underneath. Moving the transducer laterally, with a slight cranio-caudal inclination, the operator will recognize the transverse process (hyperechogenic, with a shadow cone), the pleura (hyperechogenic and moving with breathing), the intercostal muscles and the internal intercostal membrane (**Figure 12.3**). If the hyperechogenic costal margin is visible, the transducer has to be moved a few millimeters caudally in order to gain the typical image of the thoracic paravertebral space. For the paravertebral injection (**Figures 12.4**, **12.5**, **Video 12.1**) both out-of-plane and in-plane approaches are described, but only the latter allows to see the needle (SonoPlex stim Pajunk®) insertion in all its length, up to the passing under the transverse process. Unfortunately, the transverse process shadow cone does not allow to visualize the needle tip during injection, but the downward displacement of the pleura proves the correct administration of anesthetic inside the paravertebral space.

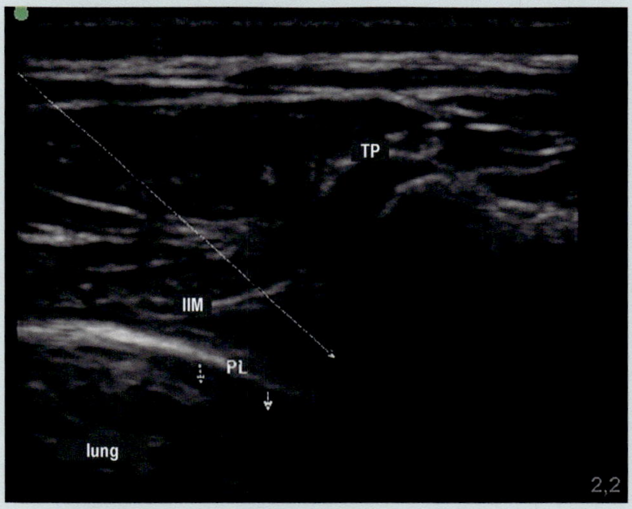

Figure 12.3 Thoracic paravertebral block sonoanatomy. IIM: internal intercostal membrane; PL: pleura; TP: transverse process.

In order to place a catheter, either a Tuohy needle (catheter-through-needle) or a catheter-over-needle system (E-Cath®) can be used; the latter has the great advantage

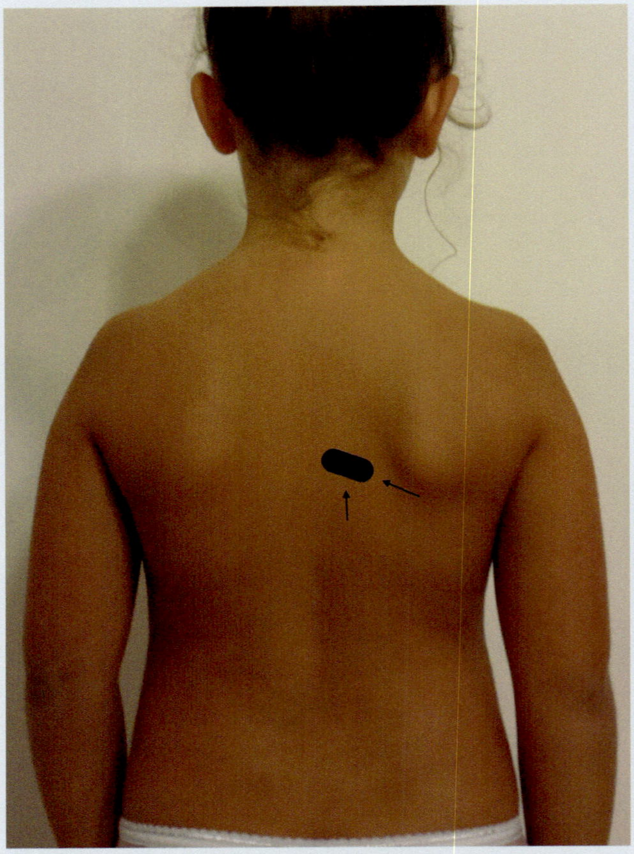

Figure 12.4 US transducer position for a mid-thoracic paravertebral block. Arrows describe the position of the needle for in-plane and out-of-plane approaches.

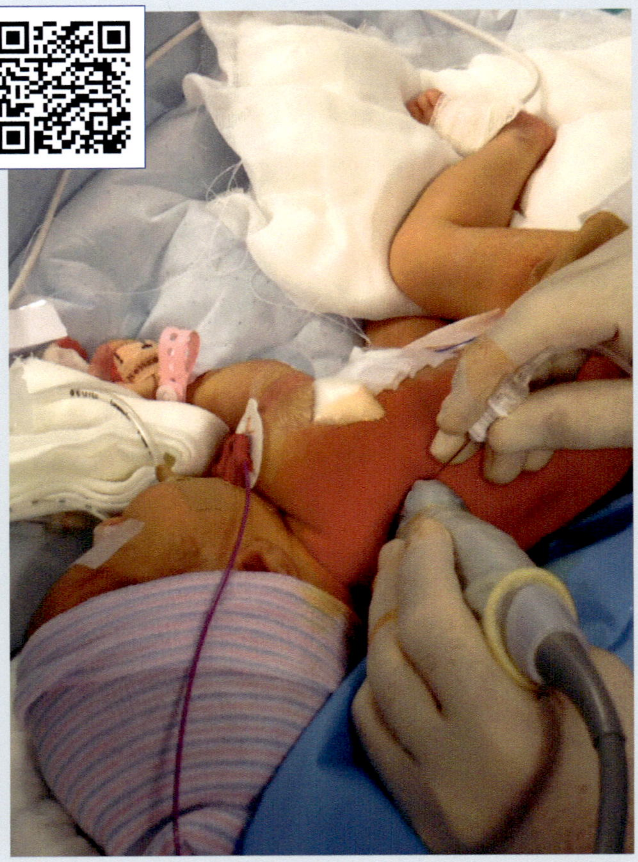

Figure 12.5 In-plane approach for a thoracic paravertebral block.

of minimizing the risk of anesthetic leakage at the insertion point, a common event in children, which often leads to catheter displacement and ineffective analgesia.
The block can be performed both as a single shot or a continuous one, even bilaterally, with a caveat on the risk of trespassing the toxic dosage.
It is known that the sympathetic block is more extended than the somatic block and that the anesthetic has a greater caudal spread from the injection site. 0.25 ml/kg of contrast medium spread radiologically for an average of 5.7 segments. In a corpse 0.5 ml/kg of methylene blue, that is injected on T12-L1 level, spread from T7 to L2.
The current Guidelines recommend not to exceed a volume of 0.5 ml/kg of 0.25% bupivacaine, levobupivacaine or 0.2% ropivacaine in the single-shot blocks and a dose by continuous infusion of 0.25 mg/kg/h of 0.125% levobupivacaine or 0.1-0.2% of ropivacaine.
In the newborn it is recommended to stop the continuous infusion after 36-48 hours.

Indications

Pediatric indications are: intraoperative and postoperative analgesic therapy for thoracotomies and thoracoscopies, for upper abdominal surgery (liver and gallbladder surgery, spleen, kidney and adrenal surgery) but also for lower abdominal surgery (inguinal hernia, for example); analgesic therapy for thoracic traumas and rib fractures.
In children, a thoracic PVB, also performed bilaterally, can be a good alternative to the thoracic epidural block for thoracic and upper abdominal surgery. Compared to

the central blocks it has fewer risks, fewer contraindications, and some advantages: a longer duration and less interference with the post-thoracotomy lung function.

Complications and contraindications

The classic technique, based on anatomic landmarks and loss of resistance test (LORT), was quite unsuccessful (10.1%) and it had complications such as pneumothorax (0.5%), intrathecal or epidural administration, hypotension (4.6%), vascular injection (3.8%), which in the past contributed to a poor circulation of the method.
Of course, the ultrasound guide has the advantage of reducing the complication rate, thanks to the direct and continuous view of the needle-anatomical structure relationship. A 2016 retrospective study reported only 6 complications out of 1500 ultrasound-guided paravertebral blocks (3 hypotensions/symptomatic bradycardia, 1 vasovagal episode, 2 plausible local anesthetic toxicities) with no pneumothorax or pleural accidental injections.
In children, little is known also of the pharmacokinetics of drugs injected in the paravertebral space. The plasmatic absorption of local anesthetics is high in this area and high doses of anesthetic (eg. in the bilateral block) can produce toxic plasmatic concentrations more frequently than with other peripheral blocks.
In infants, 1.25 mg/kg of bupivacaine, injected in the paravertebral space, produce a mean plasmatic peak of 1 μg/ml by 10-60 minutes, while a continuous infusion of 0.25 mg/kg/h bupivacaine, after 42 hours, determines a mean plasmatic concentration of 1.76 μg/ml, but – in some cases – even to potentially toxic concentrations, above 3 μg/ml.
We have to remember that local anesthetic toxicity is especially due to how quick a given plasmatic concentration is reached and that often "theoretically" toxic concentrations prove to be harmless if reached by many hours or days. In this case, a continuous infusion is safer than a multiple bolus dosing.
Some PVB contraindications are worthy of notice: paravertebral neoplasms, pleural empyema and severe bleeding disorders; these latter are limited contraindications, as the consequences of a paravertebral hematoma are not as serious as those of an epidural hematoma.

TRANSVERSUS ABDOMINIS PLANE (TAP) BLOCK

Anatomy and sonoanatomy

In children, the TAP anatomy and sonoanatomy are the same as in adults and for their close description we suggest you to refer to Chapter 7.
We briefly remind that the sensitive nerves of the anterior abdominal wall depend on the anterior branches of the intercostal nerves, on the subcostal nerves and on the first lumbar nerves that run in a neurovascular fascial plane, that is located between the internal oblique muscle (IO) and the transverse muscle (TAP).

Block target

The aim of the block is to deposit the local anesthetic in this fascial plane so that the crossing nervous structures are anesthetized.

Description of the technique

In 2001, Rafi described for the first time a local anesthetic injection in the neurovascular plane between the IO and the transverse muscles to provide analgesia for the abdominal wall. The first experiences in children date back to 2008, but the introduction of ultrasound guidance contributed to such a quick spread of this technique that nowadays it competes with central blocks for the anesthesiological management of abdominal surgery.
The use of ultrasound guidance allows to access the TAP more posteriorly (or proximally), near the lateral margin of the latissimus dorsi muscle, where the transverse muscle originates. In adults, a proximal approach to TAP seems to increase its efficacy, possibly thanks to the medial spread of the anesthetic, which draws the TAP block close to a paravertebral block.
The ultrasound-guided technique in children requires the following material: a high frequency linear probe (7-12 MHz), a sterile probe cover, sterile gel, a short bevel needle (SonoTAP®), better if with an extension, sterile drapes and an antiseptic solution to create a sterile field. Using the probe, the abdominal wall is explored laterally to the umbilicus, starting from the lateral margin of the rectus abdominis muscle. Once the external oblique muscle (EO), IO and the transverse muscle (the thinnest of the three) are displayed, the transducer is

moved laterally to the anterior edge of the latissimus dorsi muscle (**Figure 12.6**). On this level, which generally corresponds to the anterior or mid axillary line, the origin of the transverse muscle can be seen, while IO and EO can even entwine in one aponeurosis. In the in-plane technique a needle is inserted in anteroposterior direction up to the hyperechoic fascial plane between IO and transverse muscles (**Figure 12.7**). The local anesthetic injection causes the two muscles to separate, confirming the correct position of the needle (**Figure 12.7**).

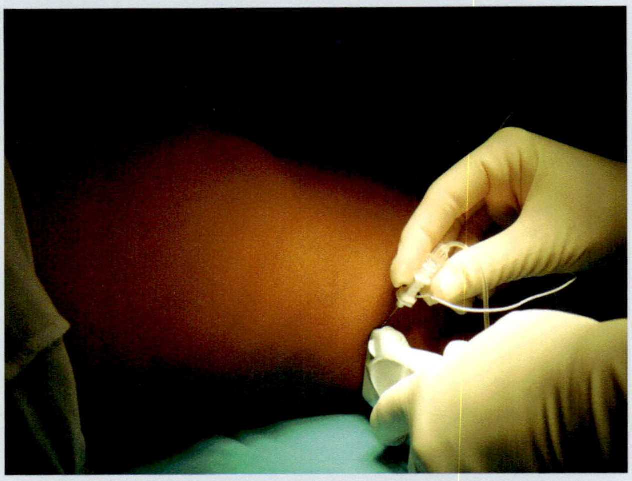

Figure 12.6 In-plane approach for a US-guided TAP block.

In children, the virtual space between the two muscles is superficial, often less than 1 cm deep, so if a large needle is used (>24-25 G) it may be difficult to correctly place the tip.

As in adults, also in children it is possible to perform this block with a more cranial and anterior, subcostal approach (**Figure 12.8**). The ultrasound probe is leaned in parallel with the costal margin and the in-plane injection follows a lateral approach. Theoretically, the anesthetic spread is more cranial compared to the classic technique, so this approach is recommended for upper abdominal surgery.

The use of volumes like 0.2-0.5 ml/kg of 0.25% levobupivacaine or 0.2% ropivacaine is recommended to perform a single TAP block.

As in the adult population, it is possible to place a catheter between the IO and the transverse muscles, performing a continuous block.

The use of 0.25-0.4 mg/kg/h of 0.1-0.125% levobupivacaine or 0.1-0.2% ropivacaine is recommended for a continuous infusion.

Indications

Indications for the TAP block in children are the same as in adults: intra and postoperative analgesia in ab-

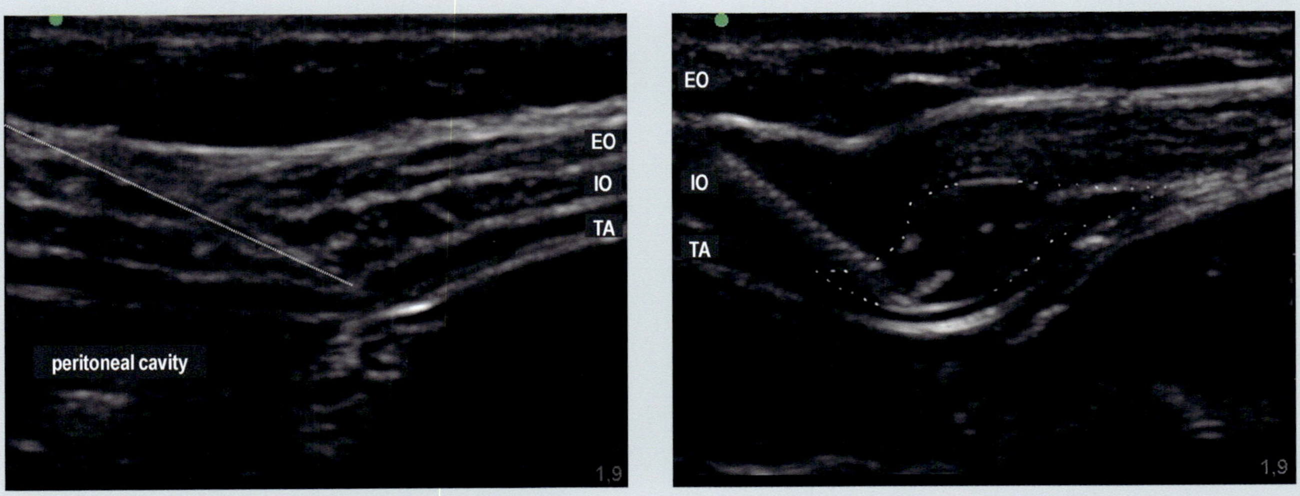

Figure 12.7 TAP block sonoanatomy. EO: external oblique muscle; IO: internal oblique muscle; TA: transversus abdominis muscle.

dominal surgery, especially if monolateral, like in kidney and urinary surgery, intestinal recanalization, colostomy, invagination, appendectomy, inguinal hernia, iliac crest harvest, laparoscopy.

A TAP block is clearly a "wall" block, because it involves only skin, muscles and parietal peritoneum and it is not as effective as a central block, especially for the visceral pain; nevertheless, it is a technique that makes intra- and postoperative pain management easier. As it is possible to leave a catheter in site to continuously administer local anesthetics in the postoperative phase, it can be an option instead of the continuous epidural one.

It is difficult to determine if the catheter placement is preferable in the pre- or postoperative phase. Theoretically, a preoperative catheter can either help the anesthetic management and allow a significant opioid sparing in the intraoperative phase, or it can be used in the postoperative phase within a multimodal analgesic program.

As a catheter placed before surgery might interfere with the surgical field, a postoperative positioning might be difficult due to an altered sonoanatomy secondary to surgical trauma and tissue swelling.

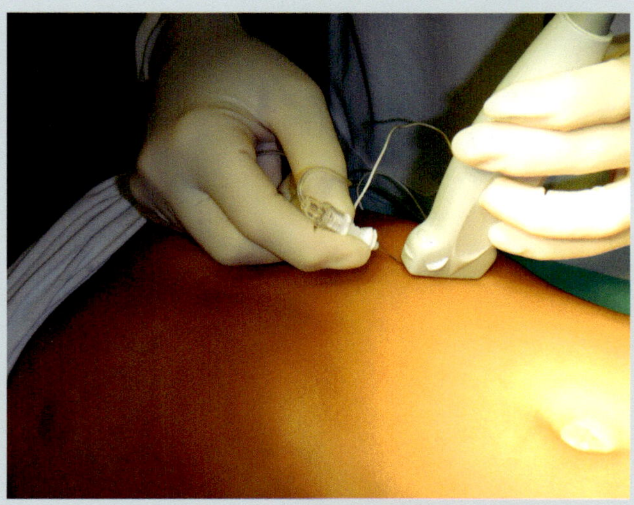

Figure 12.8 Subcostal TAP block: US transducer and needle positioning for the in-plane approach.

Complications and contraindications

TAP block is a very safe block and, on this note, the Pediatric Regional Anesthesia Network (PRAN) has recently reported only two minor complications out of 1994 cases: a vascular injection and an intraperitoneal injection.

There are no absolute contraindications to this block; if anything, the presence of infections on the injection point (**Tables 12.1**, **12.2**).

The main risk with this and other blocks, that are described in this chapter, is a local anesthetic overdose, caused by both an accidental intravascular injection and an excessive miscalculated dose. Following the recommended doses and the safety rules for the local anesthetic injections in children is the best prevention for this complication, which must always be taken into account.

In children, most peripheral blocks are very superficial, so when a catheter is placed by traditional technique (catheter-through-needle), the entry hole of the needle often allows leakage of the infused anesthetic, reducing the efficacy and causing catheter displacement. An over-the-needle catheter (E-Cath®), as described for the thoracic PVB, allows to reduce the rate of such complications (**Figure 12.9**).

ILIOINGUINAL AND ILIOHYPOGASTRIC NERVE BLOCK

Anatomy and sonoanatomy

Anatomy and sonoanatomy of the two nerves are closely described in Chapter 8, which is suggested for a more thorough dissertation.

In short, the II and IH nerves are terminal branches of the lumbar plexus and they originate from T12 and L1 metamers. At the psoas lateral margin, the nerves leave the lumbar plexus and, running in parallel, move medially and caudally into the abdominal wall 0.5-1.5 cm medially to the anterior superior iliac spine (ASIS), then between the IO and transverse muscles. The IH nerve eventually splits in two terminal branches, a lateral cutaneous branch for the gluteus, and an anterior branch for the suprapubic area. The ilioinguinal nerve – the thinnest one – reaches the round ligament (in women) or the

TABLE 12.1 INDICATIONS FOR TRUNK AND ABDOMINAL WALL BLOCKS IN CHILDREN

Surgery	PVB	ESP	Subcostal TAP	TAP	II+IH	Rectus sheath
Thoracotomy	+++	+++				
Thoracoscopy	+++	+++				
Laparoscopy	+	++	++	++		+
Colostomy	++	++	++	++		
Splenectomy	+++	+++	++	+		
Hepatectomy	+++	+++	++	+		
Nephrectomy	+++	+++	++	+++		
Pyelo-ureteroplasty	+++	++	++	+++		
Appendicectomy	+	++	+	+		
Inguinal hernia repair	+	+		++	+++	
Umbilical hernia repair						+++
Pyloromyotomy						+++
Iliac crest bone harvest	+	+		+++		

+++ strong indication; + weak indication.

TABLE 12.2 LOCAL ANESTHETIC VOLUMES AND CONCENTRATIONS FOR TRUNK AND ABDOMINAL WALL BLOCKS IN CHILDREN

Nerve block	Volume	Concentration	Continuous infusion
Thoracic paravertebral	0.5 ml/kg 20 ml max)	0.125-0.25%	0.25 mg/kg/h
ESP	0.3-0.5 ml/kg (20 ml max)	0.2-0.25%	0.1-0.3 mg/kg/h
TAP	0.2-0.5 ml/kg (20 ml max)	0.125-0.25%	0.25-0.4 mg/kg/h
II-IH	0.1-0.3 ml/kg	0.25-0.375%	
Rectus sheath	0.1 ml/kg for each side	0.25-0.375%	

spermatic cord (in men), and it takes part to the innervation of the abdominal wall, the medial part of the thigh, the lateral and cranial scrotum or labia majora (**Figure 12.10**).

Block target

The target of the block is to inject a dose of local anesthetic close to the two nerves, that are located between the IO and the transverse muscles (**Figure 12.11**).

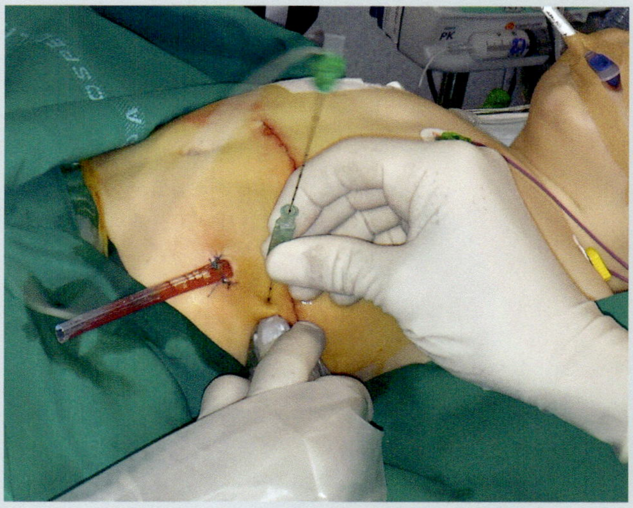

Figure 12.9 Over-the-needle catheter placement for continuous TAP block.

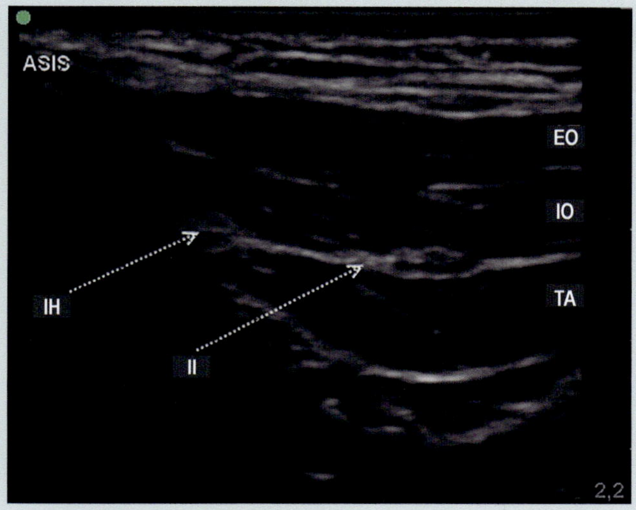

Figure 12.11 Ilioinguinal and iliohypogastric nerve block sonoanatomy. ASIS: anterior superior iliac spine; EO: external oblique muscle; IH: iliohypogastric nerve; II: ilioinguinal nerve; IO: internal oblique muscle; TA: transversus abdominis muscle.

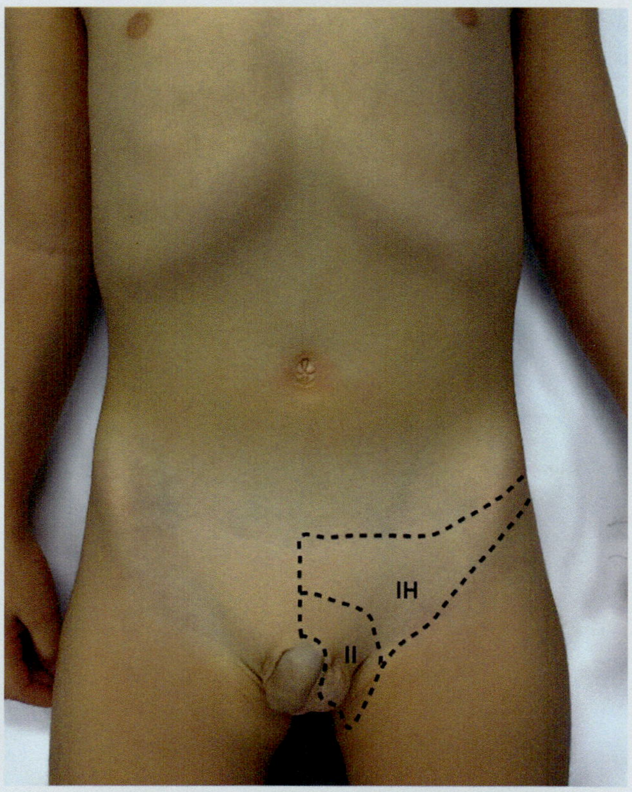

Figure 12.10 Cutaneous innervation by ilioinguinal (II) and (IH) nerves.

In case the two nerves are not visible, the anesthetic can be injected in the fascial plane between the two muscles as with TAP block.

Description of the technique

Differently from the previously described blocks, the block of the II and IH nerves has been introduced earlier in children than in adults, at the end of the 1980s. The traditional "blind" techniques for the block of the two nerves, that are described before the ultrasound introduction, are different.

The Dalens' simplified technique requires an injection by blunt needle between the lateral third and the medial third of a line connecting the anterior superior iliac spine (ASIS) to the umbilicus; with a caudal and medial direction, the needle is pushed until resistance from the IO and the transverse is appreciated. The anesthetic must be injected once a loss of resistance is perceived. Electrical stimulation is not helpful in this case, as the nerves are sensitive.

An ultrasound check on 62 blocks, performed by classic technique, found though that local anesthetic had been injected correctly around the two nerves only in 14% of cases. So, even though this block has a good safety and effectiveness profile with a traditional technique, the introduction of ultrasound guidance allowed to improve the performance, and reduce both the anesthetic dosage necessary for the block and the onset time.

The material to perform an ultrasound-guided block is the same as previously described for the PVB and the TAP blocks. The high frequency linear probe (7-12 MHz) has to be placed transversally close to the ASIS, in order to visualize the muscular planes that are part of the abdominal wall and to have a perpendicular scan of the two nerves. The EO is recognizable as the outermost, layering over the IO and the transverse muscles, that appear as hypoechogenic structures separated by their hyperechogenic aponeurosis. The peritoneal cavity is recognizable deep under the transverse muscle. To be noted, the OE muscle can be missing in about half the cases (**Figure 12.12**). The hyperechogenic ASIS with its shadow cone is a helpful anatomic landmark, as the ilioinguinal nerve runs very close (4-8 mm), while the IH nerve is rather medial (1-1.5 cm). The two nerves appear to be fuse-shaped and hyperechogenic between the two muscle bellies, but sometimes they may be hardly displayed.

The in-plane injection can be performed both with a medial or a lateral direction (the lateral one is easier in infants) (**Figure 12.12**, **Video 12.2**).

In children the nerves are very superficial, and the needle has to be inserted as close as possible to the ultrasound probe and in parallel to it. The local anesthetic injection around the two nerves has to cause the IO and transverse muscles to split, as in the TAP block.

Generally, 0.1-0.3 ml/kg local anesthetic are enough to block the two nerves and this allows to also perform a bilateral block, remaining anyway quite far from toxic doses. 0.25% bupivacaine and levobupivacaine or 0.2% ropivacaine, can be used, leaving higher concentrations for older children. If the block is correct the *onset time* is very quick (5 minutes).

Indications

Indications to this block are intra- and postoperative analgesia for any inguinal canal surgery: inguinal hernia, hydrocele (where this block should be the first choice) or cryptorchidism correction.

For the latter, this block has a limited effectiveness, due to the complex visceral innervation of the testi-

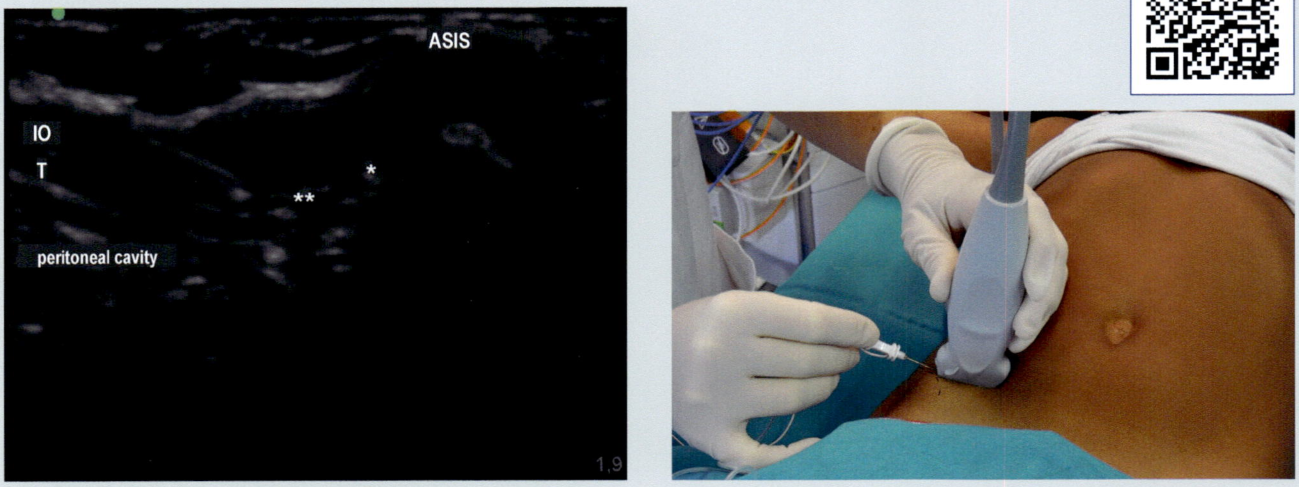

Figure 12.12 US guided iliohypogastric* and ilioinguinal** nerve block. ASIS: anterior superior iliac spine; EO, external oblique muscle; IO, internal oblique muscle; T: transversus abdominis muscle. The needle approaching the II nerve is clearly visible.

cle – involving the mediothoracic metamers – and the variable innervation of the scrotum, inconsistently relying on the ilioinguinal nerve. For both inguinal hernias and hydrocele, the II-IH block – a wall block- works as well as a caudal anesthesia.

During surgery on the inguinal canal, the surgical manipulations of deep structures (testicle, peritoneum, omentum etc.) are not covered by this block and may require a revision of the associated general anesthesia or sedation plan. When this is predictable (eg., for infants with an incarcerated hernia) the best performance is ensured by a caudal anesthesia.

In a comparison between a TAP block and a II-IH block for inguinal canal surgery, the latter proved to be superior in terms of analgesia.

Complications and contraindications

As already said, complications for this block are rare and moderate: vascular puncture or bowel puncture, which happens if the needle is advanced too deep into the abdominal wall, even more frequently with sharp tip needles. With high volumes (>0.3 ml/kg) a femoral nerve block can occur, because of the anesthetic spread to the iliac fascia. Low volumes of local anesthetic make the systemic toxicity risk irrelevant. There are no major contraindications.

RECTUS SHEATH BLOCK

Anatomy and sonoanatomy

Anatomy and sonoanatomy are the same as in the adult and for their detailed description we suggest you to refer to Chapter 9.

The rectus abdominis muscle is equally split in two on the median line by the linea alba and separated laterally from the other muscles of the abdominal wall by the linea semilunaris.

The periumbilical abdominal wall is innervated by the terminal branches of the IX, X, XI intercostal nerves. These nerves run behind the costal cartilages and then anteriorly between the IO and transverse muscles to the linea semilunaris. Here they perforate the deep rectus abdominis, run through it and reach the skin.

Block target

The aim of the block is to anesthetize the terminal branches of the intercostal nerves, which innervate the periumbilical abdominal wall when they run through the abdominal rectus muscle.

Description of the technique

The rectus sheath block was proposed in children for the first time in 1996 by Ferguson et al. for the surgical correction of the umbilical hernia.

Before the ultrasound guidance was introduced, two techniques were used, both based on superficial landmarks.

Ferguson suggested to bilaterally inject the local anesthetic into the rectus abdominis, 0.5-1 cm medially to the linea semilunaris, in order to have a cranial and caudal spread.

Courreges et al. described a double bilateral injection, both above and deep to the superficial fascia of the rectus, in order to also block the superficial fibers of the intercostal nerves, that might originate proximally to the muscle and run above it.

The material to perform an ultrasound-guided block is the same previously described for the other blocks of the abdominal wall and the trunk.

In children, as the structures to spot are superficial, a high frequency linear probe (7-12 MHz) is positioned transversally, beside the umbilicus (**Figure 12.13**); the ultrasound transducer allows to visualize the rectus muscle, as an hypoechogenic layer interposed between the peritoneum and the subcutaneous tissue, its superficial and deep fascias, which appear hyperechogenic, as the lateral margin of the rectus, intertwined with the aponeuroses of IO and transverse muscle.

The intercostal nerves cannot be directly visualized with the ultrasound, but it is sufficient to inject the local anesthetic between the muscle belly and its deep fascia, as close as possible or by its lateral margin (**Figure 12.14**).

There is no clear fascial plane between the rectus muscle and its deep fascia – as is instead present between the IO and transversus muscle-, but ultrasound guidance allows to appreciate the spread of local anesthetic between the two structures.

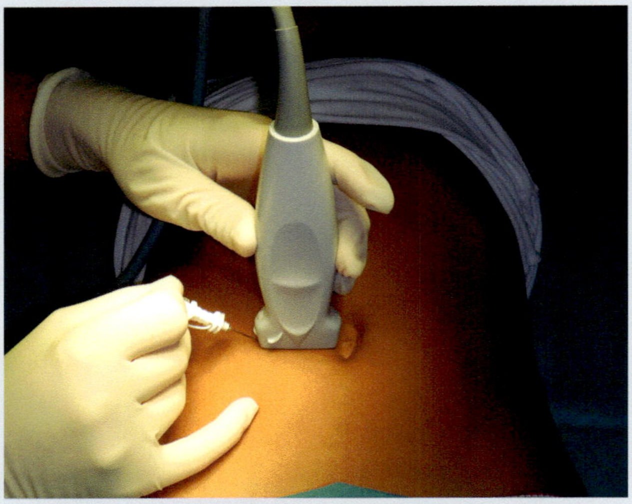

Figure 12.13 In-plane approach for the rectus sheath block.

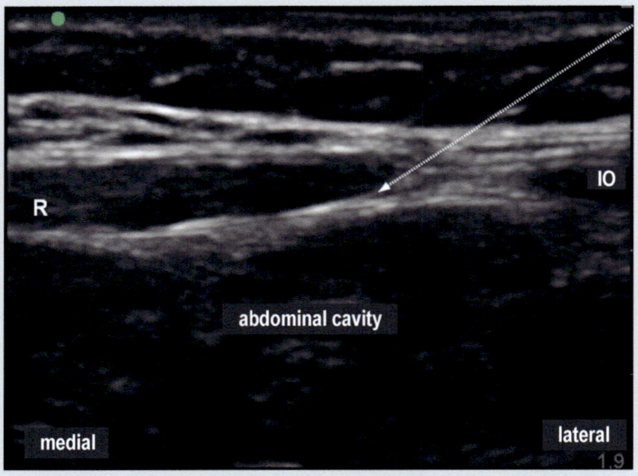

Figure 12.14 Rectus sheath block sonoanatomy. IO: internal oblique muscle; R: rectus abdominis.

The in-plane injection allows a complete visualization of the structures that are involved in the block: rectus muscle and its deep fascia, its lateral margin and the IO and transversus aponeurosis, the abdominal cavity, the needle (SonoPlex stim Pajunk®), and local anesthetic spread.

If the block is correctly performed, for each side 0.1-0.3 ml/kg of 0.25% bupivacaine/levobupivacaine or 0.2% ropivacaine is enough.

Indications

This block is indicated for intra- and postoperative analgesia in umbilical and epigastric hernia surgery, but also for pyloric stenosis surgery with periumbilical approach, for the umbilical access in laparoscopy and for all minor surgery requiring an incision along the median line. It is a wall block, as the TAP block, so it does not cover the visceral pain that may be present in the aforementioned surgeries. It is generally associated with general anesthesia in case of pyloric stenosis or of laparoscopy, but combining it with a deep sedation may be enough for umbilical surgery.

Complications and contraindications

Complications are rare and moderate: bowel injection and vascular injection with a hematoma on the abdominal wall (the inferior epigastric artery may run close to the injection point).

The use of low volumes of local anesthetic makes the risk of systemic toxicity irrelevant. There are no major contraindications.

ERECTOR SPINAE PLANE (ESP) BLOCK

Anatomy and sonoanatomy

The posterior thoracic wall consists of trapezius (TM), rhomboid (RM), erector spinae (ESM) muscles with their respective fascial planes. These muscles have insertion on the spinous and transverse processes of the vertebrae.

Sonoanatomy involves the longitudinal positioning of the ultrasound probe, proximal to the interspinous line, in order to identify the three muscle layers and the underlying acoustic shadow of the target transverse process (**Figure 12.15**).

Lateral to the transverse process the costo-transverse ligament, the paravertebral space and the pleura with its "lung-sliding" can be identified.

Block target

The target of the block is to deposit the local anesthetic (LA) in the plane between the ESM and the selected transverse process.

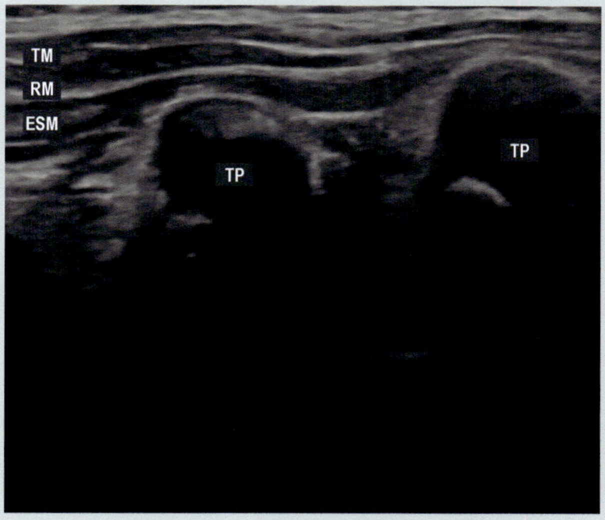

Figure 12.15 Parasagittal ultrasound view for an Erector Spinae Plane Block at the level of T5. TP, transverse process; TM, trapezius muscle; RM, rhomboid muscle; ESM, erector spinae muscle.

Description of the technique

The ESP block is an ultrasound-guided interfascial plane block first described by Forero et al. in 2016. This technique has a complex and probably multimodal mechanism of action. Therefore, the idea of this procedure as a mere alternative or simplified version of the PVB is being gradually abandoned.

The ultrasound-guided ESPB in children involves the use of a high-frequency linear probe (7-12 MHz), a sterile probe cover, sterile gel, a short bevel needle (SonoPlex stim Pajunk®), sterile drapes and an antiseptic solution.

The probe is placed in a longitudinal position lateral to the vertebral column. Above the acoustic shadow of the selected transverse process, TM, RM and ESM will be identified – from the surface to the depth.

The needle is inserted in-plane and is advanced in a cranio-caudal direction through the TM, RM, and ESM to gently contact the transverse process.

Subsequently, a volume of LA is injected verifying its spread superficially to the acoustic window of the transverse process (**Figure 12.16**).

The ESPB is an interfascial plane block, therefore its success mainly depends on the volume of LA injected. A volume of 0.1 ml/kg of LA for each dermatome seems to be necessary in order to obtain an optimal dermatomal coverage. Therefore, 0.3-0.5 ml/kg/side of 0.25% levobupivacaine or 0.2% ropivacaine would ensure diffusion and consequent analgesia for 4-5 segments.

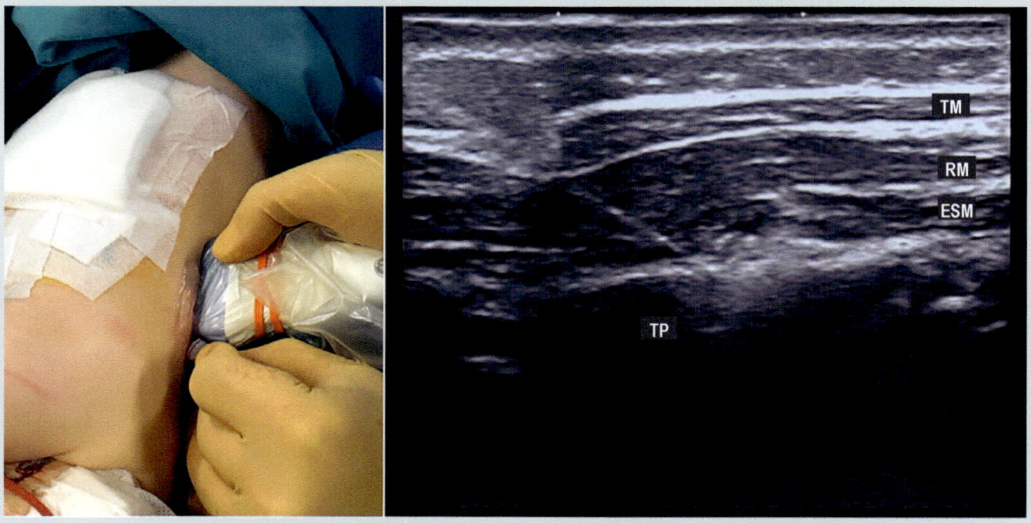

Figure 12.16 US guided Erector Spinae Plane (ESP) block. ESM, erector spinae muscle; RM, rhomboid muscle; TM, trapezius muscle; TP, transverse process. The needle approaching the transverse process is clearly visible.

Despite the anatomical analogies for ESPB at different levels, it is necessary to emphasize that ESPB in the lumbosacral region is challenging to perform and difficult to sonographically visualize, compared to thoracic applications.

Therefore, Aksu and colleagues described a new approach for lumbar erector spinae plane block that is mainly indicated for pediatric surgery.

The patient is placed in a lateral decubitus position with the block site facing up. A linear US probe is placed transversally, just cranial to iliac crest. After obtaining the classical "Shamrock" view, the probe is shifted slightly to the back to have a wider view of ESM. Using an in-plane technique, the needle is directed toward the back of the transverse process. Following a negative aspiration, 0.5 ml/kg of 0.25% levobupivacaine can be used to perform the block.

A continuous block can be performed by inserting a perineural catheter through a Tuohy needle (catether-through-needle) or catether-through-needle system (E-Cath®). To date, no infusion regimens for continuous ESPB have been codified; in our experience, we use infusions borrowed from continuous epidural and continuous PVB: 0.1-0.3 mg/kg/h of 0.1-0.125% levobupivacaine or 0.1% ropivacaine.

There are currently no pharmacokinetic data for ESPB in children and we do not know for certain whether the absorption is similar to other fascial plane blocks. This further reinforces the need to calculate the maximum allowable dosage (both in concentration and in volume) for each individual patient.

Indications

Although still limited to case reports/case series or small RCTs, the recent literature in paediatrics has highlighted how ESPB provides a good postoperative analgesia in surgeries involving incisions from T1 to L4, with no documented complications.

Complications and contraindications

Potential complications are represented by local anesthetic systemic toxicity (LAST) and the massive LA spread into the epidural space promoted by a latero-medial direction of the needle tip or by a high infusion pressure.

Lastly, the wrong identification of the target structures or the low visualization of the needle tip progression can determine the risk of accidental pleural puncture.

Contraindications to the execution of the block are: paravertebral neoplastic disease, pleural empyema, severe coagulopathies, injection site infections, allergies to LA.

RECOMMENDED READING

- Rappaport BA, Suresh S, Hertz S, et al. Anesthetic neurotoxicity – clinical implications of animal models. *N Engl J Med.* 2015;372(9):796-97.
- Ecoffey C, Lacroix F, Giaufrè E, et al. Epidemiology and morbility of regional anesthesia in children: a follow-up one year prospective survey of the French Language Society of Pediatric Anesthesiologists (ADARPEF). *Paediatr Anaesth.* 2010;20:1061-9.
- Ivani G, Suresh S, Ecoffey C, et al. The ESRA and the ASRA Joint Committee practice advisory on controversial topics in pediatric regional anesthesia. *Reg Anesth Pain Med.* 2015;40(5):526-32.
- Soni AK. Video-assisted thoracoscopic placement of paravertebral catheters: a technique for postoperative analgesia for bilateral thoracoscopic surgery. *Br J Anaesth.* 1994;72:462-4.
- Boretsky K, Visoiu M, Bigeleisen P. Ultrasound-guided approach to the paravertebral space for catheter insertion in infants and children. *Paediatr Anaesth.* 2013;23:1193-8.
- Lönnqvist PA, Hesser U. Radiological and clinical distribution of thoracic paravertebral blockade in infants and children. *Paediatr Anaesth.* 1993;3(2):83-7.
- Albokrinov AA, Fesenko UA. Spread of dye after single thoracolumbar paravertebral injection in infants. *Eur J Anaesthesiol.* 2014;31:305-9.
- Vittinghoff M, Lönnqvist PA, Mossetti V, et al. Postoperative pain management in children: Guidance from the pain committee of the European Society for Paediatric Anaesthesiology (ESPA Pain Management Ladder Initiative). Paediatr Anaesth 2018; 28:493.
- Suresh S, Ecoffey C, Bosenberg A, et al. The European Society of Regional Anaesthesia and Pain Therapy/American Society of Regional Anesthesia and Pain Medicine Recommendations on Local Anesthetics and Adjuvants Dosage in Pediatric Regional Anesthesia. Reg Anesth Pain Med 2018; 43:211.
- El Morsy GZ, El-Deeb A, El-Desouky T, et al. Can thoracic paravertebral block replace thoracic epidural block in pediatric cardiac surgery? A randomized blinded study. *Ann Card Anesth.* 2012;15(4):259-63.
- Lonnqvist PA, McKenzie J, Soni AK, Conacher ID. Paravertebral blockade, failure rate and complications. *Anaesthesia.* 1995;50:813-5.
- Pace MM, Sharma B, Anderson-dam J, Fleischmann K, Warren L, Stefanovich P. Ultrasound-guided thoracic paravertebral blockade: a retrospective study of the incidence of complications. Anesth Analg. 2016;122:1186–91.

- Cheung SLW, Booker PD, Franks R, Pozzi M. Serum concentration of bupivacaine during prolonged continuous paravertebral infusion in young infants. *Br J Anaesth*. 1997;79:9-13.
- Fredrickson M, Seal P, Houghton J. Early experience with the transversus abdominis plane block in children. *Paediatr Anaesth*. 2008;18:891-2.
- Desgranges FP, De Queiroz M, Chassard D. Continuous oblique subcostal transversus abdominis plane block: an alternative for pain management after upper abdominal surgery in children. *Paediatr Anaesth*. 2011;21:982-3.
- Long JB, Birmingham PK, De Oliveira GS, et al. TAP block in children: a multicenter safety analysis of 1994 cases from PRAN (Pediatric Regional Anesthesia Network) Database. *Anesth Analg*. 2014;119(2):395-9.
- Dalens B. Blocchi ileoinguinali e ileoipogastrici. In: Dalens B, ed. *Anestesia loco-regionale dalla nascita all'età adulta*. Milano: Fogliazza; 1995;3:201-3.
- Weintraud M, Marhofer P, Bosenberg A, et al. Ilioinguinal/iliohypogastric blocks in children: where do we administer the local anesthetic without direct visualization? *Anesth Analg*. 2008;106:89-93.
- Willschke H, Bosenberg A, Marhofer P, et al. Ultrasonographic-guided ilioinguinal/iliohypo- gastric nerve block in pediatric anesthesia: what is the optimal volume? *Anesth Analg*. 2006;102:1680-4.
- Frederickson MJ, Paine C, Hamill J. Improved analgesia with the ilioinguinal block compared to the transversus abdominal plane block after pediatric inguinal surgery: a prospective randomized trial. *Paediatr Anaesth*. 2010;20:1022-7.
- Ferguson S, Thomas V, Lewis I. The rectus sheath block in paediatric anaesthesia: new indications for an old technique? *Paediatr Anesth*. 1996;7:211-4.
- Willschke H, Bosenberg A, Marhofer P, et al. Ultrasonography-guided rectus sheath block in paediatric anaesthesia - a new approach to an old technique. *Br J Anaesth*. 2006;97:244-9.
- De Jose MB, Gotzens V, Marbrok M. Ultrasound-guided umbilical nerve block in children: a brief description of a new approach. *Paediatr Anesth*. 2007;17:44-50.
- Forero M, Adhikary SD, Lopez H, Tsui C, Chin KJ. The Erector Spinae Plane Block: A Novel Analgesic Technique in Thoracic Neuropathic Pain. Reg Anesth Pain Med. 2016;41(5):621-7.
- Ivanusic J, Konishi Y, Barrington MJ. A Cadaveric Study Investigating the Mechanism of Action of Erector Spinae Blockade. Reg Anesth Pain Med. 2018 Aug;43(6):567-571.
- Govender S, Mohr D, Bosenberg A, Van Schoor AN. A cadaveric study of the erector spinae plane block in a neonatal sample. Reg Anesth Pain Med. 2020;45(5):386-388.
- Schwartzmann A, Peng P, Maciel MA, Forero M. Mechanism of the erector spinae plane block: insights from a magnetic resonance imaging study. Can J Anaesth. 2018;65(10):1165-1166.
- Holland EL, Bosenberg AT. Early experience with erector spinae plane blocks in children. Paediatr Anaesth. 2020;30(2):96-107.
- Aksu C, Gürkan Y. Aksu approach for lumbar erector spinae plane block for pediatric surgeries. J Clin Anesth. 2018;54:74–75.
- Sauter AR, Ullensvang K, Bendtsen TF, Borglum J. The "Shamrock Method" a new and promising technique for ultrasound guided lumbar plexus block. Br J Anaesth 2013. 111.eLetter Supplement, e-publication http://bja.oxfordjournals.org/forum/ topic/brjana_el%3B9814.
- Dontukurthy S, Mofidi R. The Role of Interfascial Plane Blocks in Paediatric Regional Anaesthesia: A Narrative Review of Current Perspectives and Updates. Anesthesiol Res Pract. 2020;2020:8892537.
- Mostafa SF, Abdelghany MS, Abdelraheem TM, Abu Elyazed MM. Ultrasound-guided erector spinae plane block for postoperative analgesia in pediatric patients undergoing splenectomy: A prospective randomized controlled trial. Paediatr Anaesth. 2019;29(12):1201-1207.

CLINICAL CASE 1 – ULTRASOUND-GUIDED PARAVERTERBAL BLOCK FOR THORACOSCOPIC LUNG RESECTION

Clinic history and anamnesis An otherwise healthy toddler had a prenatal diagnosis of congenital cystic adenomatoid malformation (CCAM) of the lung, affecting her inferior left lobe.

A thoracoscopic resection of such lobe was scheduled at 12 months of life, when she had reached 9.3 kg in weight.

Technique description Under aseptic conditions, using a linear probe (7-12 Hz) with a transverse approach, we visualized the left paravertebral structures at the level of T5.

Using a 22 G 50 mm echogenic needle (Pajunk® SonoPlex) with an in-plane approach, we injected 4.5 ml of 0.25% Levobupivacaine to open the left paravertebral space, with direct visualization of the anesthetic spreading and lowering the parietal pleura.

General anesthesia was maintained with Propofol TCI (Cp 3-3.5 mcg/ml) and additional fentanyl (for a total dose of 3 mcg/kg/h) was used to control any pain due to lung manipulation.

At the end of surgery, the patient was awakened and monitored in our Post-Anesthesia Care Unit, where she received a single dose of Tramadol (1 mg/kg) to treat discomfort and unrest. She was transferred to the Surgical Ward on the same day, where she maintained a good pain control with oral paracetamol (15 mg/kg every 6 hours), with a stable 0 on FLACC evaluations.

She was discharged home on the fourth postoperative day.

Materials and methods After premedication with oral Clonidine (4 mcg/kg) 90 minutes prior to procedure, a venous access was gained (24 G cannula) and standard monitoring was applied. We induced general anesthesia with Propofol using a TCI Pedfusor protocol (with a plasmatic concentration set to 5 mcg/ml), 2.5 mcg/kg Fentanyl and 1 mg/kg Rocuronium. A 5 mm uncuffed tracheal tube was inserted and mechanical ventilation was started. A radial arterial cannula and a second venous line were also placed. The child was positioned on right side decubitus and a 5Fr Arndt bronchial blocker was positioned in the main left bronchus with fiberscopic guidance (**Figures 12.17**, **12.18**).

Conclusions The paravertebral block is a safe and effective technique to control moderate to intense pain after monolateral surgical procedures. Ultrasound guidance ensures a higher safety profile to the procedure and allows direct monitoring of the local spread of anesthetic to confirm the effectiveness of the block.

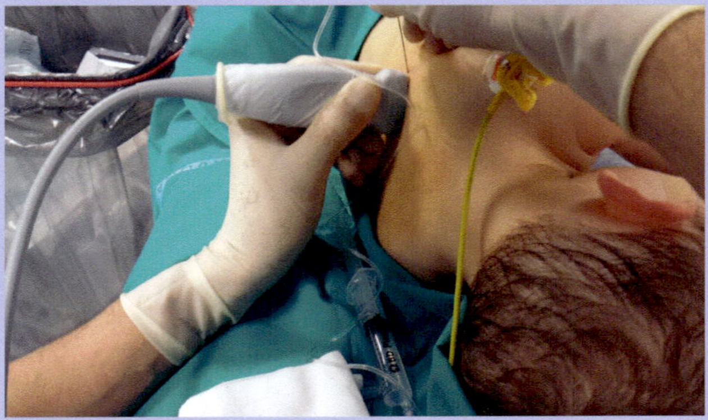

Figure 12.17 Thoracic paravertebral block by in-plane *technique* (transverse approach).

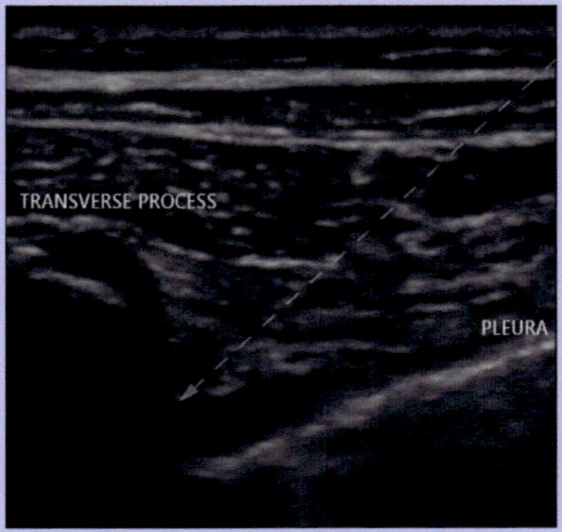

Figure 12.18 Ultrasound visualization of the paravertebral space. The tip of the needle is directed towards the paravertebral space.

CLINICAL CASE 2 – ULTRASOUND-GUIDED ILIOINGUINAL-ILIOHYPOGASTRIC NERVE BLOCK FOR INGUINAL HERNIA CORRECTION

Clinic history and anamnesis An otherwise healthy child (18 months of age, 10.6 kg in weight) was scheduled for surgical correction of a recurrent right inguinal hernia, which had a recent episode of incarceration, resolved at the time by manual reduction.

Technique description Under aseptic conditions, we positioned a linear probe (7-12 Hz) transversally, close to the right anterior superior iliac spine, in order to have a perpendicular scan of the two nerves, lying between the internal oblique and transverse muscles.

Using a 22 G 50 mm echogenic needle (Pajunk® SonoPlex) with an in-plane approach, we injected 2.5 ml of 0.25% levobupivacaine in proximity to the two nerves (**Figures 12.19**, **12.20**).

Propofol infusion was reduced to a Cet of 2-2.5 mcg/ml during surgery, and 15 mg/kg of Paracetamol was infused at the end of procedure to optimize postoperative pain management. At the end of surgery, the patient was awakened and, after a 30-minute monitoring in our Post-Anesthesia Room, discharged to the ward. During the day, he maintained a good pain control with oral paracetamol (15 mg/kg every 6 hours) and, after he got back to his usual preoperative level of activity, was discharged home in the evening.

Materials and methods After premedication with oral Clonidine (4 mcg/kg) 90 minutes prior to procedure, a venous access was gained (24 G cannula) and standard monitoring was applied. We infused Propofol using a TCI Pedfusor protocol to achieve sedation (with a plasmatic concentration set to 4 mcg/ml), together with 1 mcg/kg of Fentanyl.

Conclusions The ilioinguinal-iliohypogastric nerve block is the gold standard locoregional technique for the repair of inguinal hernias. It is a safe block, and its effectiveness allows to use it just in association with sedation, even during the surgical time.

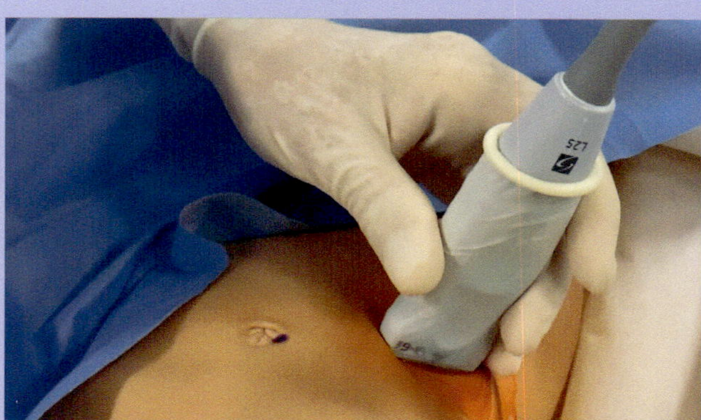

Figure 12.19 Correct position of the probe along the line connecting the anterior superior iliac spine (ASIS) to the umbilicus.

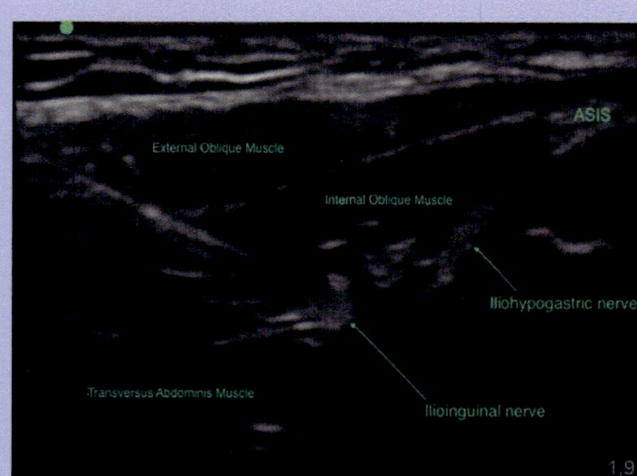

Figure 12.20 Ultrasound visualization of the ilioinguinal and iliohypogastric nerves and the needle (SonoPlex stim Pajunk®). The tip of the needle is directed towards the ilioinguinal nerve.

CHAPTER 13

Fascial plane blocks of the neck: superficial and intermediate cervical plexus block

Giuseppe Sepolvere, Cristiano D'Errico, Mario Tedesco

The cervical plexus block (CPB) provides effective anesthesia and analgesia for the head and neck region. While in the past the most common clinical use for CPB was carotid endarterectomy (CEA), it is currently performed in several head and neck surgery indications. Traditionally CPB was classified as deep (DCPB) or superficial (SCPB), but in 2004 Telford and Stoneham, based on the cadaveric study by Pandit et al., suggested the intermediate cervical plexus block (ICPB) involving a sub-investing fascial injection between the inferior surface of the sternocleidomastoid muscle (SCM) and the prevertebral fascia (PF). On this basis superficial, intermediate and deep are terms that indicate the relationship between muscles, nerves, tissue, fasciae, skin and the anatomical region in which local anesthetic is injected. In 2010, Choquet et al. refined the concept of ICPB using ultrasound technique which is used to identify important anatomical landmarks and making the procedure safer and more accurate. Particularly, understanding the cervical plexus anatomy and a detailed configuration of the cervical fasciae is essential to a successful CPB because cervical fasciae are known to have a substantial role in the diffusion of local anesthetic.

ANATOMY

The cervical plexus (CP) is formed by the anterior divisions of the second through fourth upper cervical nerves resting on the levator scapulae (LSM), longus capitis (LCM) and middle scalene muscles (MSM), covered by the sternocleidomastoid muscle (SCM). The third and fourth cervical nerves send a branch to the spinal accessory nerve while the fourth cervical nerve may send a division downward to the fifth cervical nerve and participate in the formation of the brachial plexus (BP). The fibers deriving from the superior (C1-C2) and inferior (C2-C3) roots, form a loop named ansa cervicalis (AC). The anterior rami of C3 and C4 form a loop from which the phrenic nerve rises joining C5. Moreover, the CP is known to anastomose with the spinal accessory, hypoglossal, facial, vagus and glossopharyngeal nerve such as with the sympathetic trunk (**Figure 13.1**). Crossing the SCM surface, the superficial cervical plexus (SCP) innervates the skin and superficial structures of the head, neck, and shoulder through four terminal branches: lesser occipital, great auricular, transverse cervical and supraclavicular nerves (**Figure 13.2**) The branches of the intermediate cervical plexus (ICP) lie between the inferior surface of the SCM and the superior surface of MSM, LCM and LSM. The branches of the deep cervical plexus (DCP) innervate the deeper structures of the neck, including the muscles of the anterior neck and the diaphragm, which is innervated by the phrenic nerve.

SONOANATOMY

The four terminal branches of the SCP emerge in the subcutaneous plane from the midpoint of the SCM but they are not ultrasonographically visualized. Moreover, the SCM forms a roof over the nerves of the ICP that can be visualized as a small cluster of hypoechoic nodules, not always apparent, immediately deeper the investing

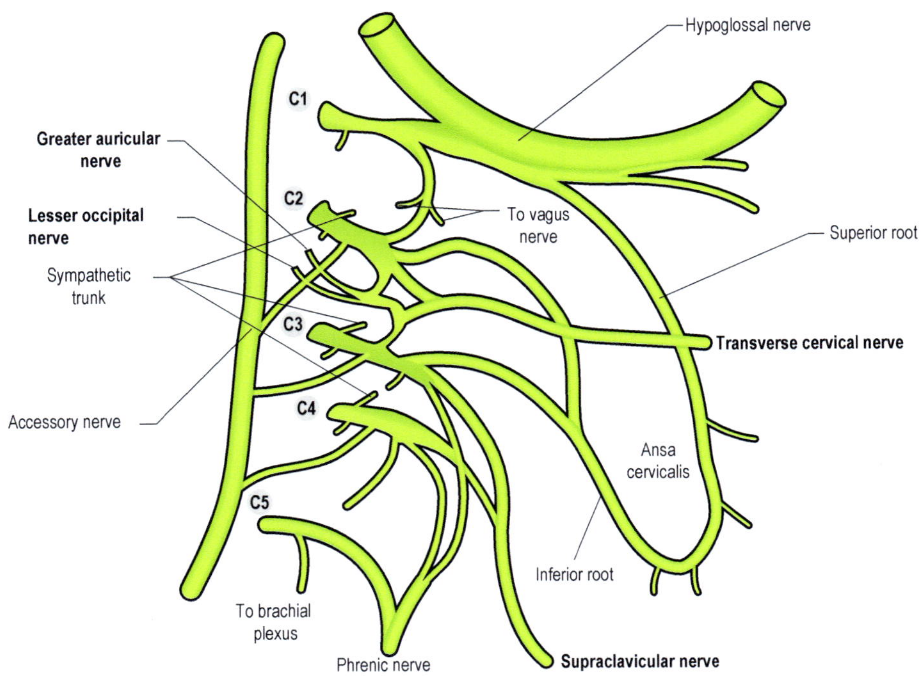

Figure 13.1 Deep and superficial cervical plexus anatomy. The cervical plexus is formed by the anterior divisions of the second through fourth upper cervical nerves that participate in the formation of the brachial plexus, ansa cervicalis, phrenic nerve. The cervical plexus is known to anastomose with the spinal accessory, hypoglossal, facial, vagus, glossopharyngeal nerve and sympathetic trunk.

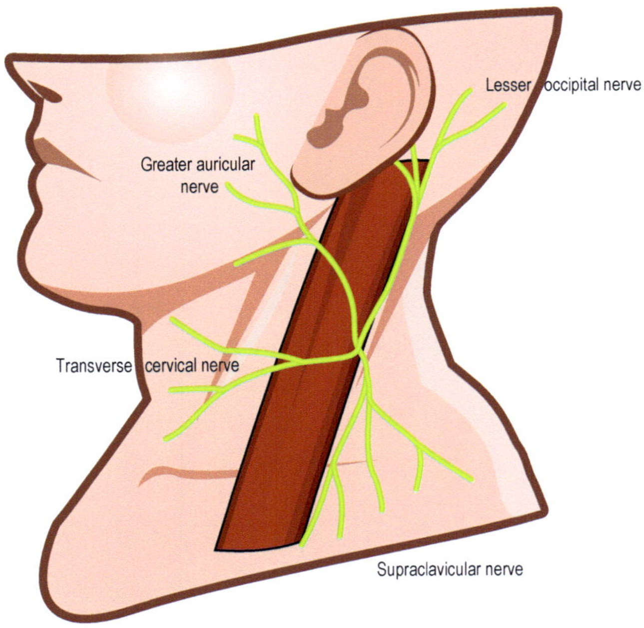

Figure 13.2 Superficial cervical plexus anatomy. Crossing the sternocleidomastoid muscle surface, the superficial cervical plexus innervates the skin and superficial structures of the head, neck, and shoulder through four terminal branches: lesser occipital, greater auricular, transverse cervical and supraclavicular nerves.

layer (IL) of the deep cervical fascia (DCF) and superficial to the PF which can be both seen as two hyperechoic linear structures. The LSM, MSM, LCM, C4 root, the anterior (AT) and posterior tubercles (PT) of transverse process (TP) may be visualized inferiorly under the PF where the DCP lies. The internal jugular vein (IJV) and carotid artery (CA) are visualized medially (**Figure 13.3**)

TECHNIQUE DESCRIPTION

Based on the ultrasound target compartment, CPB can be performed at the superficial, intermediate or deep level. The patient is placed in a supine position looking at the opposite side. A high frequencies linear probe is positioned transversely on the body of SCM at level of thyroid prominence or higher in order to visualize SCM, CA, IJV, vertebral vessels, C4 root and its TP, IL, PF, MSM, LCM and LSM. When the probe is placed too low, the BP is visualized; starting from the BP it's possible counting up the transverse processes of the cervical vertebra from C7 to C4. Via an in plane approach a 50-100 mm SonoPlex stim Pajunk® needle is inserted in a lateral to medial direction (**Figure 13.4**)

Superficial cervical plexus block

The superficial cervical plexus block is described as a subcutaneous injection at the mid-portion of the posterior border of the SCM. Via an in plane approach a 50-100 mm SonoPlex stim Pajunk® needle is inserted in a lateral to medial direction. Local anesthetic is injected above the SCM surface by a subcutaneous infiltration, targetting the four terminal branches of CP (**Figure 13.5**, **Video 13.1**).

Intermediate cervical plexus block

In 2010 Choquet et al. described the ICPB using ultrasound technique and targetting the posterior cervical space (PCS) at the C4 level. Since then many studies have been published under the name of ultrasound-guided intermediate cervical plexus block (USG-ICPB) in order to provide anesthesia/analgesia in different surgery applications. The PCS is the sub-investing fascial space between the SCM and prevertebral muscles and represents the USG-ICPB target. Via

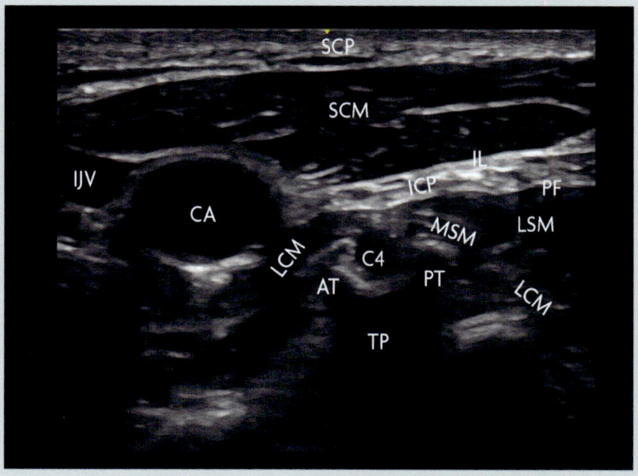

Figure 13.3 Superficial and intermediate cervical plexus sonoanatomy. The superficial cervical plexus lie over the surface of sternocleidomastoid muscle. The intermediate cervical plexus is placed under the sternocleidomastoid muscle between the investing layer and the prevertebral fascia at level of C4 root. AT: anterior tubercle; C4: C4 root; CA: carotid artery; ICP: intermediate cervical plexus; IJV: internal jugular vein; IL: investing layer; LCM: longus capitis muscle; LSM: levator anguli scapulae muscle; MSM: middle scalene muscle; PF: prevertebral fascia; PT: posterior tubercle; SCM: sternocleidomastoid muscle; SCP: superficial cervical plexus; TP: transverse process.

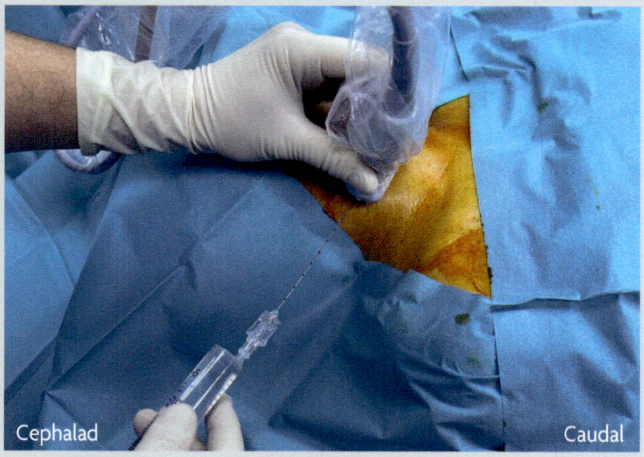

Figure 13.4 Cervical plexus block technique. The patient is placed in a supine position looking at the opposite side. A high frequencies linear probe is positioned transversely on the body of sternocleidomastoid muscle at level of thyroid prominence or higher. Via an in plane approach a 50-100 mm needle is inserted in a lateral to medial direction.

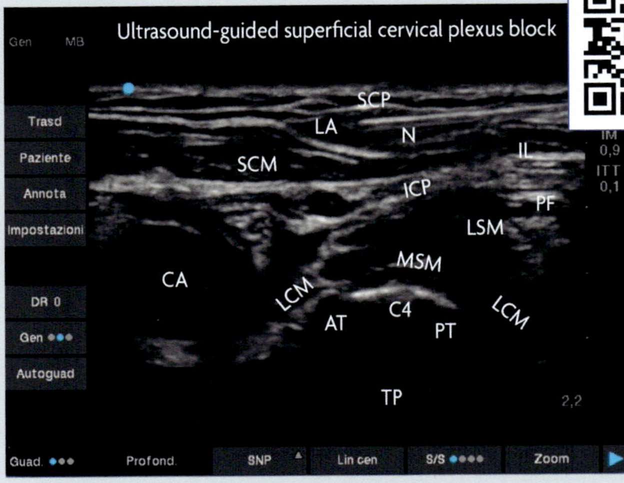

Figure 13.5 Ultrasound superficial cervical plexus block. Local anesthetic is injected above the sternocleidomastoid muscle surface targetting the four branches of superficial cervical plexus. AT: anterior tubercle; C4: C4 root; CA: carotid artery; ICP: intermediate cervical plexus; IL: investing layer; LA: local anesthetic; LCM: longus capitis muscle; LSM: levator anguli scapulae muscle; MSM: middle scalene muscle; N: needle; PF: prevertebral fascia; PT: posterior tubercle; SCM: sternocleidomastoid muscle; SCP: superficial cervical plexus; TP: transverse process.

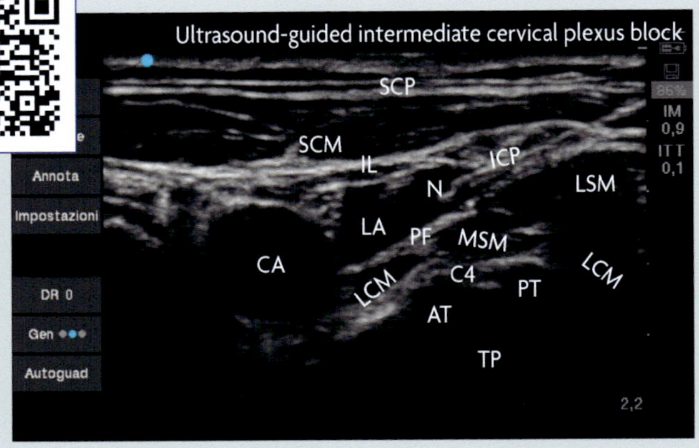

Figure 13.6 Ultrasound intermediate cervical plexus block. Local anesthetic is injected hydrodissecting the plane between the sternocleidomastoid muscle, longus capitis muscle, levator anguli scapulae muscle, middle scalene muscle and their deep cervical investing layer and prevertebral fascia. AT: anterior tubercle; C4: C4 root; CA: carotid artery; ICP: intermediate cervical plexus; IL: investing layer; LA: local anesthetic; LCM: longus capitis muscle; LSM: levator anguli scapulae muscle; MSM: middle scalene muscle; N: needle; PF: prevertebral fascia; PT: posterior tubercle; SCM: sternocleidomastoid muscle; SCP: superficial cervical plexus; TP: transverse process.

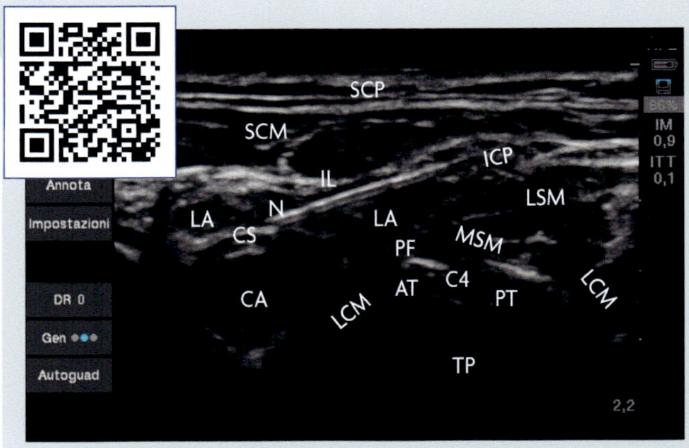

Figure 13.7 Ultrasound intermediate cervical plexus block for carotid endarterectomy. Local anesthetic is injected hydrodissecting the posterior cervical space; then the needle is advanced medially towards the carotid artery to infiltrate the carotid sheath. AT: anterior tubercle; C4: C4 root; CA: carotid artery; CS: carotid sheath; ICP: intermediate cervical plexus; IL: investing layer; LA: local anesthetic; LCM: longus capitis muscle; LSM: levator anguli scapulae muscle; MSM: middle scalene muscle; N: needle; PF: prevertebral fascia; PT: posterior tubercle; SCM: sternocleidomastoid muscle; SCP: superficial cervical plexus; TP: transverse process.

an in plane approach a 50-100 mm SonoPlex stim Pajunk® needle is inserted in a lateral to medial direction through the investing deep fascia underneath SCM keeping an eye on IJV or CA. Local anesthetic is injected hydrodissecting the interfascial plane between the SCM, LCM, LSM, MSM and their deep cervical IL and PF (**Figure 13.6**, **Video 13.1**).

Intermediate cervical plexus block and carotid endarterectomy

Carotid endarterectomy carries a significant risk of brain ischemia. The most available method for monitoring a brain injury is to keep the patient awake under regional anesthesia and ligth sedation. The CA surgery manipulation represents the most painful intraoperative period for the patient due to adventitia innervation. The USG-ICPB combined with carotid sheath infiltration is an effective and safe technique to realize an anesthetic plan. Via an in plane approach a 50-100 mm SonoPlex stim Pajunk® needle is inserted in a lateral to medial direction and local anesthetic is injected hydrodissecting the PCS. Then the needle is advanced medially towards the CA to infiltrate the carotid sheath (**Figure 13.7**, **Video 13.2**).

INDICATION AND DOSAGE

Unilateral or bilateral CPB can provide anesthesia or postoperative analgesia for head and neck surgeries such as carotid surgery, thyroidectomy, minimally invasive parathyroidectomy, tympanomastoid surgery, anterior cervical discectomy and fusion, infratentorial and occipital craniotomy, pinnaplasty or otoplasty, lymph node excision, central venous catheters and portacaths, tracheostomy. It can also be used as a sole anesthetic modality for external ear surgery. CPB can also be used as an adjuvant block for shoulder, clavicle, breast and upper chest wall surgeries, particularly by blocking the supraclavicular branches. The ICPB could provide more profound analgesia or anesthesia for deep structures such as the CA or deeper muscles that may have a visceral distribution of pain (**Figure 13.8**, **Table 13.1**) Higher concentrations of local anesthetic are used to achieve an anesthetic plan while smaller concentrations to ensure intra and postoperative analgesia. The CPB represents a fascial compartment block for which at least 20 ml of local anesthetic are required to obtain the interfascial plane hydrodissection. Levobupivacaine and Ropivacaine are usually adopted to get both an anesthetic plan and a long-lasting analgesia. Due to their short action, mepivacaine and lidocaine are used to achieve an anesthetic plan for fast surgery. The dosages and volumes of the most common local anesthetic are shown in the **Table 13.2**.

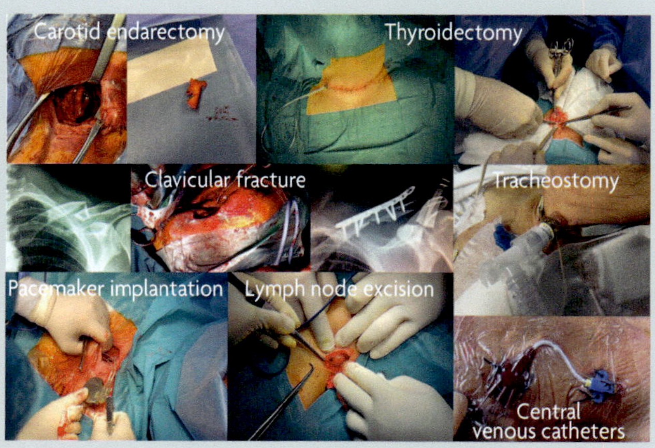

Figure 13.8 Main indications of intermediate and superficial cervical plexus block.

COMPLICATIONS AND CONTRAINDICATIONS

Although both blocks are essentially targeting the same branches of CP, ICPB may produce some adverse events that SCPB do not produce. ICPB could lead to paralysis of recurrent laryngeal nerve block (hoarse voice) and potentially interscalene brachial plexus block particularly when larger volumes and higher concentrations are used. The phrenic nerve paralysis (sensation of breathlessness) may occur depending on the permeability characteristics of PF. On this basis, using 0.2 ml/kg of 0.25% ropivacaine at the C4-5 intervertebral level, ICPB do not cause ipsilateral hemidiaphragmatic paresis. This may imply that the effect of the ICPB on the phrenic nerve is not significant probably due to the protective nature of PF. Further complications are represented by infection, local hematoma, intravascular injection, local anesthetic systemic toxicity, nerve injury. Inadvertent subarachnoid or epidural anesthesia, glossopharyngeal, vagus, hypoglossal and accessory nerves paralysis are expected complications deriving from deep cervical plexus block or from the use of high volume and concentration of local anesthetic. Horner's syndrome (blurred vision, eyelid droop) does not produce any clinical consequence in itself, but it is an unpleasant side effect, although it may not be described as a complication. Contraindications for a cervical plexus block include patient refusal, local infection, previous surgery or radiation therapy to the neck. The main complications and contraindications of CPB are described in the **Table 13.3**.

CHRONIC PAIN

The USG-ICPB provides long-lasting analgesia during the postoperative period and may mitigate the development of neuropathic persistent postoperative pain (PPP) after carotid CEA. SCPB can provide postoperative analgesia for thyroid surgery. Herpes produces painful skin lesions whose pain sometimes continues becoming postherpetic neuralgia. On this

TABLE 13.1 CERVICAL PLEXUS BLOCK INDICATIONS

Local anesthetics	
Carotid surgery	Ensures an adequate monitoring of cerebral blood flow during cross-clamping of the carotid artery in awake patient
Tympanomastoid surgery	Combined with the auricular branch of the vagus (nerve of Arnold) avoids the need for opiates
Pinnaplasty or otoplasty	Intra and postoperative pain management
Lymph node excision	Intra and postoperative pain management
Clavicular surgery or fractures	May require intermediate cervical plexus block and its combination with interscalene block
Central venous catheters	Tunnelled central venous catheters for renal replacement therapy
Central venous catheters, portacaths, pacemaker implantation	Inserted into the subclavian or jugular veins, may require combination with Pecs 1 block for pain management below the clavicle
Tracheostomy	Pay close attention on safety profile of performing bilateral blocks and risks of respiratory distress due to phrenic nerve or recurrent largyngeal nerve block
Thyroidectomy	Intra and postoperative pain management
Emergency department	Para-cervical muscle spasm/pain, acromionclavicular joint injuries, radicular pain, rotator cuff disorder

TABLE 13.2 CERVICAL PLEXUS BLOCK DOSAGES AND VOLUME

Cervical plexus block	Dosage and volume
Anesthesia	Levobupivacaine 0.5% 20 ml
	Mepivacaine 1.5% 20 ml
	Ropivacaine 0.75% 20 ml
	Lidocaine 1.5% 20 ml
Analgesia	Levobupivacaine 0.25% 20 ml
	Ropivacaine 0.375% 20 ml

TABLE 13.3 CERVICAL PLEXUS BLOCK COMPLICATIONS AND CONTRAINDICATIONS

Cervical plexus block complications	Contraindications
Recurrent laryngeal nerve block: Hoarse voice	Patient refusal, local infection, previous surgery or radiation therapy to the neck
Interscalene brachial plexus block: Upper arm anesthesia	
Phrenic nerve paralysis: Sensation of breathlessness	
Infection, local hematoma, intravascular injection, local anesthetic systemic toxicity, nerve injury	
For higher local anesthetic volume and concentrations and for deep cervical plexus block: • Inadvertent subarachnoid or epidural anesthesia • Glossopharyngeal paralysis (difficulty swallowing, impairment of taste over the posterior one-third of the tongue and palate, impaired sensation over the posterior one-third of the tongue, palate, and pharynx, an absent gag reflex and dysfunction of the parotid gland) • Vagus paralysis (palatal and pharyngeal paralysis, laryngeal paralysis, abnormalities of esophageal motility, gastric acid secretion, gallbladder emptying, heart rate and other autonomic dysfunction) • Hypoglossal paralysis (ipsilateral deviation of the tongue and disphagia) • Accessory nerves paralysis (trapezium muscle paralysis is not recognized immediately after injury)	
Horner's syndrome: Blurred vision, eyelid droop	

basis, SCPB can help patients by relieving the pain involving the C3 dermatome level. ICPB with steroid injections is effective in refractory chronic neck and upper back pain from a whiplash injury. Due to its location, SCP is an anatomical site with the potential risk of fibrosis, radiotherapy-associated retraction phenomena or neuroma formation. Interventional treatments performed under ultrasound guidance allow therapies such as radiofrequency ablation. Platelet Rich Fibrin (PRF) could potentially cause an additive effect between neuromodulation and the hydrodissection caused by the infiltration of substances within a fibrotic area.

RECOMMENDED READING

- Avidan A. Horner's syndrome is not a complication of a brachial plexus block. *Regional Anesthesia & Pain Medicine.* 2004;29:378.
- Barone M, Brigand C, Sonnek T, et al. Intermediate cervical plexus block for cervical esophagus diverticulectomy. *Acta Anaesthesiologica Belgica.* 2015;66:59–61.
- Choquet O, Dadure C, Capdevila X. Ultrasound-guided deep or intermediate cervical plexus block: the target should be the posterior cervical space. *Anesthesia & Analgesia.* 2010;111:1563–4.
- Girard F, Quentin C, Charbonneau S, et al. Superficial cervical plexus block for transitional analgesia in infratentorial and occipital craniotomy: a randomized trial. *Canadian Journal of Anaesthesia.* 2010;57:1065–70.
- Guay J, Grabs D. A cadaver study to determine the minimum volume of methylene blue or black naphthol required to completely color the nerves relevant for anesthesia during breast surgery. *Clinical Anatomy.* 2011;24:202–8.

- James A, Niraj G. Intermediate Cervical Plexus Block: A Novel Intervention in the Management of Refractory Chronic Neck and Upper Back Pain Following Whiplash Injury: A Case Report. *A&A Practice.* 2020 Apr;14(6):e01197. doi: 10.1213/XAA.0000000000001197. PMID: 32784315.
- Kesisoglou I, Papavramidis T, Michalopoulos N, et al. Superficial selective cervical plexus block following total thyroidectomy: a randomized trial. *Head & Neck.* 2010;32:984–8.
- Kim HY, Soh EY, Lee J, et al. Incidence of hemi-diaphragmatic paresis after ultrasound-guided intermediate cervical plexus block: a prospective observational study. *Journal of Anesthesia.* 2020 Aug;34(4):483-490. doi: 10.1007/s00540-020-02770-2. Epub 2020 Mar 31. PMID: 32236682
- Kim JS, Joe HB, Park MC, et al. Postoperative analgesic effect of ultrasound-guided intermediatecervical plexus block on unipolar sternocleidomastoid release with myectomy in pediatric patients with congenital muscular torticollis: a prospective, randomized controlled trial. *Regional Anesthesia Pain & Medicine.* 2018;43:634–40.
- MĐdro P, DĐbrowska A, Jarecki J, et al. Anaesthesia for carotid endarterectomy. Ultrasound-guided superficial/intermediate cervical plexus block combined with carotid sheath infiltration. *Anaesthesiology Intensive Therapy.* 2016;48:234–8.
- Mariappan R, Mehta J, Massicotte E, et al. Effect of superficial cervical plexus block on postoperative quality of recovery after anterior cervical discectomy and fusion: a randomized controlled trial. *Canadian Journal of Anaesthesia.* 2015;62:883–90.
- Martusevicius R, Swiatek F, Joergensen LG, et al. Ultrasound-guided locoregional anaesthesia for carotid endarterectomy: a prospective observational study. *European Journal of Vascular and Endovascular Surgery.* 2012;44:27–30.
- Mayhew D, Sahgal N, Khirwadkar R, et al. Analgesic efficacy of bilateral superficial cervical plexus block for thyroid surgery: meta-analysis and systematic review. *British Journal of Anaesthia.* 2018;120:241–51.
- Orduña Valls JM, Soto E, Ferrandis Martínez M, et al.. Cervical plexus as anatomical target for the treatment of postoperative cervical neuropathic pain. *Journal of Pain Research.* 2019 Apr 16;12:1217-1221. doi: 10.2147/JPR.S184306. PMID: 31114303; PMCID: PMC6489597.
- Pandit JJ, Dutta D, Morris JF. Spread of injectate with superficial cervical plexus block in humans: an anatomical study. *British Journal of Anaesthia.* 2003;91:733–5.
- Paraskevas GK, Natsis K, Nitsa Z, et al. Unusual morphological pattern and distribution of the ansa cervicalis: a case report. *Romanian Journal of Morphology and Embryology.* 2014;55:993–6.
- Perisanidis C, Saranteas T, Kostopanagiotou G. Ultrasound-guided combined intermediate and deep cervical plexus nerve block for regional anaesthesia in oral and maxillofacial surgery. *Dentomaxillofacial Radiology.* 2013;42:29945724
- Petrucci E, Cofini V, Pizzi B, et al. Intermediate Cervical Plexus Block in the Management of Persistent Postoperative Pain Post Carotid Endarterectomy: A Prospective, Randomized, Controlled, Clinical Trial. *Pain Physician journal.* 2020 Jun;23(3):237-244. PMID: 32517389.
- Pintaric TS, Hocevar M, Jereb S, et al. A prospective, randomized comparison between combined (deep and superficial) and superficial cervical plexus block with levobupivacaine for minimally invasive parathyroidectomy. *Anesthesia & Analgesia.* 2007;105:1160–3.
- Ritchie MK, Wilson CA, Grose BW, et al. Ultrasound-guided greater auricular nerve block as sole anesthetic for ear surgery. *Clinical Practice.* 2016;6:856.
- Rössel T, Kersting S, Heller AR, et al. Combination of high-resolution ultrasound-guided perivascular regional anesthesia of the internal carotid artery and intermediate cervical plexus block for carotid surgery. *Ultrasound in Medicine & Biology.* 2013;39:981–6.
- Rössel T, Kersting S, Heller AR, et al. Combination of high-resolution ultrasound-guided perivascular regional anesthesia of the internal carotid artery and intermediate cervical plexus block for carotid surgery. *Ultrasound in Medicine & Biology.* 2013;39:981–6.
- Sait Kavaklı A, Kavrut Öztürk N, Umut AyoĐlu R, et al. Comparison of combined (deep and superficial) and intermediate cervical plexus block by use of ultrasound guidance for carotid endarterectomy. *Journal of Cardiothoracic and Vascular Anesthesia.* 2016;30:317–22.
- Saranteas T, Paraskeuopoulos T, Anagnostopoulou S, et al. Ultrasound anatomy of the cervical paravertebral space: a preliminary study. *Surgical and Radiologic Anatomy.* 2010;32:617–22.
- Seidel R, Schulze M, Zukowski K, et al. Ultrasound-guided intermediate cervical plexus block. Anatomical study. *Anaesthesist.* 2015 Jun;64(6):446-50. German. doi: 10.1007/s00101-015-0018-6. Epub 2015 May 27. PMID: 26013020.
- Shakespeare TJ, Tsui BC. Intermittent hoarseness with continuous interscalene brachial plexus catheter infusion due to deficient carotid sheath. *Acta Anaesthesiologica Scandinavica.* 2013;57:1085–6.
- Shin HY, Kim DS, Kim SS. Superficial cervical plexus block for management of herpes zoster neuralgia in the C3 dermatome: a case report. *Journal of Medical Case Reports.* 2014 Feb 19;8:59. doi: 10.1186/1752-1947-8-59. PMID: 24548417; PMCID: PMC3942766.
- Shoja MM, Oyesiku NM, Shokouhi G, et al. A comprehensive review with potential significance during skull base and neck operations, Part II: glossopharyngeal, vagus, accessory, and hypoglossal nerves and cervical spinal nerves 1-4. *Clinical Anatomy.* 2014;27:131–44.
- Telford RJ, Stoneham MD. Correct nomenclature of superficial cervical plexus blocks. *British Journal of Anaesthesia.* 2004;92:775.
- Winnie AP, Ramamurthy S, Durrani Z, et al. Interscalene cervical plexus block: a single-injection technic. *Anesthesia & Analgesia.* 1975;54:370–5.
- Woldegerima YB, Hailekiros AG, Fitiwi GL. The analgesic efficacy of bilateral superficial cervical plexus block for thyroid surgery under general anesthesia: a prospective cohort study. *BMC Research Notes.* 2020 Jan 28;13(1):42. doi: 10.1186/s13104-020-4907-7. PMID: 31992341; PMCID: PMC6986007.

CLINICAL CASE 1 – INTERMEDIATE CERVICAL PLEXUS BLOCK IN A PATIENT AFFECTED BY RIGHT CAROTID STENOSIS AND BULLOUS EMPHYSEMA

Clinical history and anamnesis We report a case of a patient affected by severe chronic pulmonary disease (COPD) and recurring transitory ischemic attack (TIA) due to a right carotid soft plaque stenosis (**Figure 13.9 A**). The patient was admitted to Intensive Care Unit (ICU) after the third TIA without any neurological deficit or respiratory distress despite the computed tomography scan (CT-scan) showing radiologic signs of bullous emphysema (**Figure 13.9 B**).

Technique description Under aseptic conditions via in-plane approach, using a linear probe, a 22 G 100 mm echogenic SonoPlexstim Pajunk® needle was inserted to perform a right intermediate cervical plexus block (US-ICPB) 20 minutes before surgical incision. 10 ml of levobupivacaine 0,5% were injected between the investing layer (IL) and the paravertebral fascia (PF) at level of C4. 7 ml of levobupivacaine 0.5% were injected surrounding the carotid artery (CA) and carotid sheath (CS) (**Figure 13.10 A, B**). No periprocedural complications were recorded. Spontaneous ventilation was maintained, and the patient was cooperative during the carotid clamping (**Figure 13.10 C-E**). No pain was reported (numerical rating scale 0) during surgery. No respiratory depression or pulmonary complications were recorded. Oxygen saturation was >97%, partial pressure of arterial oxygen was >90 mmHg, and partial pressure of arterial carbon dioxide was 41 mmHg. Patient reported a good 24 hour postoperative analgesia (numerical rating scale <3). No nonsteroidal anti-inflammatory agents or opioids were administered.

Materials and methods The patient was scheduled to undergo carotid endarterectomy (CEA) and written informed consent to the procedure was obtained. He received a light sedation via continuous intravenous dexmedetomidine (0.7 mg/kg/h) and supplemental oxygen was administered (8 l/min of oxygen flow) to obtain a SpO_2 of 99%. Continuous verbal contact, vital and respiratory parameters (Hr, Invasive blood pressure, Sao_2%) were monitored.

Conclusions Ultrasound intermediate cervical plexus block can be considered a safe and effective technique for patients undergoing carotid endarterectomy affected by severe chronic pulmonary disease and bullous emphysema, keeping them awake in spontaneous breathing, avoiding respiratory complications deriving from endotracheal intubation and general anesthesia.

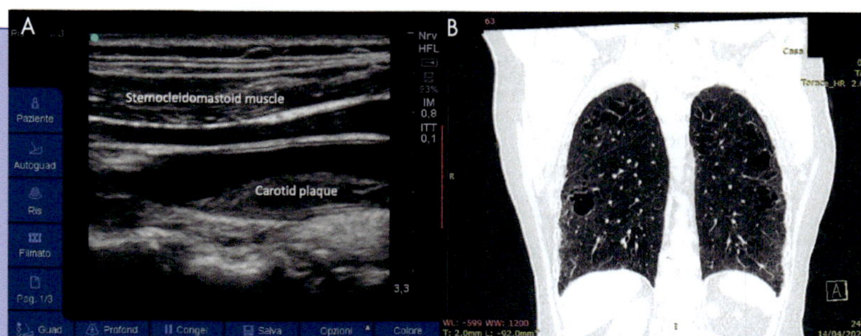

Figure 13.9 A Long axis view of right carotid plaque. **B** Computed tomography scan shows the radiologic signs of severe chronic pulmonary disease and bullous emphysema.

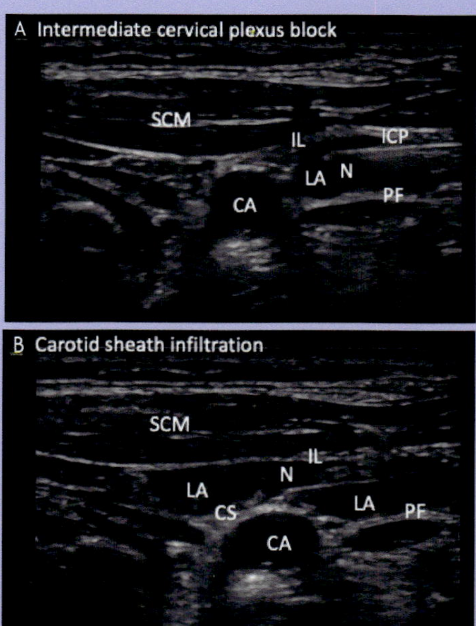

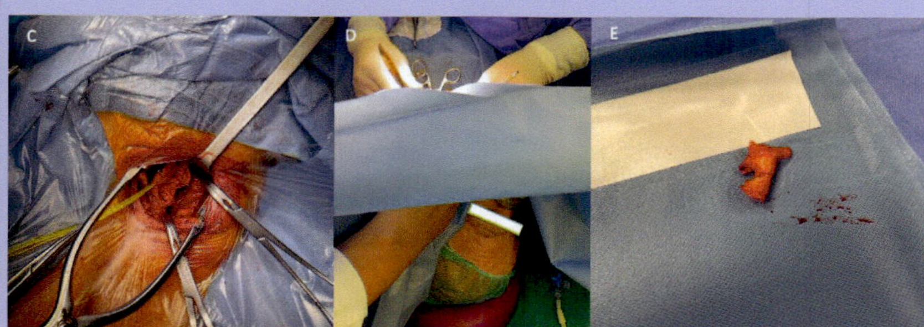

Figure 13.10 A Intermediate cervical plexus block. **B** Carotid sheath infiltration. **C** Carotid clamping. **D** Spontaneous breathing. **E** Carotid plaque. CA: carotid artery; CS: carotid sheath; ICP: intermediate cervical plexus; IL: investing layer; LA: local anesthetic; N: needle; PF: prevertebral fascia; SCM: sternocleidomastoid muscle.

CLINICAL CASE 2 – PECS 1 AND INTERMEDIATE CERVICAL PLEXUS BLOCK IN A PATIENT AFFECTED BY ALZHEIMER'S DISEASE AND SECOND-DEGREE ATRIOVENTRICULAR BLOCK MOBITZ TYPE 1

Clinical history and anamnesis We report a case of a patient affected by advanced Alzheimer's disease, second-degree atrioventricular block Mobitz type 1, blood hypertension, renal chronic disease, diabetes type 1. Previous operations: coronary artery bypass grafting, left carotid stenting. The patient's family referred several lipothymic and syncopal episodes for which he was scheduled to undergo to pacemaker implantation.

Materials and methods Written informed consent to the procedures was obtained. The patient received light sedation via continuous intravenous dexmedetomidine (0.7 mg/kg/h) and supplemental oxygen was administered (3 l/min of oxygen flow). Vital and respiratory parameters (Hr, ECG, Non-invasive blood pressure, SaO_2%) were monitored.

Technique description Under aseptic conditions, using a linear probe and a 22 G 100 mm echogenic SonoPlex stim Pajunk® needle in-plane approach, a combined Pecs 1 and intermediate cervical plexus block (US-ICPB) were performed. 10 ml of ropivacaine 0,5% were injected between pectoralis major (PMM) and pectoralis minor muscles (pmm). 10 ml of levobupivacaine 0.5% were injected under the sternocleidomastoid muscle (SCM) between the investing layer (IL) and prevertebral fascia (PF) (**Figure 13.11**). No periprocedural complications were recorded. Spontaneous ventilation was maintained and no respiratory depression or pulmonary complications were recorded. Oxygen saturation was >98 (**Figure 13.12**).

Conclusions Despite Pecs 1 is considered an effective anesthetic technique for pacemaker implantation, it does not completely anesthetize the clavicular skin region in which the device is usually placed. On this basis, an intermediate cervical plexus block is required to block the supraclavicular branches or cervical plexus. The combination of two regional techniques ensures a complete anesthesia for pectoral and clavicular region and represents a safe procedure also in critically ill patients.

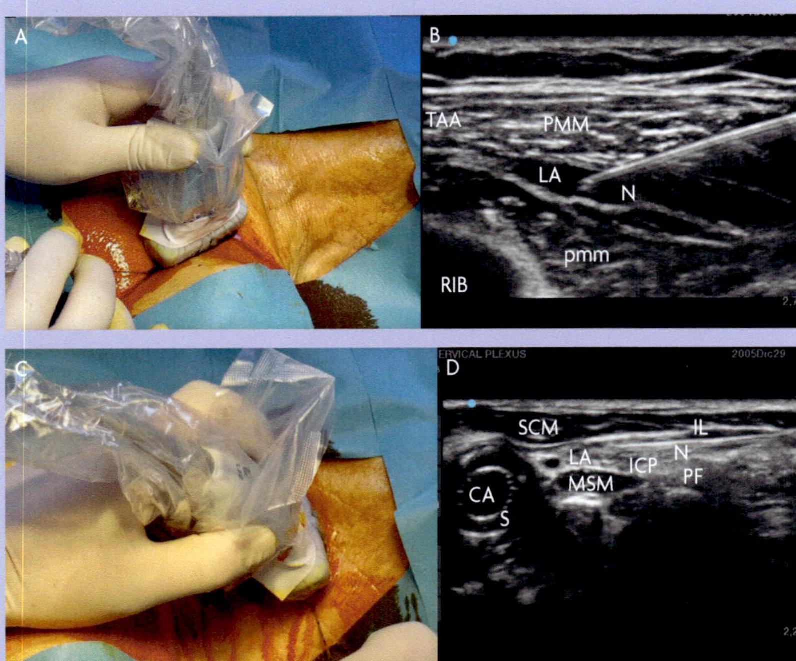

Figure 13.11 A Pecs 1: probe and patient position, needle insertion. **B** Pecs 1 block: local anesthetic is injected between pectoralis major and pectoralis minor muscles. **C** Intermediate cervical plexus block: probe and patient position, needle insertion. **D** Intermediate cervical plexus block: local anesthetic is injected between the investing layer and prevertebral fascia. CA: carotid artery; ICP: intermediate cervical plexus; IL: investing layer; LA: local anesthetic; MSM: middle scalene muscle; N: needle; PF: prevertebral fascia; PMM: pectoralis major muscle; pmm: pectoralis minor muscle; RIB: rib; S: carotid stent; SCM: sternocleidmoastoid muscle; TAA: thoracoacromial artery.

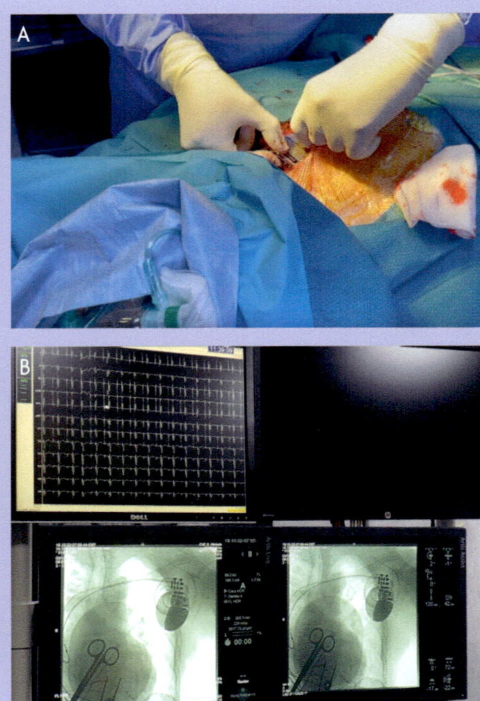

Figure 13.12 A Pacemaker implantation and spontaneous breathing. **B** Pacemaker X-ray control.

CHAPTER
14

Local infiltration analgesia (LIA) and continuous wound infusion (CWI)

Fabio Costa, Giuseppe Pascarella, Danilo Canzio, Fausto D'Agostino, Andrea Tognù

Basic principles of LIA and continuous wound infusion

LIA and CWI consist of direct infiltration of the surgical site with local anesthetic (LA) or infusion of LA through a catheter directly placed into the surgical wound. They are effective, safe and easy to perform. Their effectiveness goes beyond the sodium channel blockade of peripheral nerves.

Postoperative pain results from:

1. **Nerve fibers** that are innervating the site of the incision, retraction or suturing **generate impulses**;
2. **Inflammatory mediators**, at the surgical site **sensitize** uninjured and injured **nerve fibers**;
3. Pain circuits in the **spinal cord become sensitized**, then have an increased response to stimuli that are noxious and can transform the responsiveness to stimuli that are not painful, for example light touch or gentle pressure.

With LIA and CWI, LA affect these factors:

- Wound **LA** infiltration **attenuate generation and propagation of injury-induced discharges;**
- **LA suppress** some phases of the **inflammation**, **inhibiting local sensitizing responses** (anti-inflammatory properties of local anesthetics have been clearly demonstrated);
- **Central sensitization is inhibited** in some neuronal pathways activated by inflammation, also attenuated by the reduced peripheral sensitization itself.

In addition, LA plasmatic reabsorption, leads to systemic concentrations sufficient to relieve postoperative pain and suppress processes that would eventually escalate pain in the days following surgery.

Given these considerations, LIA and CWI seem to be a rational approach to reduce the afferent nociceptive barrage and thereby pain and stress responses while preserving motor function.

History of LIA and CWI

In the early 1900s Fulde and Capelle had the intuition to irrigate the surgical wound with LA to allow both pain control and postoperative mobilization, developing, in 1930, the first CWI system. It has been experimented with throughout the 20th century and resulted safe and effective in several clinical settings. Though, LIA and CWI started to spread just over a decade ago, after the development of multi-holed catheters designed to infuse LA over a wider area. Standard epidural catheters, previously used, were not found to be equally effective. Development of portable infusion pumps enhanced capability to continue the regional wound infusion effectively for days. Nowadays, pumps prefilled with sterile LA, ready to infuse, are available. They allow faster procedures with minimum manipulation further reducing the risk of wound infection (**Figure 14.1**).

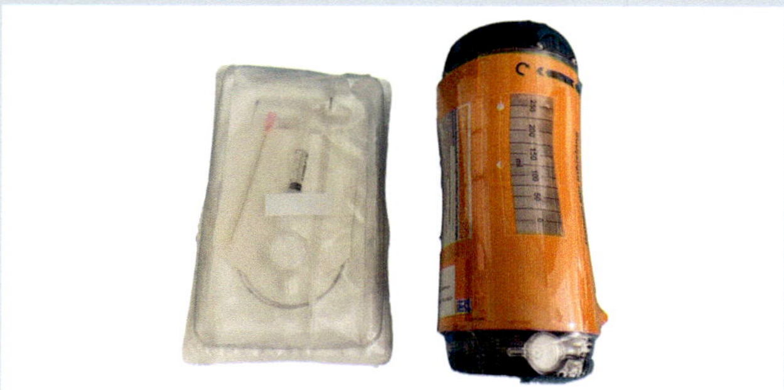

Figure 14.1 Ropivacaine Readyfusor (BioQ Pharma, San Francisco, California, US) – ready to infuse pump, prefilled with sterile LA.

ANATOMY AND SONOANATOMY

Anatomy for LIA and CWI mainly coincide with the surgical wound and the catheters are placed by the surgeons under direct vision, so there is not a sono-anatomy.

The main planes for catheter positioning are summarized in **Table 14.1**.

For abdomino-pelvic surgeries, a preperitoneal plane, between the parietal peritoneum and the transversalis fascia, along the full length of the wound is the most effective (**Figure 14.2**).

For other procedures, there is not a recommended specific plane for placing a catheter.

For breast surgery, the catheter is usually placed at the top of the wound above or below the pectoralis major muscle. A second catheter in the axillary region may be useful for axillary node dissection.

For thoracotomies, sub-pleural and inter-pleural catheter placement showed poorer results, compared with intercostal or sub-serratus catheters. For cardiac surgery the catheter is generally placed over the sternal closure. Eljezi et al put a double catheter on both

TABLE 14.1 PLANES FOR CATHETER PLACEMENT IN DIFFERENT TECHNIQUES

CWI for abdomino-pelvic surgery	Preperitoneal
CWI for breast surgery	
Simple mastectomy	Top of the scar (drain at the bottom)
Inplant subpectoral	Subpectoral plane at the top (drain at the bottom)
CWI for cardiothoracic surgery	
Thoracotomy	Interpleural – Intercostal Deep serratus plane close to rib reapproximation
Sternotomy	Presternal midline Two catheters pecto-intercostal plane both sides
Shoulder	Subacromial space Glenohumeral space
Hip	Intrarticular, close to femoral head
Knee	Intrarticular, close to tibial component and posterior capsule, ending close to medial condile

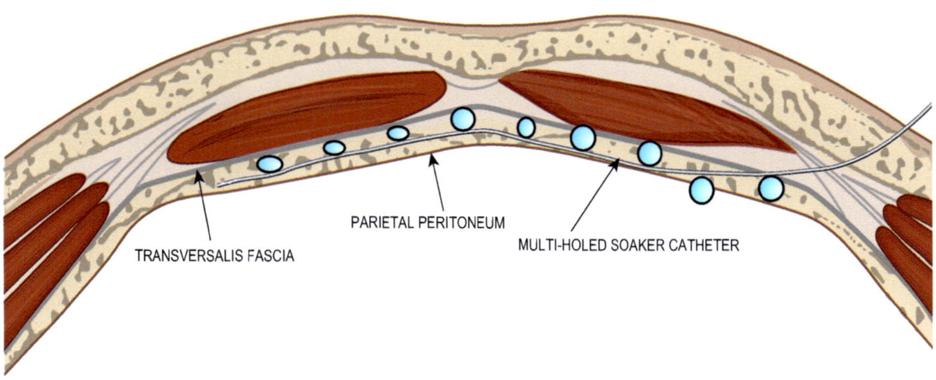

Figure 14.2 Preperitoneal catheter in the plane between transversalis fascia and parietal peritoneum.

sides of the sternum, between the deep fascia of the pectoralis major muscle and the fascia of the outer intercostal muscle, aiming to involve the anterior cutaneous branches of the intercostal nerves; Dowling et al described a technique in which two catheters connected to a single pump were placed on the midline as showed in **Figure 14.3**. For the other procedures, either sub-fascial or subcutaneous catheter placement are described.

For orthopedic procedures, single shot LIA consists in direct infiltration of specific periarticular structures (**Table 14.2**).

It is usually performed by the surgeon under direct vision. Del Buono et al, described an ultrasound guided LIA for hip surgeries, performed by the anesthesiologist: an anterior infiltration between the iliopsoas muscle and the ilio-femoral ligament; a posterior infiltration between the quadratus femoris muscle and the posterior hip capsule (**Figure 14.4**). The technique resulted in a complete analgesia comparable to the LIA performed by the surgeon.

For periarticular LIA a distinction between points of injection (**Table 14.2**) and site for catheter placement (**Table 14.1**), is necessary.

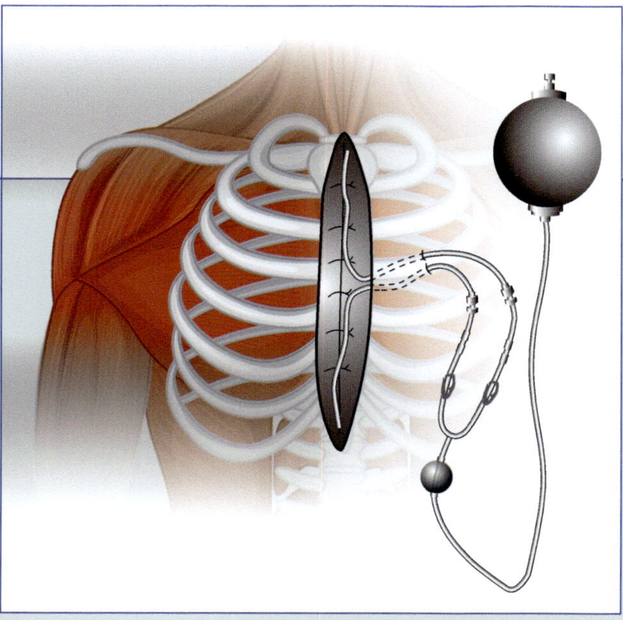

Figure 14.3 Dowling 2003 – double presternal catheter for CWI after cardiac surgery.

Shoulder: tissues surrounding the glenoid, rotator capsule and cuff around the humerus and skin incision are the target structures for local infiltration; catheter either in the sub-acromial or the gleno-humeral space.

Hip: deep and superficial fascia, tissues around the rim of the acetabulum, external rotators (gluteus medius, maximus and minimus muscles, quadratus femoris muscle, obturator muscle), gluteus maximus tendon, subcutaneous layer and skin; catheter tunnelled into the hip joint with the tip near the femoral head.

Knee: posterior capsule (posterior femoral condyles), collateral ligaments, cruciate ligament, circularly around prosthesis, subcutaneous layer and skin; catheter either proximal or lateral to the incision, tunnelled into the joint along the posterior capsule, tip behind medial condyle.

TECHNIQUE DESCRIPTION (SINGLE SHOT AND CONTINUOUS)

The basic common procedures for LIA and CWI may be applied to every field of application.

Basics of LIA

LIA consists in an injection of a high volume of a diluted LA, with or without adjuncts, directly in the

TABLE 14.2 PERIARTICULAR LIA – ANATOMIC TARGET STRUCTURES

Shoulder	• Tissues surrounding the glenoid • Rotator capsule and cuff around the humerus • Skin incision
Hip joint	• Deep and superficial fascia • Tissues around the rim of the acetabulum • External rotators (gluteus medius, maximus and minimus muscles, quadratus femoris muscle, obturator muscle) • Gluteus maximus tendon • Subcutaneous layer and skin
Knee joint	• Posterior capsule (posterior femoral condyles) • Collateral ligaments • Cut cruciate ligament • Circularly around the prosthesis • Subcutaneous layer and skin

tissues (or around them) identified as responsible for the postoperative nociception for a specific surgical procedure. LIA is commonly performed by the surgeon at the end of the procedure, before the skin closure. Specific target points for the injections are described in the previous paragraph. Main technical features of LIA relate to infection prevention and are the following:

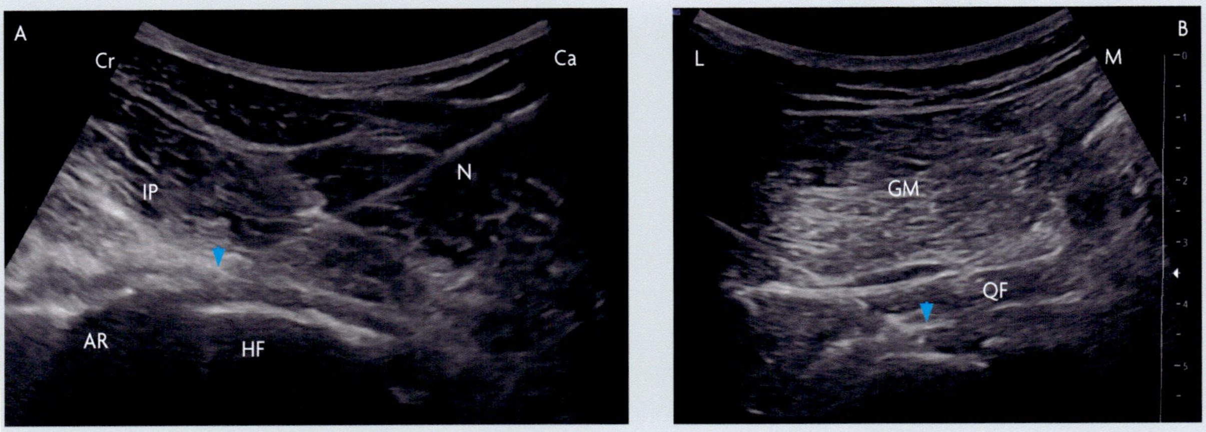

Figure 14.4 Del Buono 2019 – Ultrasound guided LIA of the hip. **A** Anterior. **B** Posterior; AR: acetabular rime; Ca: caudal; Cr: cranial; GM: gluteus maximus muscle; HF: head of femur; IP: iliopsoas muscle; L: lateral; M: medial; N: needle; QF: quadratus femoris muscle; arrowhead: injection point.

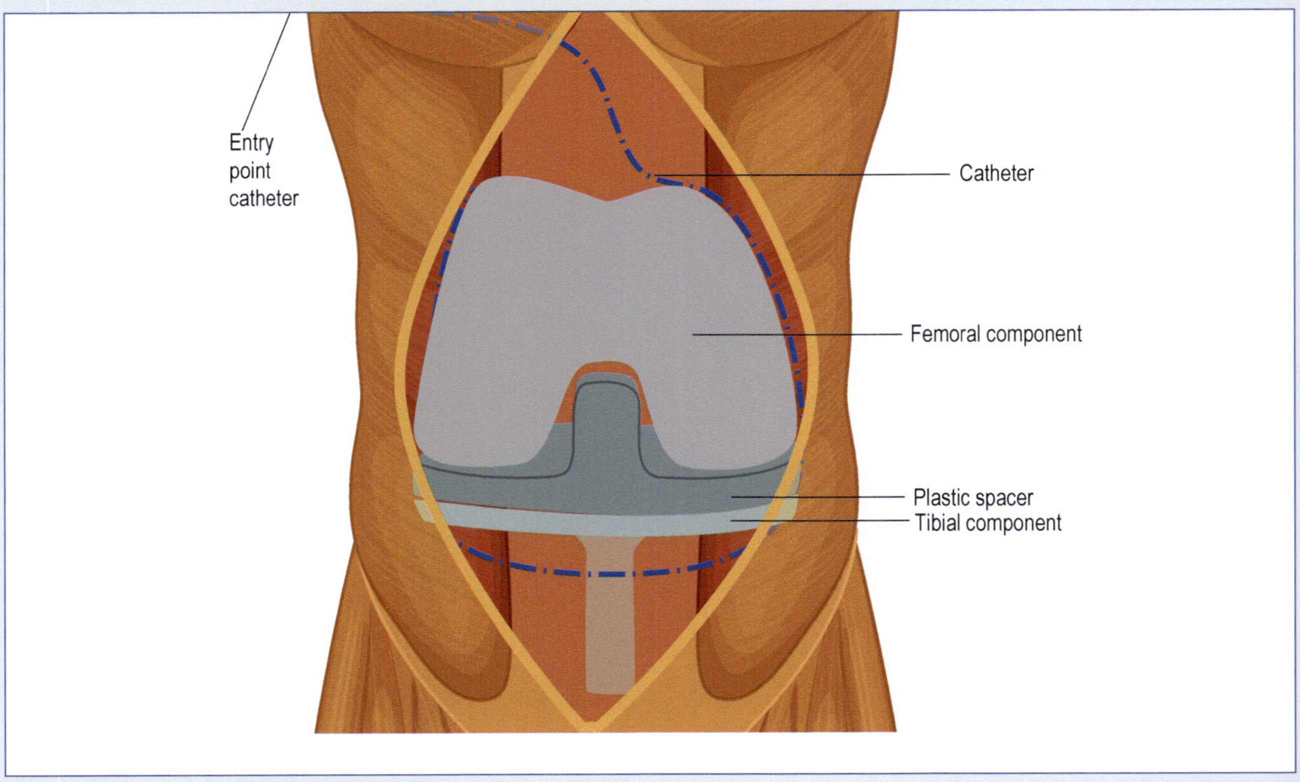

Figure 14.5 Catheter placement for continuous periarticular LIA after knee arthroplasty.

- LIA mixture has to be sterile, it should be prepared with all the precautions avoiding any possible contamination of the solution;
- INJECTIONS must be performed with a sterile needle;
- an ANTIBACTERIAL FILTER should be placed between the syringe and the needle before the injection.

Basics of CWI

CWI is a prolonged instillation of LA inside the wound, through a multi-hole catheter, usually inserted by the surgeon at the end of the procedure. The following steps of the procedure should be observed:

1. Choice of catheter EXIT-SITE:
    - far enough (2-3 cm) from the wound to avoid the wound medication to involve it (**Figure 14.6**);
    - usually either at the top or at the bottom of the wound; or at the middle side. To facilitate catheter insertion and positioning.
2. Selection of CATHETER:
    - multi-holed specifically designed catheters are preferred. They allow the maximum LA distribution into the wound;
    - catheter length must be adequate to obtain a proper positioning along the whole wound and an adequate catheter dressing.
3. Catheter INSERTION:
    - a specifically designed percutaneous peel apart introducer should be preferred (**Figure 14.6**), catheter through needle technique may also be chosen. As alternatives either the use of epidural catheters, inserted through the Thuoy needle or of a thin multi-holed drain tube inserted with the aid of a Kelly clamp from the inside of the wound have been described.
4. Catheter POSITIONING:
    - the catheter holes should be positioned in the middle of the wound. If the catheter length exceeded the wound length, it should be coiled inside the wound. All catheter holes must lay inside the wound.
5. Catheter SECUREMENT:
    - securement should avoid accidental dislodgement, especially during patients movements. A coil at the exit site Is recommended (**Figure 14.7**). Either suturing or adhesive transparent dressings are described. Tissue adhesives may be useful in reducing catheter movements and exit site leakage.
6. DRAIN:
    - if a drain was necessary, it should be placed as far away as possible from the catheter (**Figure 14.8**). In those cases, intermittent boluses of LA, followed by temporary drain closure, may be advantageous in comparison with continuous infusion.

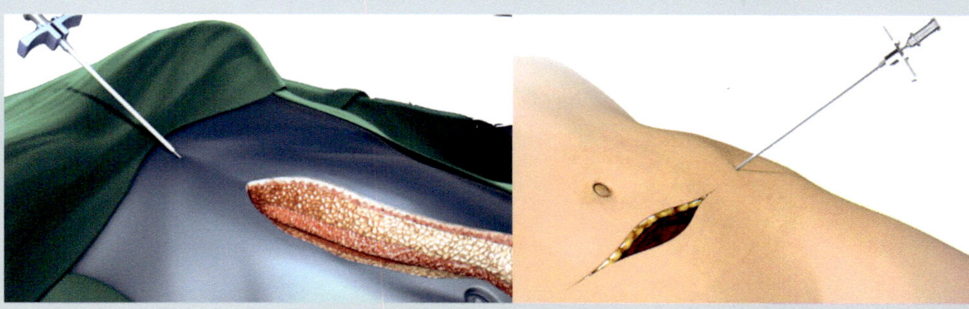

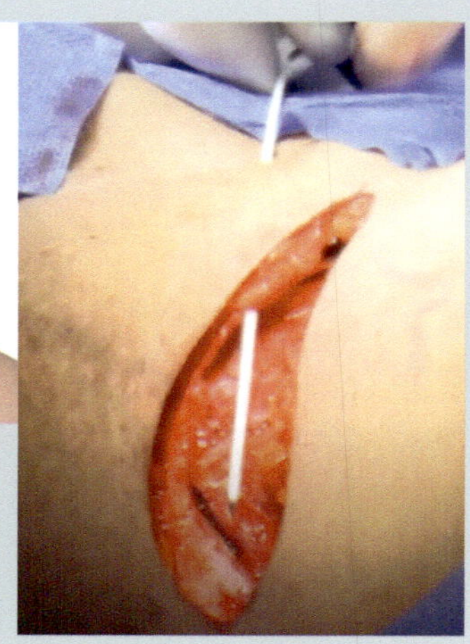

Figure 14.6 Peel-apart introducer inserted below transversalis fascia.

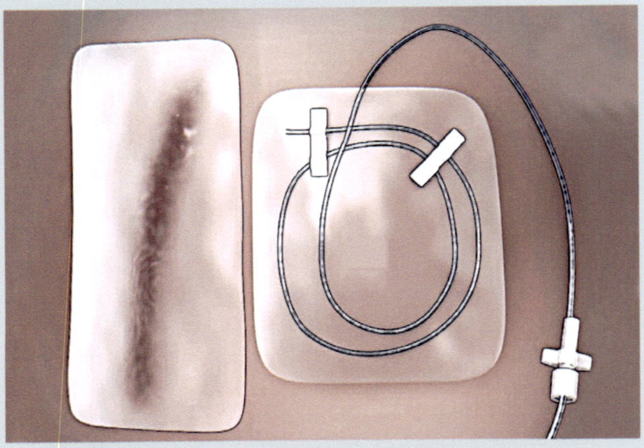

Figure 14.7 Catheter securement and dressing.

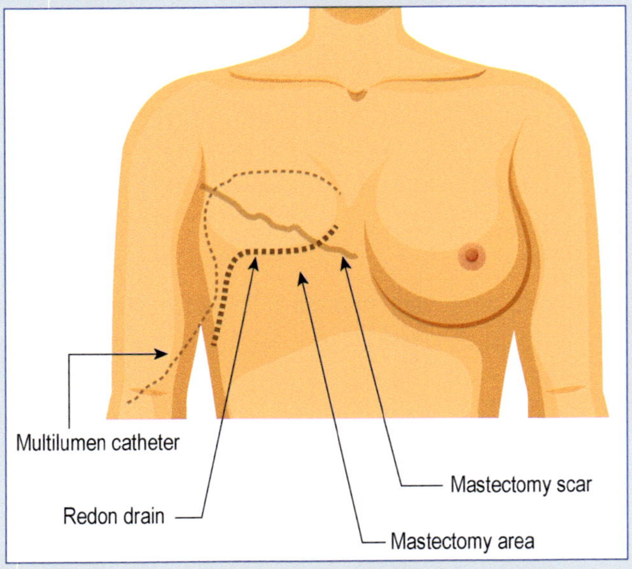

Figure 14.8 Beguinot 2020 – CWI catheter and drain in the same wound after mastectomy.

Video 14.1 Preperitoneal wound catheter placement.

7. PRIMING:
   - catheter priming and starting bolus are mandatory before wound closure in order to verify proper catheter positioning and to obtain initial analgesic effect before surgery ending.

8. DRESSING:
   - Sterile, semipermeable, transparent dressings are recommended, however, any kind of dressing can been used, either to cover the exit site or to stabilize the catheter over the patient's skin.

9. INFUSION:
   - Various infusion regimens have been described. Continuous infusion, as well as intermittent or on demand boluses have been effectively used (**Video 14.1**).

INDICATIONS AND DOSAGES

Indications

LIA and CWI are effective in reducing postoperative pain, opioid consumption, hospitalization and to improve rehabilitation in several clinical settings in which they could be considered indicated. Though, indications and dosages have not been completely defined yet. For some procedures, LIA and CWI are not recommended because of their poor contribution to patient's analgesia.

Main fields of application were analyzed in a recent review by Paladini et al. (2020) and a meta-analysis of 121 RCTs by Huang et al (2021). They are summarized in **Table 14.3**, together with a brief summary of available levels of evidence (LoE) and grades of recommendation (GoR).

Less frequently LIA and CWI have been used in plastic surgery procedures such as abdominoplasty or breast reconstructions. Either continuous infusion or intermittent boluses are safe and effective, though the analgesic effect is modest.

LIA and CWI are promising for spine surgeries, from the single-level lumbar discectomy to the more complex spinal fusion procedures.

There are encouraging reports about applications in pediatric surgery.

Dosages

Local anesthetics

The first and main purpose of LIA and CWI is to achieve a sensory block in the wound area for as long as possible, thus long acting molecules are preferred. The most used are 0.2 to 0.5% ropivacaine and 0.25

TABLE 14.3 INDICATIONS FOR LIA AND CWI* AND SUMMARY OF RECOMMENDATIONS

FIELD OF APPLICATION	SPECIFIC SURGERIES	SUMMARY OF RECCOMENDATIONS
Orthopedic	Shoulder replacement	Comparable to nerve blockade
	Knee replacement	EL high – GoR strong
	Hip replacement	Not recommended
	Spine fusion	Single shot EL high – GoR strong
	Shoulder arthroscopy and rotator cuff repair	Not enough data
Upper and lower limb	Carpal tunnel release Hand lacerations Ankle and foot surgery Revascularization and amputation of lower limb	Not enough data
Abdomino-pelvic	C-section	Single shot or CWI – Grade A
Laparotomic	Hysterectomy	Single shot – Grade A CWI not recommended
	Radical prostatectomy	Single shot – Grade B CWI not recommended
	Colo-rectal	CWI preperitoneal as alternative to TEA Grade B
	Gastrectomy	EL low to moderate – GoR weak
	Liver surgery	EL moderate – GoR strong
	Pancreatic surgery	EL moderate – GoR weak
Laparoscopic	Colorectal Gastric bypass Living donor nephrectomy	Not enough data
Breast		
Minor surgeries	Breast lump excision	Grade A
Major surgeries	Wide local excision and reduction mammoplasty Mastectomy with or without reconstruction Radical mastectomy Axillary node dissection	Grade A (added to regional blocks)
Cardiothoracic	Thoracotomy	EL high – GoR strong
	Sternotomy	Not enough data
	Thoracoscopy	Not enough data

*Paladini et al., 2020.

to 0.5% levobupivacaine and bupivacaine. Ropivacaine and levobupivacaine should be preferred as they have a higher safety profile. New slow release preparations of LA are under investigation. First data on liposomal bupivacaine are controversial and inconclusive.

Adjuvants

In order to prolong sensory block for LIA, many drugs have been used as adjunct to the LA. Efficacy and dosages are summarized in **Table 14.4**. Sometimes epinephrine has been included in order to delay LA clearance from the local site due to the epinephrine-induced vasoconstriction.

Delivery rates, modalities and duration of treatment

(summarized in **Table 14.5**)

Catheter priming and starting bolus consist of a 10 ml bolus of LA through the catheter already placed before closing the wound, to check the spread of LA into

TABLE 14.4 EFFICACY AND REPORTED DOSAGES OF THE MOST USED ADJUVANTS IN LIA AND CWI

ADJUVANT	DOSAGE	PROVED EFFECTIVE	PROMISING	NOT RECOMMENDED
Clonidine	30 to 250 μg	✓		
Dexmedetomidine	0.5 to 5 μg/kg	✓		
Fentanyl	10-100 μg		✓	
Morphine	2-5 mg			✓
Meperidine	50 mg			✓
Buprenorphine	0.5 μg/kg		✓	
Ketorolac	30-60 mg		✓	
Meloxicam	7.5 mg			✓
Diclofenac	20 mg/48h		✓	
Dexamethasone	8-16 mg		✓	
Methylprednisolone	40 mg			✓
Ketamine	0.5 to 2 mg/kg			✓
Magnesium sulfate	500 to 6000 mg or 80 mg/kg		✓	

TABLE 14.5 DELIVERY RATES, MODALITIES AND DURATION OF TREATMENT

FIELD OF APPLICATION	MODALITY	DELIVERY RATE	DURATION
Orthopedic procedures			
Shoulder, hip, knee	Single shot: 80-120 ml: target tissues and skin incision mainly ropivacaine 0.2% Infusion through catheter	2-6 ml/h – PCA	24-72 h
Abdomino-pelvic surgery			
Colorectal and general surgery Gynecology (C-section, hysterectomy)	10 ml starting bolus through the wound catheter Infusion through one or two catheters ropivacaine 0.2%; levobupivacaine 0.25%; bupivacaine 0.25%	Infusion 2-6 ml/h Intermittent bolus 15-20 ml/4-6h	24-48 h
Breast surgery	10 ml starting bolus through the wound catheter Infusion through catheter ropivacaine 0.2%; levobupivacaine 0.25%; bupivacaine 0.25%	Infusion 2-5 ml/h Intermittent bolus 15-20 ml/4-6h	24-48 h
Cardiothoracic surgery Thoracotomy Sternotomy	10 ml starting bolus through the wound catheter Infusion through catheter ropivacaine 0.2%; bupivacaine 0.25%	0.1 ml/kg/h 3-6 ml/h	24-120 h

the wound. After the skin closure, the infusion starts at a rate between 3 and 6 ml/h and continued for 24-72 hours.

COMPLICATIONS AND CONTRAINDICATIONS

Problems associated with LIA and CWI are rare, however potential complications and related safety strategies must be taken into account.

One of the main concerns about CWI is the potential for **wound infection**. LA are bacteriostatic, therefore the risk for local infections is small and the incidence of infections is less than 0.1%. Nevertheless, adopting a sterile technique is recommended and use of a sterile, prefilled pump such as Readyfusor system is preferable compared to self-built infusion systems and self-prepared mixtures. Use of strict aseptic procedures for all top-ups and refills are also recommended.

Delayed wound healing is another feared problem potentially related to CWI. Indeed, LA may influence the process of wound healing, but what is more important is to rule out any adverse effect of LA on mechanical strength of the scar. Studies concluded that lidocaine, bupivacaine and ropivacaine do not produce any significant harm to the tissue cicatrization.

Long term exposure to LA may result in several **tissues toxic effects**. Skeletal muscles exposed to LA displayed myotoxic effects. However, only a few concerning cases have been seen, but effects may be clinically relevant. Risk factors included higher concentrations, prolonged exposure, and use of bupivacaine. LA may also lead to tendinotoxic effects, decreasing tendons biomechanical strength with a potential development of fatty degeneration. Lidocaine showed more cytotoxic effects compared with ropivacaine and bupivacaine. Current data suggest that toxicity may not affect postoperative function. Although, caution must be used for LIA and CWI especially for shoulder surgeries. Cartilage tissue seems to be highly susceptible to LA. Some studies have showed cytotoxicity of LA on chondrocytes that increases from ropivacaine to mepivacaine to bupivacaine in a time-dependent and concentration-dependent manner. For LIA and CWI, concentrations lower than 0.25% of bupivacaine, 0.5% of ropivacaine, and 0.5% of mepivacaine did not reveal significant chondrotoxicity and are recommended.

Since CWI requires prolonged administration of quite high volumes of LAs, **local anesthetic systemic toxicity (LAST)** is a potentially lethal complication that must be always considered. Despite no cases have ever been reported with LIA and CWI, close attention to the drug selection and the total dose must be paid. Ropivacaine 0.2 to 0.5% should be preferred, hepatic and renal function should be assessed.

The most common complication of a regional anesthesia technique is its failure. CWI effectiveness may be affected by **catheter and pumps related problems** also. Catheter dislodgment, catheter kinking and obstruction, leakage from exit site, pump disconnection, pump malfunction have been reported as cause of ineffectiveness. Elastomeric pumps may be inaccurate and deliver inappropriate amounts of LA. Electronic pumps could be more precise, but need batteries and programming. Drug delivery systems with spring mechanism such as Readyfusor may combine easiness of elastomeric pumps to accuracy of electronic pumps.

RECOMMENDED READING

- Abrão, J, Antunes MB, Garcia LV. Local Anesthetics Infiltration and Wound Healing Process. 2019. Available from: doi:10.5772/intechopen.89278.
- Bai JW, An D, Perlas A, et al. Adjuncts to local anesthetic wound infiltration for postoperative analgesia: a systematic review. Reg Anesth Pain Med. 2020 Aug;45(8):645-655. Available from: doi: 10.1136/rapm-2020-101593.
- Beguinot M, Monrigal E, Kwiatkowski F, et al. Continuous wound infiltration with ropivacaine after mastectomy: a randomized controlled trial. J Surg Res. 2020 Oct;254:318-326. Available from: doi: 10.1016/j.jss.2020.05.006.
- Capelle W. Die bedentung des wundschmerzes und seiner ausschaltung fur dan ablauf der atmung bei laparotomierte. Dtsch Z Chir. 1935;246:466–485
- Del Buono R, Pascarella G, Costa F, et al. Ultrasound-guided local infiltration analgesia for hip surgery: myth or reality? Minerva Anestesiol. 2019 Nov;85(11):1242-1243. Available from: doi: 10.23736/S0375-9393.19.13701-7.
- Dowling R, Thielmeier K, Ghaly A, et al. Improved pain control after cardiac surgery: results of a randomized, double-blind, clinical trial. J Thorac Cardiovasc Surg. 2003 Nov;126(5):1271-8. doi: Available from: doi:10.1016/s0022-5223(03)00585-3.

- Eljezi V, Imhoff E, Bourdeaux D, et al. Bilateral sternal infusion of ropivacaine and length of stay in ICU after cardiac surgery with increased respiratory risk: A randomised controlled trial. Eur J Anaesthesiol. 2017 Feb;34(2):56-65. Available from: doi: 10.1097/EJA.0000000000000564.
- Goerig M, Gottschalk A. Beginning of continuous wound infusion with local anesthetics: with special emphasis on the contributions from Walter Capelle and Ewald Fulde. Anaesthesist. 2017;66 (7):518–529. Available from: doi:10.1007/s00101-017-0285-5.
- Gupta A. Wound infiltration with local anaesthetics in ambulatory surgery. Curr Opin Anaesthesiol. 2010 Dec;23(6):708-13. Available from: doi: 10.1097/ACO.0b013e32833f0dd7.
- Haller Y, Gantenbein AR, Willimann P, et al. Systemic ropivacaine diminishes pain sensitization processes: a randomized, double-blinded, placebo-controlled, crossover study in healthy volunteers. Pain Ther. 2014;3(1):45-58. Available from: doi:10.1007/s40122-013-0021-z.
- Hollmann MW, Durieux ME, Fisher DM. Local Anesthetics and the Inflammatory Response: A New Therapeutic Indication?. Anesthesiology. 2000;93:858–875 Available from: doi: 10.1097/00000542-200009000-00038.
- Honda, H., Gotoh, M., Kanazawa, T., et al. Effects of lidocaine on torn rotator cuff tendons. J. Orthop. Res. 2016; 34: 1620-1627. Available from: doi: 10.1002/jor.23153
- Huang XZ, Zhao JH, Gao P, et al. Continuous wound infiltration with local anesthetic is an effective and safe postoperative analgesic strategy: a meta-analysis. Pain Ther. 2021;10(1):525-538. Available from: doi:10.1007/s40122-021-00241-4
- Hussain N, McCartney CJL, Neal JM, et al. Local anaesthetic-induced myotoxicity in regional anaesthesia: a systematic review and empirical analysis. Br J Anaesth. 2018 Oct;121(4):822-841. Available from: doi: 10.1016/j.bja.2018.05.076.
- Jacobs A, Lemoine A, Joshi GP, et al. PROSPECT guideline for oncological breast surgery: a systematic review and procedure-specific postoperative pain management recommendations. Anaesthesia. 2020 May;75(5):664-673. Available from: doi: 10.1111/anae.14964.
- Lassen K, Marielle ME, Coolsen C, Karem S. Guidelines for perioperative care for pancreaticoduodenectomy: Enhanced Recovery After Surgery (ERAS) Society recommendations. Clinical Nutrition. 2012. Available from: doi.org/10.1016/j.clnu.2012.08.011.
- Liu SS, Richman JM, Thirlby RC, et al. Efficacy of continuous wound catheters delivering local anesthetic for postoperative analgesia: a quantitative and qualitative systematic review of randomized controlled trials. J Am Coll Surg. 2006 Dec;203(6):914-32. Available from: doi: 10.1016/j.jamcollsurg.2006.08.007.
- Mattila I, Pätilä T, Rautiainen P, et al. The effect of continuous wound infusion of ropivacaine on postoperative pain after median sternotomy and mediastinal drain in children. Paediatr Anaesth. 2016 Jul;26(7):727-33. Available from: doi: 10.1111/pan.12919.
- Melloul E, Hübner M, Scott M. et al. Guidelines for Perioperative Care for Liver Surgery: Enhanced Recovery After Surgery (ERAS®) Society Recommendations. World J Surg. 2016; 40, 2425–2440. Available from: doi:10.1007/s00268-016-3700-1.
- Mortensen K, Nilsson M, Slim K, et al. Consensus guidelines for enhanced recovery after gastrectomy: Enhanced Recovery After Surgery (ERAS®) Society recommendations. Br J Surg. 2014 Sep;101(10):1209-29. Available from: doi: 10.1002/bjs.9582.
- Pace V, Gul A, Prakash V, et al. Wound Infiltration with Levobupivacaine, Ketorolac, and Adrenaline for Postoperative Pain Control after Spinal Fusion Surgery. Asian Spine J. 2020 Sep 3. Available from: doi: 10.31616/asj.2020.0107.
- Paladini G, Di Carlo S, Musella G, et al. Continuous Wound Infiltration of Local Anesthetics in Postoperative Pain Management: Safety, Efficacy and Current Perspectives. Journal of pain research. 2020 Jan 31;13:285-294. Available from: doi:10.2147/JPR.S211234.
- Pawel F, Tadeusz M, Mikko H, et al. Continuous Ropivacaine infusion offers no benefit in treating postoperative pain after cardiac surgery. Journal of Cardiothoracic and Vascular Anesthesia. 2019 Feb; 33(2):378-384.
- Porter AC, Behrendt NJ, Zaretsky MV, et al. Continuous local bupivacaine wound infusion reduces oral opioid use for acute postoperative pain control following myelomeningocele repair. Am J Obstet Gynecol MFM. 2021 Mar;3(2):100296. Available from: doi: 10.1016/j.ajogmf.2020.100296.
- Rhee SM, Chung NY, Jeong HJ, et al. Subacromial local anesthetics do not interfere with rotator cuff healing after arthroscopic repair. Am J Sports Med. 2018 Apr;46(5):1097-1105. Available from: doi: 10.1177/0363546517753827.
- Roofthooft E, Joshi GP, Rawal N, et al. PROSPECT guideline for elective caesarean section: updated systematic review and procedure-specific postoperative pain management recommendations. Anaesthesia. 2021 May;76(5):665-680. Available from: doi: 10.1111/anae.15339.
- Roy CF, Azzi AJ, Davison P. Review of Wound Infusion With Local Anesthetics in Plastic Surgery. Annals of Plastic Surgery. 2019 Dec;83(6):110-117. Available from: doi: 10.1097/SAP.0000000000001916.
- Strichartz GR. Novel ideas of local anaesthetic actions on various ion channels to ameliorate postoperative pain. Br J Anaesth. 2008 Jul;101(1):45-7. Available from: doi: 10.1093/bja/aen101.
- Thornton PC, Buggy DJ. Local anaesthetic wound infusion for acute postoperative pain: a viable option?. BJA: British Journal of Anaesthesia. November 2011;107(5):656–658.

CLINICAL CASE 1 – LONG TERM ANALGESIA WITH CWI FOR HIP FRACTURE REPAIR IN A JOUNG PATIENT

Clinical history and anamnesis We report the use of continuous wound infiltration for postoperative analgesia in a 19-year-old patient (height 1.65 m, weight 75 kg, BMI 27.55), ASA physical status 1, undergoing surgery for femoral neck fracture.

Materials and methods Written informed consent was obtained. A peripheral venous access (18 g) was obtained and standard monitoring were applied. GA was induced with propofol 150 mg, rocuronium 50 mg and remifentanil TCI with a target of 2 ng/ml at effector site and maintained with sevoflurane 2%, remifentanil TCI (2-3 ng/ml at effector site) and rocuronium as required. Vital and respiratory parameters (HRHR, MAP, SaO_2% and expired CO_2) were monitored.
Multimodal analgesia was given through administration of dexamethasone 4 mg, acetaminophen 1 g and ketorolac 30 mg. No other analgesic was added during the surgery.

Technique description At the end of surgery, before awakening, a 150 mm multi-holed catheter (Painfusor Baxter®) was placed on the surgical wound and, after a starting bolus of ropivacaine 0.5 % 20 ml, a continuous infusion of 0.2 % ropivacaine (5 ml/h) through elastomeric pump was administered for 120 hours postoperatively (**Figure 14.9**).
No supplementary opiates nor other local anesthetic agents were administered. Additionally, no complications of the technique were recorded.

Results Postoperative pain scores, measured in a 0-10 numerical rate scale (NRS), were recorded in Post-anesthesia care unit (PACU) (T_0), at 2(T_1)-6 (T_2)-12 (T_3)-24 (T_4)-36 (T_5)-48 (T_6)-72 hours (T_7) and at 1 week (T_8) after surgery. NRS revealed to be respectively 4 (T_0), 3 (T_1), 2 (T_2), 2 (T_3), 2 (T_4), 0 (T_5), 0 (T_6), and 0 (T_7) and patient did not require any additional analgesic during the whole postoperative period, as no severe pain was observed. At 6th day postoperatively, continuous wound infiltration was stopped and the catheter was removed without any complication. Patient showed to be extremely satisfied by this analgesic technique.

Discussion and conclusions This above described case shows how continuous wound infiltration with local anesthetic is able to provide an effective postoperative analgesia after hip fracture surgery, reducing systemic analgesic consumption and preserving hip motor function. Furthermore, the absence of any side effect underlines the safety of this procedure, rather than other regional anesthesia techniques, i.e. epidural anesthesia or continuous peripheral blocks. Future trials and high quality evidence will be needed to confirm these results and eventually suggest continuous wound infiltration as the first-choice technique orthopedic surgery.

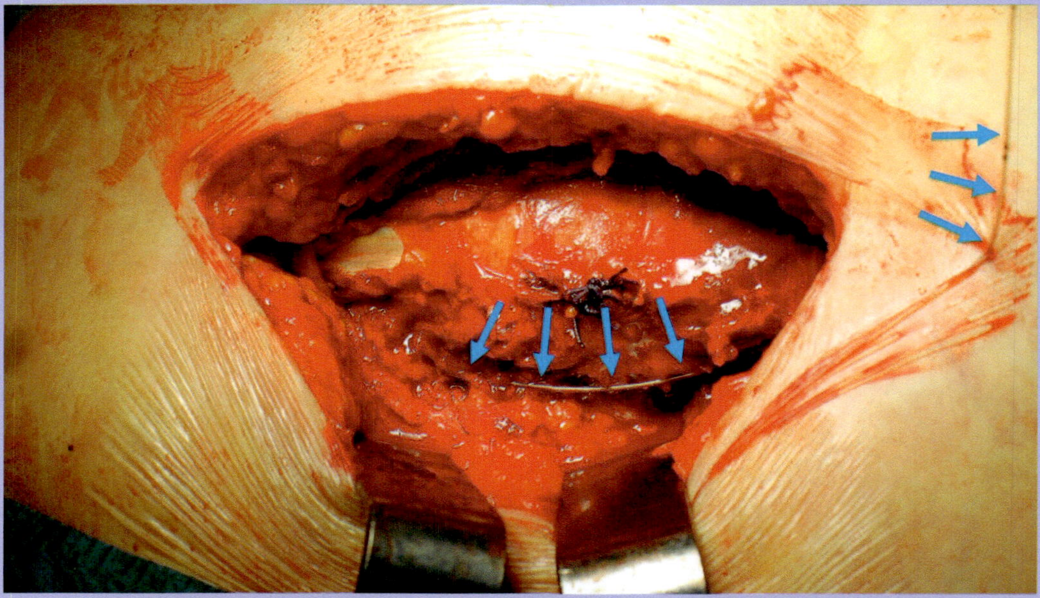

Figure 14.9 Catheter placement for continuous wound infiltration multi-holed catheter placed on surgical wound.

CLINICAL CASE 2 – OPIOID (ALMOST) FREE ANESTHESIA/ANALGESIA FOR LAPAROTOMIC HYSTERECTOMY

Clinical history and anamnesis We report a case of opioid sparing perioperative management for a laparotomic hysterectomy in a in a 49-year-old ASA 2 woman suffering from multiple uterine myoma.

Technique description At the end of the surgery, after closure of the parietal peritoneum, the surgeon inserted a 20-Gauge multi-holed 16 cm soaker catheter, approximately 3 cm laterally to the edge of the incision through a peel-away introducer (**Video 14.2**). The catheter was positioned between the previously closed parietal peritoneum and the transversalis fascia, along the full length of the wound (Ropivacaine 0.2% – ReadyFusOR – BioQ Pharma). Before to close the fascia, a 10-ml bolus of 0.75% plain ropivacaine was administered through the catheter, then fascia and skin were sutured and the catheter secured to the skin. The prefilled pump, preset to deliver a 5 ml/h during 48 h was connected immediately thereafter. The catheter was covered with a transparent dressing. After 1 hour of infusion, a local anesthetic leakage from the catheter exit site was noticed. The dressing was changed and few drops of N-butyl-2 cyanoacrylate glue were deposited at the leakage site (**Figure 14.10**).

Video 14.2 Spinal anesthesia + CWI.

Postoperative pain management consisted in oral administration of: acetaminophen 1 g TID; etoricoxib 90 mg QD; tramadol oral drops 50 mg in case of NRS score exceeding 4/10.

During the 48 hours observation period, NRS always ranged between 1 and 2 with a maximum value of 3 by the spinal anesthesia wearing off time, approximately 4 hours after the block execution. No other opioids were needed, Neither PONV episodes, nor wound complications occurred.

Materials and methods Written informed consent was obtained. A peripheral venous access (18 g) was obtained and standard monitoring was applied. I.V. acetaminophen 1g, dexamethasone 16 mg and ketorolac 30 mg were administered preoperatively as pre-emptive analgesia. After ultrasound spine evaluation, a segmental thoracic spinal anesthesia was performed at T11-T12 intervertebral space with pencil point 27 G spinal needle, hyperbaric 0,5% bupivacaine 15 mg were administered with the addition of fentanyl 0,02 mg as adjuvant. After 35% oxygen supplementation with venturi face-mask, moderate sedation with propofol TCI 0,8 Y/ml was administered along the 90 minutes of surgery.

Conclusions Association of opioid sparing anesthetic techniques (such as spinal anesthesia) and CWI could lead to optimal perioperative management and according to ERAS protocols requirements a PAIN/PONV FREE postoperative period, allowing the patient to early refeed and ambulate and allowing eventually an earlier and safe home discharge.

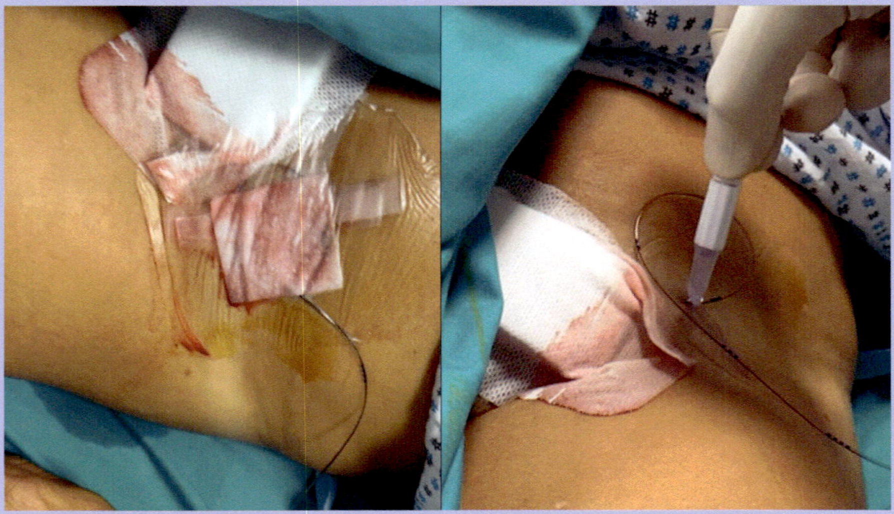

Figure 14.10 Leakage from catheter exit site, fixed with tissue adhesive.

CHAPTER 15

Fascial plane blocks and neuraxial blocks: two planets not so far apart

Roberto Starnari, Carmine Pullano

In recent years, the operative applications of neuraxial blocks have been constantly expanding beyond their already well-known anesthetic use for legs, lower abdomen, and pelvis surgery.

All the neuraxial anesthesias from single-shot spinal to continuous thoracic spinal and from epidural to combined spinal-epidural have now found application in previously considered off-limits surgical specialties previously considered off-limits such as all major surgery of the upper abdomen, some thoracic procedures, and even in the laparoscopic and robotic modalities.

At the same time, the recent refinements of para-neuraxial fascial planes blocks have not only confirmed their prominent efficacy as analgesic methods but have also inspired the development of some interesting potentiality for obtaining of a partial thoracoabdominal surgical anesthesia.

On this basis, the possibility of exploiting the association of a neuraxial technique with one or more fascial plane blocks is now under evaluation. The goal is to achieve a multimodal synergy favoring improved results for both anesthetic and analgesic approaches in comparison to the two taken individually.

PLANET NEURAXIAL – PUSHING THE LIMITS

Epidural anesthesia (EA) is the neuraxial method that has undergone fewer changes regarding technique and materials over the years, its application being usually restricted to an anesthetic and analgesic complement in combined general-epidural anesthesia.

Nevertheless, epidural has been successfully used for a long time as sole anesthesia for many types of major surgery and even in unusual areas such as upper limb or neck, along with being employed in laparoscopic surgery.

Moreover, it has been shown that the advantages of the epidural are all the more evident when they are not overtaken by the disadvantages of associated general anesthesia, like V/Q mismatch, atelectasis, diaphragmatic postoperative dysfunction, increased incidence of pulmonary infections, delirium, cognitive dysfunctions, residual effects of muscle relaxant and other anesthetic drugs.

While guaranteeing all the advantages of neuraxial anesthesia compared to general or combined general-epidural anesthesia, the epidural does however show some limitations in comparison to spinal anesthesia such as slower onset, lesser dense, homogeneous and reliable quality of the block, higher quantity of employed anesthetic, lesser ease of execution and greater traumatism.

On the other hand, in comparison to spinal block, the epidural has fewer consequences on hemodynamic and a safer spread profile. These advantages can be maintained by adding a single-shot spinal to an epidural, both in reduced doses, compensating for respective drawbacks and obtaining a successfully **combined spinal-epidural anesthesia** (CSEA).

As for **spinal anesthesia** (SA), its applications have been widely reinterpreted thanks not only to the new materials and drugs employed but above all to the new discoveries in terms of safety.

SA has always been burdened with the concern of possible damage to the spinal cord when the puncture is performed above L1-L2, even though the technique has been applied at the thoracic level since its introduction and has continued for decades without encountering any particular problems.

As confirmation of this longtime clinical empirical experience, MRI investigations have described the favorable anatomical situation of the perimedullary structures at the thoracic level, suggesting the practicality and safeness of a puncture executed with prudence and adequate technique.

Moreover, recent evidence suggests that the use of ultrasound for neuraxial procedures increases the success rate and ease of execution of the block, reduces the risk of trauma, and, therefore, can further increase safety.

It can thus be said that subarachnoid puncture at the thoracic level of the spine can now be considered in experienced hands as a reliable method, reasonably safe, and remarkably advantageous.

Thanks to the overcoming of the classic anatomical safety limits, it is possible to obtain advantageous metameric anesthesia with the consequent extension of the technique in applications no longer limited to the lower abdomen and lower limbs and with peculiar characteristics particularly suitable for critically ill patients.

PLANET NEURAXIAL – FOCUSING THE EFFECT, GETTING SEGMENTAL

Segmental or **metameric spinal anesthesia** is the kind of procedure in which the deposition of the anesthetic is made exactly at the more appropriate point of the thoracic spine to cover the surgical needs with the least amount of anesthetic and without including in the block other areas not affected by the intervention.

This helps to avoid the side effects of the anesthetic block covering an unnecessarily large area, often obtained with less reliable and in other respects more dangerous methods, such as the use of gravity through positioning the patient to redirect averagely bigger doses of anesthetic made at the lumbar level.

This concept applies both to single-shot SA and also to the spinal component of the SEA combined technique performed at the thoracic level but finds its best expression when applied to continuous spinal anesthesia (CSA).

Continuous lumbar spinal anesthesia (CLSA) was already successfully performed for anesthesia and analgesia in high-risk patients undergoing abdominal, orthopedic, vascular, and obstetric surgery, but in all cases the catheter was placed at a lumbar level below L3.

While allowing the extension of the length of anesthesia, the insertion of the catheter at a lumbar level implies the necessity of much larger doses of a local anesthetic to obtain the coverage of the thoracic segments affected by abdominal surgery and it is therefore burdened with the relative drawbacks already described for lumbar single-shot spinal anesthesia.

Segmental single-shot **thoracic spinal anesthesia** (TSA) was also already used for abdominal surgery in critical patients.

Although it is a convenient method for using a smaller amount of anesthetic at the desired level, as a single shot technique it cannot modulate the dose and extend the length of anesthesia.

On the contrary, placing the catheter directly at the level of the thoracic segmental field of surgical interest allows for an actual metameric targeted **continuous thoracic spinal anesthesia** (CTSA).

The most prominent advantages of this technique are a drastic reduction of the anesthetic dosage with fewer collateral effects, the modulation of a much more precise and dense quality of anesthesia, and the extension of its duration to as long as required.

CTSA is the technique that brings together and maximizes all the advantages of the other neuraxial anesthesias while limiting their disadvantages.

PLANET NEURAXIAL – CONTINUOUS THORACIC SPINAL ANESTHESIA (CTSA)

In our experience, CTSA has allowed the carrying out of hundreds of major abdominal and urological surgeries in critically ill geriatric patients, both elective and emergent, limiting the impact on the functionality of the different organs and systems, reducing the adverse outcomes, and avoiding recourse to postoperative hospitalization in intensive care.

Further advantages were the almost total absence of delirium, the lower incidence of respiratory infections, the more rapid recovery of intestinal transit, and the greater general satisfaction of patients.

There was no need to convert to general anesthesia in any case, including in the most critical where considerable blood loss occurred or the patient was severely respiratory and cardiac compromised.

Although our experience of applying this technique to critically ill patients with high anesthetic risk is confirmed and supported in several previous more generic works, further research is needed to validate its efficacy and safety.

From a security point of view, thoracic spinal puncture assumes knowledge of the different anatomy of the spine at that level. The use of ultrasound may help establish the most convenient needle direction and measure the depth of the intrathecal space, increasing the safety level of the procedure.

In all cases, it is advisable to play it safe during puncture and adopt a step-by-step needle advancement technique by checking the flowing out of the cerebrospinal fluid every 2 mm (**Video 15.1**).

Once in the intrathecal space, the catheter is then introduced through the needle for a length of 4-5 cm, tested, fixed, and ready to use.

Upon induction, the minimum effective dose is obtained by administering micro boluses and verifying the level reached in 2-3 minutes after each. Whichever anesthetic is used, boluses of 2-2.5 mg are equally appropriate.

Concentrations of 0.2-0.25% are equally effective as those of 0.5%, with likely less hemodynamic and motor block impact.

If hypobaric boluses are required, these can be obtained by diluting the anesthetic with double distilled water (i.e. ropivacaine 1% – 1 ml diluted to 5ml → ropivacaine 0.20% hypobaric).

Video 15.1 Continuous Spinal Anesthesia.

During maintenance, the top-ups are administered either every 45-60 minutes or as needed when pain or discomfort for the patient appears, allowing a very rapid resolution. Again the dose is typically 2-2.5 mg.

Video laparoscopic surgery performed under CSA does not generally require changes in the management of the anesthetic doses except for paying particular attention to the coverage of C3-C4-C5 to avoid shoulder pain due to pneumoperitoneum (especially for operations in the upper-middle abdomen) (**Table 15.1**).

In case of lack of spinal catheters or lack of confidence with the spinal technique, it is still possible to obtain appreciable results by performing CSEA preferably according to the two-space puncture technique.

The spinal anesthetic dose can be conveniently reduced by 1/3 compared to a single shot dose when delivering spinal-epidural anesthesia.

The epidural dose is reduced by at least two thirds compared to an entire surgical dosage. It is also convenient to use reduced concentrations (0.2%-0.25%-0.3%) in a volume of 10 ml for both the initial bolus and the top-up.

Given the higher latency of the effect, the management of epidural top-ups, unlike spinal ones, always requires a scheduled administration that avoids a possible gap in anesthesia with prolonged discomfort for the patient and the surgeons.

Usually, 45-60 minutes between top-ups is appropriate.

For video laparoscopic surgery, CSEA can be performed with the following variations to the protocol for open surgery:

- the spinal is performed one or two spaces below;
- the initial epidural dose is doubled and administered in two boluses.

PLANET NEURAXIAL – SEDATION AND POSTOPERATIVE ANALGESIA

Sedation is an important complement to neuraxial anesthesia and is essential for operation success.

For this purpose, the patient should remain at ease at all the time, not necessarily asleep, and above all not deprived of the cough reflex and the ability to swallow. He should be able to communicate spontaneously or on request for every need.

TABLE 15.1 CONTINUOUS SPINAL AND SPINAL-EPIDURAL ANESTHESIA

SURGERY	CONTINUOUS SPINAL (open and laparoscopic surgery) starting doses	SPINAL-EPIDURAL (open surgery) starting doses	SPINAL-EPIDURAL (laparoscopic surgery) starting doses
• **LIVER – GALLBLADDER** • **SPLEEN – PANCREAS** • **ADRENAL** • **KIDNEY – URETER**	**T8-T9** prot. 1	EPIDURAL **T7-T8** prot. 2	EPIDURAL **T7-T8** prot. 5
		SPINAL **T8-T9** prot. 3	SPINAL **T9-T10** prot. 6
	Manipulation of the central diaphragmatic dome, lesser omentum, liver ligaments, and gallbladder* Unilateral surgery with subcostal or lumbotomy incision***		
• **DISTAL ESOPHAGUS** • **STOMACH** • **DUODENUM – JEJUNUM**	**T8-T9** prot. 1	EPIDURAL **T7-T8** prot. 2	EPIDURAL **T7-T8** prot. 5
		SPINAL **T8-T9** prot. 3	SPINAL **T9-T10** prot. 6)
	Manipulation of the central diaphragmatic dome and lesser omentum*		
• **ILEUM** • **RIGHT COLON**	**T9-T10** prot. 1	EPIDURAL **T8-T9** prot. 2	EPIDURAL **T8-T9** prot. 5
		SPINAL **T9-T10** prot. 3	SPINAL **T10-T11** prot. 6
• **TRANSVERSE COLON** • **DESCENDING COLON** • **SIGMOID COLON** • **RECTUM**	**T10-T11** prot. 1	EPIDURAL **T9-T10** prot. 2	SPINAL **T10-T11** prot. 3
		EPIDURAL **T9-T10** prot. 5	SPINAL **T11-T12** prot. 6
	Manipulation of sigmoid colon-rectum**		
• **BLADDER** • **PROSTATE – TESTICLES** • **UTERUS – OVARIES**	**T11-T12** prot. 1	EPIDURAL **T10-T11** prot. 2	EPIDURAL **T10-T11** prot. 5
		SPINAL **T11-T12** prot. 3	SPINAL **T12-L1** prot. 6
	Manipulation of the bladder neck**		
• **HIP**	**L1-L2** prot. 1	EPIDURAL **T12-L1** prot. 2	
		SPINAL **L1-L2** prot. 4	
	Unilateral surgery***		
• **KNEE**	**L3-L4** prot. 1	EPIDURAL **L2-L3** prot. 2	
		SPINAL **L3-L4** prot. 4	
	Unilateral surgery***		
• **VASCULAR** **Aortobifemoral bypass**	**T11-T12** prot. 1	EPIDURAL **T10-T11** prot. 2	
		SPINAL **T11-T12** prot. 4	
• **VASCULAR** **Femoropopliteal bypass**	**L2-L3** prot. 1	EPIDURAL **L1-L2** prot. 2	
		SPINAL **L2-L3** prot. 4	
	Unilateral surgery***		

WARNING:
The information provided in this table is derived from the authors' decades of experience and intended for use by skilled anesthetists fully aware of the risks and benefits of the procedures described.
Doses are subject to variations up to 10-15% plus or minus depending on the type of patient and his clinical condition.
The level of punctures may vary by one intervertebral space without significant differences in outcome. A variation of the order of two spaces or more requires the consequent adaptation of the doses and/or type of anesthetic and/or length of the introduction of the catheters (normally 4-5 cm into epidural or intrathecal space).

Prot. 1: HB, B, L, R = 2-2.5 mg boluses until desired spread is reached – **Prot. 2**: LD = 40 mg (test dose) + B, L = 20 mg or R = 30 mg
Prot. 3: HB, B, L = 8 mg or R = 10 mg – **Prot. 4**: HB, B, L = 6-8 mg or R = 8-10 mg – **Prot. 5**: LD = 40 mg (test dose) + B, L = 20 mg x 2 or R = 30 mg x 2 – **Prot. 6**: HB, B, L = 6 mg or R = 8 mg

LD = Lidocaine; HB = Hyperbaric Bupivacaine; B = Bupivacaine; L = Levobupivacaine; R = Ropivacaine

*Manipulation of the central diaphragmatic dome, lesser omentum, liver ligaments, gallbladder, and laparoscopic surgery requires the sensitive block of C3-C4-C5. This can be obtained at the beginning or during surgery with one or more hypobaric boluses in continuous spinal and with an initial double epidural bolus (20 ml of 0.20-0.25% solution) in the spinal-epidural. The epidural coverage of eventual diaphragmatic pain during surgery can be attempted with lidocaine 1% 200 mg.

**Manipulation of organs and viscera below the pelvic pain line requires the sensitive block of S2-S3-S4.
This can be obtained by performing saddle anesthesia with hyperbaric bupivacaine 5 mg given before the planned dose.

***Both continuous spinal and the spinal component of the combined spinal-epidural anesthesia may be delivered selectively to reduce hemodynamic consequences.

Good sedation can be obtained with the intravenous administration of appropriate drugs but, in our experience, the intrathecal and epidural routes of administration of selected adjuvants have proved to be safer and more suitable.

The neuraxial route produces a rather peculiar quality of sedation, without real hypnosis, with the maintenance of the main reflexes and perfect immobility, the absence of snoring, and paradoxical breathing.

It involves lower depressive effects on blood pressure and breathing, greater homogeneity of the sedative effect and absence of residual effects. There is also a noticeable reduction of drug doses with relative independence from the variable factors that influence the pharmacokinetics of the same intravenous drug.

We looked for adjuvants able to enhance the action of local anesthetics without collateral effects and with additional benefits, for example a reduction of postoperative nausea and vomit, reduction of shivering, anti-delirium activity and hemodynamic stabilization. In our experience, we have found ketamine, midazolam, dexmedetomidine, and dexamethasone to fulfill these requirements.

Delivered in boluses or continuous infusion by intrathecal and/or epidural route, they have met all our expectations without showing unwanted side effects and symptoms of neurological damage.

Spinal and epidural catheters also allow the administration of effective postoperative **neuraxial analgesia**.

The analgesic infusion should begin intraoperatively by replacing the sedative infusion and meshing with an anesthetic cover that is still effective, therefore no later than 15 minutes after the last expected or necessary top-up and in any case not less than 30 minutes before the planned end of the intervention.

Whenever possible before starting the infusion, a previous check of the initial reappearance of legs motility is advisable for extra safety.

In our experience the intrathecal analgesic infusion consists of levobupivacaine 40 mg (or ropivacaine 60 mg) + midazolam 5 mg in 50 ml at an infusion rate starting from 1 ml/h to a maximum of 2 ml/h.

The epidural analgesic infusion consists of levobupivacaine 0.125% + midazolam 0.075 mg/ml at an infusion rate of 5-6 ml/h.

Ketamine, midazolam, dexmedetomidine, and dexamethasone free from dangerous excipients are safe drugs regarding local neurotoxicity. Although neuraxial utilization of these drugs is now considered after long-time research and wide application, it is still commonly regarded as off-label. Further research is therefore needed to confirm the efficacy and safeness of this utilization.

FASCIAL PLANE BLOCK (FPB) PLANET – NOT JUST ANALGESIA

The FPB are becoming increasingly popular, especially as intraoperative and postoperative analgesic support to general anesthesia.

On the other hand, anesthesia is still a clear prerogative of spinal and epidural blocks for most surgical procedures, even though these methods may bring serious complications, such as epidural hematoma, nerve injury, and hypotension.

Moreover, they cannot be used for patients on anticoagulant or antiaggregant treatment and cannot take full advantage of the aid of ultrasounds.

In an attempt to reproduce the action of the neuraxial blocks with fewer side effects, the approaches to the closest area to the spine, the paravertebral space, thus started being investigated.

The **paravertebral block** (PVB) has hitherto been employed as the sole anesthesia for some limited types of surgery.

Over neuraxial anesthesia, it has the advantage of visualization of the needle position using ultrasonography, besides the possibility of being used in patients assuming anticoagulants or antiplatelets.

Nevertheless, it is still associated with a risk of serious complications, such as pneumothorax, hypotension, or nerve injury.

Recently, many studies have thus focused on FPB as technically easier and safer approaches to the paravertebral space for anesthetic purposes. The possible anesthetic qualities of the FPB are not yet well understood. However, studies on their efficacy on visceral pain are beginning to define this potential role where the ***erector spinae* plane (ESP) block** is primarily involved.

Some suggest that ESP block provides analgesic efficacy comparable to PVB.

This similar effect is likely due to the amount of anesthetic that starting from between the transverse process and the erector spinae muscle diffuses via the anteriorly directed pathway to the paravertebral space through the superior costotransverse ligament, thus reaching the fascial compartments defined by the endothoracic fascia where it can potentially block not only the ventral and dorsal rami of spinal nerves but also the rami communicantes that transmit sympathetic fibers.

The ESP block was shown to be effective for referred shoulder pain following laparoscopic interventions, thus suggesting a possible role in the anesthetic coverage of all those structures generating painful impulses conducted by the phrenic nerve, such as the central part of the diaphragmatic peritoneum, the gallbladder, the hepatic ligaments, and the lesser omentum in the abdomen, along with in the thorax, diaphragmatic and mediastinal pleura, and pericardium.

FUSION ANESTHESIA – SAFETY IN NUMBERS

Based on all the previous considerations and relying on the experimental finding that conduction along a nerve fiber is inversely proportional to the length of the fiber exposed to the anesthetic, it seemed logical to us to combine two different forms of nerve block in distinct parts of the same afferent pathway, exposing a longer length of it to the anesthetic. We therefore started investigating the use of neuraxial blocks in association with FPB, choosing PVB and ESP blocks that we saw as offering some level of visceral coverage and as a result being potentially useful for our thoracoabdominal surgery. A result Fusion anesthesia was born.

In our experience, we have conducted dozens of interventions for major surgery, for the most part laparoscopic, under different combinations of neuraxial anesthesia and FPB. The advantages found are reduction of the neuraxial loading dose, reduction of the onset time, thinning of the top-ups and reduction of single doses, longer duration of single-shot neuraxial with the possibility of avoiding the need for a spinal or epidural catheter, lower hemodynamic impact deriving from reduced neuraxial doses, lower incidence of patchy or missing segments blocks, saving on opioids, reduced motor block and reduced workload in the wards.

Disadvantages are the need for posterior extra punctures, the need for accurate calculation of the maximum feasible total dose of anesthetic, availability of ultrasound equipment and lengthening of execution times.

The following is the protocol used in our experience. The ESP block technique involves bilateral puncture between T4 and T10 (depending on the intervention) with 0.2-0.25% levobupivacaine or 0.3-0.375% ropivacaine in quantities of 20-25 ml per side (depending on association with PVB). The PVB technique involves bilateral puncture between T4 and T10 (depending on the intervention) with 0.2-0.25% levobupivacaine or 0.3-0.375% ropivacaine in a quantity of 7-20 ml per side (depending on association with ESP). PVB and ESP block have been variably associated with SA, EA, and CTSA depending on surgical needs (**Table 15.2**). The adjuvant used for both blocks is one of the following: clonidine 2 mcg/kg, dexamethasone 4-8 mg, dexmedetomidine 0.5-1 mcg/kg. However, the utilization of these drugs for FPBs still requires further research.

We have never encountered such problems as having to heavily modify the anesthetic conduct or convert locoregional anesthesia into general anesthesia.

Particularly evident was the contribution of ESP block in preventing referred shoulder pain during pneumoperitoneum, with only very few exceptions.

Pain-free manipulation of high abdominal and endothoracic structures with limited use of the neuraxial catheter was also made possible, as demonstrated by carrying out an Ivor-Lewis surgery in spontaneous breathing (C. Pullano personal communication).

In some cases of laparoscopic surgery converted to open, the PUB + ESP block combination alone was sufficient to provide the necessary anesthetic coverage since the neuraxial catheter was used only for adjuvant drugs. This confirms the still poorly investigated individual potential of FPB as sufficient aids for surgical anesthesia.

TABLE 15.2 FUSION ANESTHESIA

SURGERY	BLOCK	LEVEL	ROPIVACAINE OR L-BUPIVACAINE	
LAPAROSCOPIC UPPER ABDOMEN	NEURAXIAL	T6-T8	see **Table 15.1***	see **Table 15.1***
	ESP**	T4-T7	0.3% 20 ml/side	0.2% 20 ml/side
	PVB (optional)	T6-T8	0.3% 10 ml/side	0.2% 10 ml/side
LAPAROSCOPIC LOWER ABDOMEN	NEURAXIAL***	T6-T8	see **Table 15.1***	see **Table 15.1***
	ESP	T4-T7	0.3% 20 ml/side	0.2% 20 ml/side
	PVB	T6-T8	0.3% 10 ml/side	0.2% 10 ml/side
XIPHOID-PUBIC LAPAROTOMY	NEURAXIAL***	T8-T10	see **Table 15.1***	see **Table 15.1***
	ESP	T6-T9	0.3% 20 ml/side	0.2% 20 ml/side
	PVB	T8-T10	0.3% 10 ml/side	0.2% 10 ml/side
XIPHOID-UMBILICAL LAPAROTOMY – SUBCOSTAL INCISION LUMBOTOMY	NEURAXIAL****	T6-T9	see **Table 15.1***	see **Table 15.1***
	ESP	–	–	–
	PVB	T6-T9	0.375% 15 ml/side	0.25% 15 ml/side
UMBILICAL-PUBIC LAPAROTOMY – PFANNENSTIEL INCISION	NEURAXIAL***	T9-T11	see **Table 15.1***	see **Table 15.1***
	ESP	below T9	0.3% 20 ml/side	0.2% 20 ml/side
	PVB	T9-T11	0.3% 10 ml/side	0.2% 10 ml/side
VIDEO-ASSISTED THORACIC SURGERY (VATS)	NEURAXIAL	–	–	–
	ESP****	T5	0.375% 20 ml/side	0.25% 20 ml/side
	PVB****	T5	0.375% 10 ml/side	0.25% 10 ml/side

ESP = *Erector spinae* plane; FPB = Fascial plane block; PVB = Paravertebral block.
*Doses in Table 15.1 can be reduced by up to 30% in the Fusion mode.
**ESP allowing coverage of diaphragmatic pain.
***Neuraxial needing completion with the adjunct of a saddle block of the sacral roots.
****Neuraxial anesthesia may be lateralized and/or the FPB performed singly in case of one side surgery.

In conclusion, our experience of Fusion anesthesia as the association of a neuraxial block with one or more FPBs (especially ESP block and PVB) has shown the possibility of obtaining certainty of the anesthetic plan with less hemodynamic impact, analgesic stability in the postoperative period, and the saving or avoidance of opioid drugs at the price of a slight increase in the complexity of the procedure.

Although still poorly supported by literature, Fusion anesthesia seems to be an extremely valid method in patients with high anesthetic risk.

The prospect of avoiding general anesthesia and the intensive care hospitalization of critically ill patients is one of the main advantages given the most recent trends in optimizing the perioperative period. In addition, during pandemics reducing intensive care bed occupancy is even more valuable. In addition, in times of pandemics, saving in intensive care bed occupancy is even more valuable.

We hope that further research and in-depth studies of safety and efficacy will bring new developments to this promising method so these two planets of the locoregional galaxy will orbit more and more in tune in the future.

RECOMMENDED READING

- Castellani D, Starnari R, Faloia L, et al. *Radical cystectomy in frail octogenarians in thoracic continuous spinal anesthesia and analgesia: a pilot study*. Ther Adv Urol. 2018 Sep 3;10(11):343-349. doi: 10.1177/1756287218795427. PMID: 30344646; PMCID: PMC6180380.
- Chin KJ, Malhas L, Perlas A. *The Erector Spinae Plane Block Provides Visceral Abdominal Analgesia in Bariatric Surgery: A Report of 3 Cases*. Reg Anesth Pain Med. 2017 May/Jun;42(3):372-376. doi: 10.1097/AAP.0000000000000581. PMID: 28272292.
- Ellakany M. *Comparative study between general and thoracic spinal anesthesia for laparoscopic cholecystectomy*. Egypt J Anaesth. 2013;29:375–81.
- Fortuna A. Jonnesco. *One century of thoracic spinal anesthesia history*. Rev Bras Anestesiol. 2011 Jan-Feb;61(1):128-34; author reply 130-7. doi: 10.1016/S0034-7094(11)70014-9. PMID: 21334515.
- Gülçin Ö, Kaya M, Gonca T. *Continuous spinal anaesthesia and analgesia in high-risk patients undergoing abdominal surgery*. Indian Journal of Surgery, April 2006, Volume 68; Issue 2: 73-79.
- Hung WC, Chen WH, Shih YH, et al.. *Epidural anesthesia for laparoscopic bariatric surgery: a case report*. Springerplus. 2015 Jul 17;4:363. doi: 10.1186/s40064-015-1153-x. PMID: 26203409; PMCID: PMC4504868.
- Hutton M, Brull R, Macfarlane AJR. *Regional anaesthesia and outcomes*. BJA Educ. 2018 Feb;18(2):52-56. doi: 10.1016/j.bjae.2017.10.002. Epub 2017 Nov 27. PMID: 33456810; PMCID: PMC7807931.
- Imbelloni LE, Quirici MB, Ferraz Filho JR, et al. *The anatomy of the thoracic spinal canal investigated with magnetic resonance imaging*. Anesth Analg. 2010 May 1;110(5):1494-5. doi: 10.1213/ANE.0b013e3181d5aca6. Epub 2010 Mar 19. PMID: 20304985.
- Kalagara H, Nair H, Kolli S et al. *Ultrasound Imaging of the Spine for Central Neuraxial Blockade: a Technical Description and Evidence Update*. Curr Anesthesiol Rep 11, 326–339 (2021). https://doi.org/10.1007/s40140-021-00456-3.
- Karmakar MK, Chin KJ. *Spinal Sonography and Applications of Ultrasound for Central Neuraxial Blocks*. In: Hadzic A. eds. Hadzic's Textbook of Regional Anesthesia and Acute Pain Management, 2e. McGraw Hill; 2017. Accessed December 01, 2021. https://accessanesthesiology.mhmedical.com/content.aspx?bookid=2070&sectionid=157603239
- Kim DH, Kim SJ, Liu J, et al. *Fascial plane blocks: a narrative review of the literature*. Reg Anesth Pain Med. 2021 Jul;46(7):600-617. doi: 10.1136/rapm-2020-101909. PMID: 34145072.
- Kumar CM, Corbett WA, Wilson RG. *Spinal anaesthesia with a micro-catheter in high-risk patients undergoing colorectal cancer and other major abdominal surgery*. Surgical Oncology 2008; 17: 73-79.
- Kwon HM, Kim DH, Jeong SM, et al. *Does Erector Spinae Plane Block Have a Visceral Analgesic Effect?: A Randomized Controlled Trial*. Sci Rep. 2020 May 21;10(1):8389. doi: 10.1038/s41598-020-65172-0. PMID: 32439926; PMCID: PMC7249264.
- Megahed MAF, Magdy IAA. *Case report and review of literature: Thoracic epidural as a sole anesthetic technique in laparoscopic myomectomy*, Egyptian Journal of Anaesthesia, Volume 32, Issue 3, 2016, 435-43, ISSN 1110-1849, https://doi.org/10.1016/j.egja.2016.05.005.
- Onishi E, Toda N, Kameyama Y, et.al. *Comparison of Clinical Efficacy and Anatomical Investigation between Retrolaminar Block and Erector Spinae Plane Block*. Biomed Res Int. 2019 Mar 28;2019:2578396. doi: 10.1155/2019/2578396. PMID: 31032339; PMCID: PMC6458933.
- Paliwal NWl, Ingle J, Lawhale S, Dhakulkar A. *Segmental spinal vs general anaesthesia in patients undergoing laparoscopic cholecystectomy: A comparative study*. MedPulse International Journal of Anesthesiology. June 2020; 14(3): 77-83. http://medpulse.in/Anesthsiology/index.php.
- Raft J, Chin KJ, Richebé P. *Erector spinae plane (ESP) block with a transverse in-plane approach for management of referred shoulder pain after laparoscopic cholecystectomy*. J Clin Anesth. 2019 Aug;55:100-101. doi: 10.1016/j.jclinane.2018.12.024. Epub 2018 Dec 31. PMID: 30.
- Raymond SA, Steffensen SC, Gugino LD, et al. *The role of length of nerve exposed to local anesthetics in impulse blocking action*. Anesth Analg. 1989 May;68(5):563-70. PMID: 2785778.
- Shatri G, Singh A. *Thoracic Segmental Spinal Anesthesia*. 2021 Jul 23. In: StatPearls [Internet]. Treasure Island (FL): StatPearls Publishing; 2021 Jan–. PMID: 34283453.
- Spannella F, Giulietti F, Damiani E, et al. *Thoracic continuous spinal anesthesia for high-risk comorbid older patients undergoing major abdominal surgery: one-year experience of an Italian geriatric hospital*. Minerva Anestesiol. 2020 Mar;86(3):261-269. doi: 10.23736/S0375-9393.19.13896-5. Epub 2019 Sep 3. PMID: 31486624.

- Swain A, Nag DS, Sahu S, et al. *Adjuvants to local anesthetics: Current understanding and future trends*. World J Clin Cases. 2017 Aug 16;5(8):307-323. doi: 10.12998/wjcc.v5.i8.307. PMID: 28868303; PMCID: PMC5561500.
- Thavaneswaran P, Rudkin GE, Cooter RD, et al. *Brief reports: paravertebral block for anesthesia: a systematic review*. Anesth Analg. 2010 Jun 1;110(6):1740-4. doi: 10.1213/ANE.0b013e3181da82c8. Epub 2010 May 6. PMID: 20448076.
- Toledano RD, Van de Velde M. *Epidural Anesthesia and Analgesia*. In: Hadzic A. eds. Hadzic's Textbook of Regional Anesthesia and Acute Pain Management, 2e. McGraw Hill; 2017. Accessed December 03, 2021. https://accessanesthesiology.mhmedical.com/content.aspx?bookid=2070&sectionid=157600760
- van Zundert AA, Stultiens G, Jakimowicz JJ et al. *Laparoscopic cholecystectomy under segmental thoracic spinal anaesthesia: a feasibility study*. Br J Anaesth. 2007 May;98(5):682-6. doi: 10.1093/bja/aem058. Epub 2007 Mar 19. PMID: 17371777.
- VeliĐkoviĐ I, Pujic B, Baysinger CW, et al. *Continuous Spinal Anesthesia for Obstetric Anesthesia and Analgesia*. Front Med (Lausanne). 2017 Aug 15;4:133. doi: 10.3389/fmed.2017.00133. PMID: 28861414; PMCID: PMC5559441.
- Vincenzi P, Starnari R, Faloia L, et al. *Continuous thoracic spinal anesthesia with local anesthetic plus midazolam and ketamine is superior to local anesthetic plus fentanyl in major abdominal surgery*. Surg Open Sci. 2020 Jul 17;2(4):5-11. doi: 10.1016/j.sopen.2020.07.002. PMID: 32885157; PMCID: PMC7453121.
- Waegerle JD. *Combined spinal-epidural anesthesia/analgesia*. CRNA. 1999 Nov;10(4):155-64. PMID: 10723293.

CLINICAL CASE 1 – LAPAROSCOPIC CHOLECYSTECTOMY UNDER ERECTOR SPINAE PLANE (ESP) BLOCK AND SPINAL ANESTHESIA

Clinical history and anamnesis We report the use of bilateral ultrasound-guided ESP block combined with single-shot spinal anesthesia for laparoscopic cholecystectomy in a 70 year-old male (height 190 cm, weight 90 kg) suffering from chronic obstructive pulmonary disease (COPD).

Materials and methods After written informed consent was obtained, peripheral venous access was placed and standard monitoring was applied. Supplemental oxygen was administered by Venturi-mask with continuous expired CO_2 ($ceCO_2$) monitoring. Vital and respiratory parameters (Hr, MaP, SaO_2%, and $ceCO_2$) were monitored.

Technique description Under aseptic conditions, using a convex probe and a 22 G needle with an in-plane approach, a bilateral ESP block was performed at T4 level with 20 ml of ropivacaine 0.375% for each side. After 30 minutes, dorsal anesthesia in the T2-T9 territory was present. T8-T9 spinal anesthesia was performed with a 24 G Quincke needle and ropivacaine 10mg plus dexmedetomidine 10 mcg was administered.

Pinprick test confirmed a complete T2-T12 block and it was possible to perform the planned surgery without the need for additional opioids or anesthetic drugs for a total duration of 25 minutes (**Figure 15.1**).

Conclusions According to the Fusion anesthesia concept, the combination of an ESP block with spinal anesthesia made it possible to perform a laparoscopic cholecystectomy in a COPD patient without the need for general anesthesia and IV drugs to cover diaphragmatic pain, besides a probable postoperative intensive care hospitalization.
This possibility is one of the main advantages given the most recent trends in the optimization of the perioperative period. In addition, in times of pandemics, cutting the occupancy of intensive care beds occupancy is even more valuable.
In conclusion, although still poorly supported by literature, Fusion anesthesia appears as an extremely valid method in patients with high anesthetic risk.
Nonetheless, its application, as well as the use of adjuvants in both neuraxial and fascial blocks, require further studies to confirm their efficacy and safety.

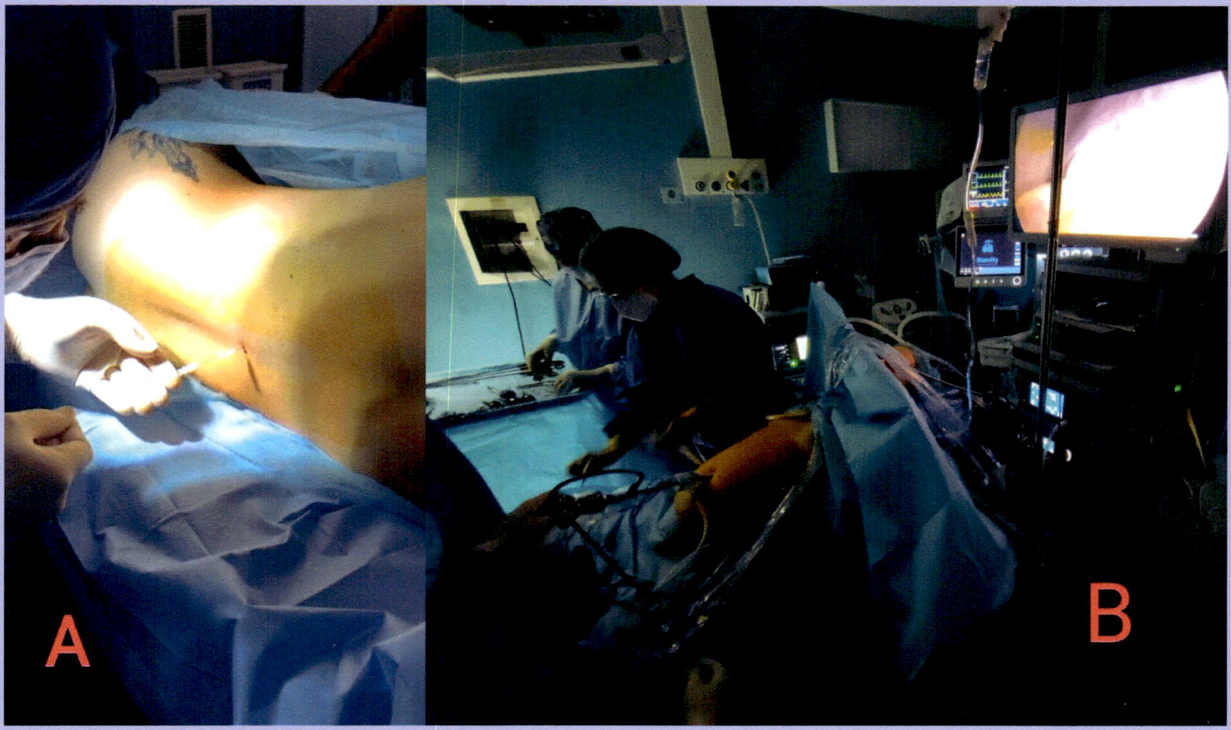

Figure 15.1 A Spinal anesthesia performed at T8-T9. **B** Patient breathing spontaneously in Venturi mask despite 30° head-up position and pneumoperitoneum.

CLINICAL CASE 2 – LAPAROSCOPIC SIGMOIDECTOMY WITH BILATERAL ESP BLOCK PLUS BILATERAL PVB AND SADDLE SPINAL

Clinical history and anamnesis A case of sigmoid neoplasia in laparoscopic surgery in an 88-year-old patient suffering from chronic obstructive pulmonary disease, conducted under saddle spinal anesthesia with L2-L3 puncture, two ESP blocks, and two ultrasound-guided PVBs.

Materials and methods Once the patient's informed consent was obtained, the patient's vital parameters (HR, NIBP, SaO_2, $EtCO_2$) were monitored.

Technique description Under aseptic conditions, with linear probe and 22 G needle, we performed ESP block at T7 bilaterally with the in-plane technique, and bilateral PVB at T6 using the in-plane technique and para-sagittal probe.
We administered 20 ml of 0.3% ropivacaine for each ESP block and 8 ml of 0.3% ropivacaine for each PVB.
After 25 minutes, having ascertained the presence of bilateral anesthesia in the T2 to T12 dermatomes with pin-prick test, a spinal puncture was performed at L2-L3 with Whitacre 25 G and administration of hyperbaric bupivacaine 5 mg followed by dexmedetomidine 12 mcg.
The three-hour surgery was completed with the intravenous infusion of dexmedetomidine at 0.4-0.6 mcg/kg/h (**Figure 15.2**).

Conclusions The combination of bilateral ESP and bilateral PVB according to the Fusion anesthesia concept produces in most cases extensive anesthesia of the wall and viscera which allows abdominal interventions to be completed with the possibility of laparoscopy without the patient experiencing diaphragmatic pain. The manipulation of the pelvic viscera, not covered by the combination of the two blocks, requires the execution of a saddle block or a caudal block to cover the sacral roots.
In this case, it was possible to perform a laparoscopic sigmoidectomy in a COPD patient without the need for general anesthesia and a postoperative intensive care hospitalization.
This possibility is one of the main advantages given the most recent trends in the optimization of the perioperative period.
In addition, in times of pandemics, cutting down on occupancy of intensive care beds is even more valuable.
In conclusion, although still poorly supported by literature, Fusion anesthesia appears as an extremely valid method in patients with high anesthetic risk.
Nonetheless, its application, as well as the use of adjuvants in both neuraxial and fascial blocks, require further studies to confirm their efficacy and safety.

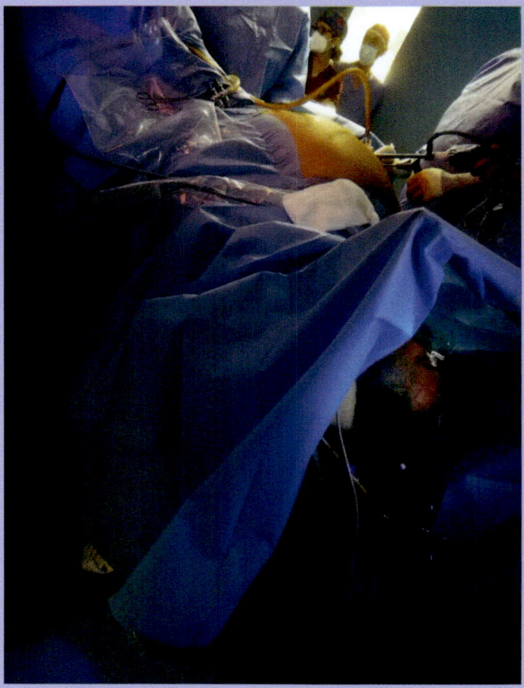

Figure 15.2 Patient breathing spontaneously in Venturi mask despite 30° head-down position and pneumoperitoneum.

Ultrasound-guided regional anesthesia simulation

Pierfrancesco Fusco, Gianmarco Petroni, Francesca Angelucci

Learning a new technique is not an easy goal, especially when we talk about ultrasound-guided blocks, in which we have to improve not only ultrasound but also anesthesiologists' knowledge.

The success of a nerve block depends on various factors: the knowledge about materials and equipment, a deep knowledge about sonoanatomy, about the use of ultrasound, and on a good hand-eye coordination.

In the past the learning of a new techniques was done on the patients.

Today, is not possible to do so because of the possible complications and the medico-legal issues. Moreover, the need for greater efficiency in the operating theatre often prevents having enough time to acquire necessary notions.

For all of these reasons, the possibility to reproduce or "simulate" anesthesiology techniques is becoming more important in order to allow the operator to learn and improve techniques that until today were possible to perform only on patients.

Simulators for central-neuraxial blocks have existed for a long time. They allow to improve the execution of epidural and spinal blocks (that, as we know, do not need ultrasounds), while recently dummy-simulators are available for peripheral nervous blocks, that have many limits, especially from a technologic and software point of view, and that are improvable.

The fundamental point to acquire the execution capacity for ultrasound-guided block, is to be familiar with needle and probe. This is made possible using echogenic simulators, made of silicone material, which faithfully reproduce nerves and vases. The possibility to exercise the needle orientation relative to the probe helps to improve the needle-probe relationship and hand-eye coordination, that is essential for the successive execution of blocks on patients. In recent years, highly efficient simulators have been available that allow the medical doctor to safely practice in order to acquire the hand-eye coordination skills, which are well-known to be indispensable to perform the ultrasound-guided nerve block.

While the advantage of initial training with a simulator is evident, on the other hand, simulators are not available for every type of nerve block. Therefore, the acquisition of specific skills on the patient is limited, especially for blocks of recent introduction.

This is extremely true for recently introduced wall and fascial blocks, that are technically more difficult to execute than peripheral nerve blocks.

Although the use of some coarse "handcrafted" simulators were produced, with encouraging results, but is recent the introduction of the first fascial block simulator.

BlockSim™ represents an innovative and revolutionary, one of a kind, high fidelity system to simulate ultrasound guided fascial blocks (**Figure A1.1**).

This new simulator is equipped with a high fidelity sensor for visualization, on a virtual monitor, needle and probe movements, and, over more, accurate reproduction of fascial block reproduction. BlockSim™ allows to acquire and practice technique competences in a safe, controlled and reproducible location, with no risk for the patients. What is more, it allows to reproduce the block many times, meanwhile allowing to have extremely realistic tactile feedback during execution of the procedure, and to reproduce clinical scenarios (**Figure A1.2**).

All of this will allow the anesthesiologist to have a safer approach to the patients and to the execution of fascial block, thanks to the acquisition of manual skills and the high-fidelity block reproduction derived from the new simulator.

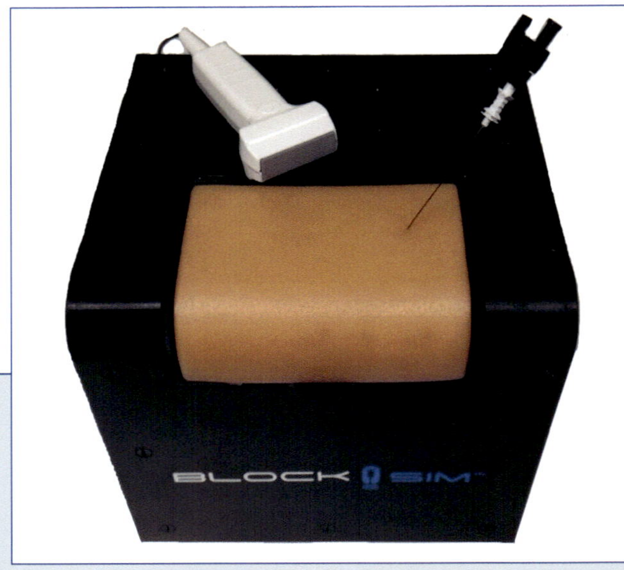

Figure A1.1 Simulator of ultrasound guided fascial blocks.

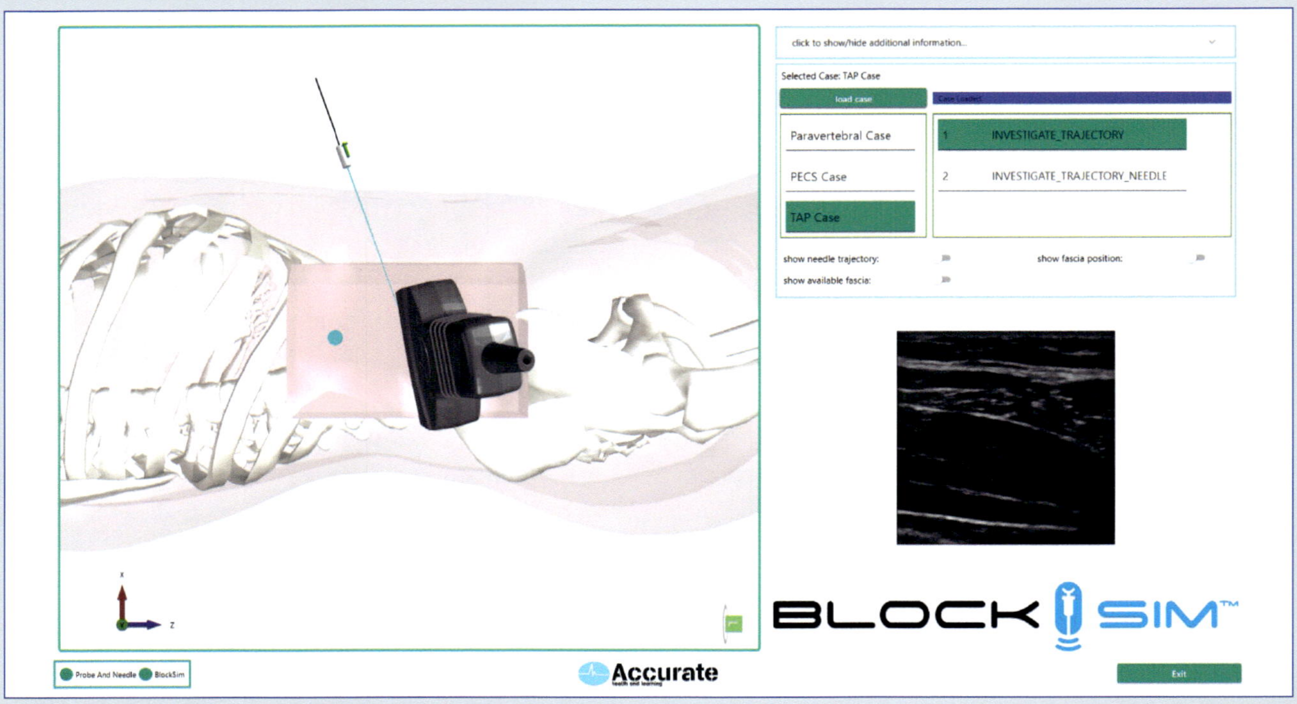

Figure A1.2 Simulation of the TAP Block through the BlockSim™ system.

Regional anesthesia in the COVID-19 era

Francesca De Sanctis, Pierfrancesco Fusco

COVID-19 has been a problem for global health since March 11 2020, when the pandemic was declared, changing medical practice forever and offering opportunities for growth and improvement for health systems in various subspecialties including anesthesia. During the first months of the pandemic, in the attempt to limit the spread of infection and to preserve healthcare resources, one commonly used strategy was to postpone elective surgery, reserving anesthetic only for urgent and emergency surgery, but we now have a better awareness of the disease and other weapons to fight against it, first of all vaccines. Living with the virus we are often required to perform surgical interventions (elective or emergent) in COVID-19 patients with varying degrees of pulmonary and systemic impairment.

All the guidelines of the main international anesthesia societies agree in recommending the use of locoregional anesthesia (LRA) when and if possible, within an anesthesiological plan tailored to the patient, after carrying out a preanesthesiological evaluation of the patient with blood tests, anamnestic collection, clinical and laboratory classification, including the severity of the infectious pathology. The clinical presentation following human infection with SARS-CoV-2 ranges from a mild upper respiratory tract infection to a severe acute respiratory distress syndrome and sepsis. The consequences can be lethal, particularly in the elderly or those with comorbidities such as hypertension, cardiac failure and diabetes.

Reasons why regional anesthesia (RA) is preferable are many, but the most important is certainly the airway management while minimizing manipulation because these are aerosol generating procedures (AGP) (e.g. bag mask ventilation, airway suction, intubation and extubation). We know that the transmission of the virus occurs mostly via respiratory droplets and fomite. These are the procedures at highest risk of droplet spreading, especially if the patient coughs or sneezes, with risk of contagion 6.6 times greater, if not performed in a negative pressure room, or if the air exchange is not sufficient to ensure an abatement of viral load in the environment. Therefore the proximity to the patient, the duration of exposure and the amount of air exchange, are all issues to be considered in addition to the question of aerosol spreading.

The main guidelines in this regard also provide recommendation tools on how to perform these procedures under adequate protective personal equipment (PPE). The role of regional anesthesia is reaffirmed, including peripheral nerve block, neuraxial and fascial blocks in order to achieve a relative preservation of respiratory function in these patients, who present a various degrees of respiratory failure. In these cases a supplementation of oxygen for surgical intervention performed under regional anesthesia, is often necessary, which can be implemented by means of nasal cannulas, facial masks (preferable), or high flow systems. Always remember to make the patient wear a surgical mask throughout the surgery, during transport to the recovery room, and throughout the intra-hospital transport on dedicated paths.

Other important advantages of regional anesthesia are: providing better intra and postoperative analgesia with consensual reduction of perioperative consumption of sedative and opiate drugs, which have direct and indirect depressive effect on respiratory and immune function. This could lead to: a theoretical reduction of pulmonary complications due to temporary depression of respiratory function during general anesthesia, with or without muscle paralysis; reduction of postoperative nausea and vomiting; early discharge from the surgery room; safety of health personnel and reduction of cost for PPE. Regional anesthesia also helps in saving time and reducing personnel exposure, minimizing movements during patient positioning if blocks are performed with simple and unique patient positioning.

RECOMMENDATIONS AND PRACTICAL CONSIDERATIONS FOR REGIONAL ANESTHESIA

The clinical experience of these two years teaches us that exist specific conditions to keep under control and that the good anesthesiologist must have experience in managing complications related to RA:

1. Failed block: anesthesiologist should test the block before surgery and be able to rapidly and safely perform adequate sedation, or convert to general anesthesia if needed, using institutional PPE guidelines and an induction technique that minimizes the risk of aerosolization.
2. LAST: recognize clinical features and early treatment of LAST, ask for help and additional personnel if necessary; manage LAST as per international guidelines.
3. Specific to RA technique, Brachial plexus blocks (interscalene, supra and infra-clavicular and axillary). Major complications of these blocks include pneumothorax and diaphragm palsy. The most experienced operator should always perform the ultrasound-guided block in direct visualization of the needle tip and check for pleural sliding both during and after the execution. Diaphragmatic palsy, occurring for anesthetic spreading over C3-C5 roots of phrenic nerve, could sometimes but not always be avoided using strategies such as modifying local anesthetic volume and concentration or modifying the injection site of interscalene block. Useful tips could be that of performing only suprascapular, inflaclavear and axillary block.
4. Spinal and epidural analgesia. Apply routine indications and contraindications for spinal anesthesia, caution should be exercised on dosage of local anesthetics when attempting to reduce duration of anesthesia as conversion to general anesthesia is less desirable, however no dose adjustment for spinal and epidural anesthesia is commonly necessary. Check clotting time and INR (<1.5) as trombocytopenia is frequent in these patients. Although it is still controversial, be aware that parturients are likely to have intraoperative hypotension more frequently than other patients, so manage vasopressor accordingly to avoid free drip of CSF after dural puncture in order to minimize the risk of encephalitis and meningitidis reported in COVID-19. Management of PDPH involves conservative strategies, consider blood patch and avoid sphenopalatine ganglion block as it can be classified as AGP.

Ideally patients should be sedated (preferably with dexmedetomidine) but collaborative, with spontaneous breathing, not coughing and wearing surgical mask. Administer supplemental oxygen if needed through nasal cannulae or, better, via facial mask, monitor respiratory rate and consider continuous capnography, avoid certain blocks, and most importantly, be ready to perform emergent airway intervention and/or general anesthesia in case of block failure or surgical complication.

FOCUS ON INTERFASCIAL PLANE BLOCKS

Both in the COVID-19 era and previously, the interfascial block plays a very important role in multimodal and opioid sparing analgesia. It guarantees a postoperative period as free as possible from pain, administering systemically as few opiates as possible thus avoiding the main systemic side effects: sedation, bradypnea, risk of respiratory arrest due to overdose, constipation and nausea. Similarly, even more so in COVID-19 patients, what is desirable is to reduce the use of systemic adjuvants such as cortisones (dexamethasone in the first place) for their immunosuppressive effect, or hypotensive agents such as clonidine etc., which all have undesirable effects in a patient who is fighting against an acute infection. Amongst other advantages the use of these techniques may also allow the avoidance of hospitalization in intensive care and reduce the duration of the patient's stay both in the operating room at the end of the intervention, and in the recovery room. In addition, with these wall blocks the single shot is often enough to provide adequate post-operative pain control without the need to administer other drugs, adjust infusions or recharge catheter infusion pumps.

For the execution of these blocks in COVID-19 patients it is good practice to use only long-acting anesthetics and chosen adjuvants preferably in the fascial plane.

Use of the ultrasound is mandatory, in-plane approaches should be preferred and atraumatic eco-reflective blunt needles should be used. The success of the fascial block, once the hydrodissection of the fascial plane has been performed, is confirmed by the V-sign, a sign of the correct opening of the fascial plane ready to accommodate the local anesthetic along which it makes its way. Placing an interfascial catheter connected to a Patient-Control Analgesia (PCA) device pump, if available, is an even better method. A problem of major concern is patient positioning. For patient safety the anesthesiologist should perform blocks that require fewer position changes, and block must be executed if bilateral. This is the procedure in upper abdomen and thoracic surgery, in particular breast surgery, where blocks such as bilateral ESPB, PSB or PECS I and PECS II are often required and used for anesthesia and analgesia accompanied by a good sedation plan. For the middle and lower abdomen valid options could be TAPB, QLB I and QLB II, Rectus sheath RSB, ESPB, Ileoinguinal and Ileoipogastric Block, alone or together according to the surgical incision and to the procedure itself. These are safe and effective options in elective but also in emergent surgery, as shown by Guven Erturk et al who performed combined TAP block and Rectus Sheat Block (RSB) for an emergency ileostomy in a patient with COVID-19 pneumonia, avoiding general anesthesia or spinal anesthesia and achieving sensory blockage of the abdominal wall. The patient required systemic analgesia only during peritoneal and intestinal manipulation and intravenous ketamine and fentanyl were administered. Ng et al performed TAP+ RS + ilioinguinal and ileoipogastric block in surgical revision for a loop colostomy. Since COVID-19 patients are often given low molecular weight heparin (e.g. enoxaparine) or fondaparinux, to treat or to prevent thromboembolic complications of the infection, there is a real risk of bleeding. This is the reason why deep compartment blocks such as PVB or QLB III should be avoided; neurological complications could be severe and the site of bleeding could be difficult to compress or to treat without surgical or radiological intervention. So safer, more superficial and easier to perform blocks should be the first options.

As already mentioned LAST should be, immediately and quickly treated, but avoided if at all possible by using a low concentration and normal/high volume of anesthetics.

PREOPERATIVE

PATIENT ASSESSMENT

- Adequately screen all patients with SARS-CoV-2 test.
- Team briefing with surgical equipe, discuss the surgical plan, duration and manage strategies for overcoming complications, eventual tourniquet.
- Access electronic health record and obtain informed written consent, provide alternative choices and discuss the advantages of proposed regional technique
- Check laboratoristic (especially platelet count and clotting) and radiological exams.

EQUIPMENT

- The operating room closest to the entrance of the surgery block must be reserved to COVID-19 patients, equipped with a negative pressure ventilation system or with at least frequent air exchange.
- Bring everything you need, including necessaire to manage anesthesiological and/or surgical complications inside the operating room.
- Equipment that can be found near the patient's airways (videoendoscopic column, ventilators, monitors, ultrasound) must be protected with transparent covers.
- Proceed with dressing in protective mask (surgical, FFP2, FFP3), water-repellent gown, visor, double glove, overshoes. Even if the LRA procedures do not generate aerosol, the use of PPE for aerosol generating procedures must be considered in anticipation of complications/failure of the LRA, that require the anesthesiologist to rapidly manage the airways.
- The patient, after disinfecting the hands with ethyl solution and after wearing a surgical mask, directly accesses the operating room.
- Always use the probe cover, possibly long, and clean the probe at the end of each procedure (no chlorhexidine).
- The necessary drugs should be brought inside the operating room in plastic bags and disposed of at the end of the intervention, along with needles and other disposable devices.
- The anesthesiological report and the operative check list must be filled in, using paper materials specifically for that purpose or, better yet, on a dedicated PC.

INTRAOPERATIVE

TIPS

- The patient enters the operating room, after sanitizing the hands, equipped with a surgical mask, following special intra-hospital paths to transport COVID-19 positive patients.
- Insert at least one large caliber vascular access, preferably two, and any arterial catheter.
- Provide oxygen supplementation preferably using mask with reservoir, start multiparametric monitoring with capnography to be connected directly to the patient by placing HEPA filter to the ventilator or CO_2 line.
- To avoid further contamination of the environment and health personnel, have the LA techniques performed by experienced personnel.

INTRAOPERATIVE

- Choose an adequate sedation plan to keep the patient breathing spontaneously, avoiding apnea or bradypnea, conditions that would predispose emergency intervention on the airways, especially in symptomatic patients for dyspnea and impaired respiratory function.
- Choose an adequate block for the coverage of myotomes, dermatomas and osteotomas, and possible use of tourniquet. Provide for any supplementation for visceral analgesia.
- LRA should be performed with the usual doses of local anesthetic (LA); carefully calculate the dosage of the drug to avoid complications such as LAST or possible ascent of a neuroaxial block. Consider the use of adjuvants to prolong blockade and potentiate analgesic effects while avoiding systemic opioids.
- Always prefer ultrasound-guided techniques that involve fewer changes in the patient's position to execute.

STEP BY STEP EXECUTION

- You should prepare a sterile kit containing: gauze, disinfectant and saline solution in special containers; disposable syringes preloaded with physiological solution to perform hydrolocation of the needle and hydrodissection of the fascial plane; 20 ml syringes preloaded with the anesthesiological mixture to be used; atraumatic eco-reflective needles (of different sizes from 50 mm-80 mm-120 mm Gauge), catheter kit; fixing and dressing material; preloaded syringe for local anesthesia of the skin at the point of entry of the needle. Then proceed to sterile dressing of the anesthesiologist operator and patient positioning.
- Proceed with skin disinfection and prepare surgical field. Probe dressing with long sterile probe cover.
- Take a first look at the block. Identify the nervous target/fascial plane to be blocked. Provide anesthesia of the skin plane.
- Insert the needle, favoring in-plane approaches, so as to visualize the path of the needle. Advance towards the fascial plane andonce the passage through the fascial connective structure is appreciated, proceed with suction maneuver and injection of saline solution for hydrodissection test of the plane. If confirmed, proceed with injection of the desired local anesthetic.
- Follow with ultrasound, the correct opening of the fascial plane and the expansion of the local anesthetic pocket, possibly changing the position of the needle to allow a wider and more uniform opening of the same plane. Then retract the needle andmedicate the puncture area.
- Perform contralaterally block if necessary.
- If deemed appropriate, insert catheter and connect to PCA system.

POST BLOCK ISSUES

- The effectiveness of the LRA must be properly tested before the start of surgery and another block potentially performed.
- Carefully monitor the patient, checking for signs and symptoms of LAST, proceed with surgery.

POSTOPERATIVE

RECOVERY

- Recovery and postoperative monitoring must take place in the operating room to avoid contamination of other areas, then transfer the patient to the destination ward.
- Ensure that instructions on the management of postoperative pain, adverse effects related to blockage or anesthesia are clear and understood by the ward staff.
- Prescribe a rescue pain medication.

EQUIPMENT DECONTAMINATION

- Dispose of and decontaminate equipment including ultrasound carefully using appropriate materials (quaternary ammonium chloride disinfectant).
- The sanitization of the patient paths and the operating room, the sterilization of reusable materials and the disposal of waste must be regulated and carried out according to company operating procedure.
- If continuous peri dural or perinervous infusion has been chosen, use devices (elastomers, electronic pumps) and infusion regimens that limit the number of the ward staff coming into contact with the patient.

CHRONIC PAIN MANAGEMENT IN COVID-19 PATIENTS

Chronic pain patients, especially elderly patients and those with multiple comorbidities, immunosuppressed for chronic therapies, are more susceptible to COVID-19. Oncologic pain is a common chronic condition that is notoriously difficult to manage; patients often show poor response to analgesic medications or experience intolerable adverse effects. Furthermore, during the COVID-19 pandemic, oncologic patients affected by SARS-CoV-2 infection reported an increase of pain, often due to the infection itself or to the discontinuation of pain therapies. Many immunological changes occur, as previously mentioned, in patients suffering from COVID-19, so, in their Joint Statement, ASRA/ESRA recommend not changing ongoing opioid treatment regimens in the absence of documented changes in pain and/or function. They also recommend careful monitoring of patients on transdermal opioids, as the rate of absorption in case of high fever can be unpredictable. Moreover, since the use of non-steroidal anti-inflammatory drugs may mask or reduce symptoms like fever or myalgias, they recommend that all patients who have been prescribed or use non-steroidal anti-inflammatory drugs on a regular basis, to continue using and to promptly report mild fever or new myalgia. In this setting, locoregional anesthesia could be a useful tool to manage chronic pain, improving pain relief, eliminating side effects related to the conventional therapies and reducing the need of close follow-up. With regard to procedural treatments, the same guidelines distinguish between urgent and semi-urgent procedures. Among the urgent, and therefore non-deferrable procedures, they include the management of IntraTecal Pump devices, recommending refill to avoid withdrawal pain and management of devices and neurostimulators that must be maintained and/or removed in case of infections. Among the semi-urgent procedures are those for the treatment of intractable cancer pain, acute Herpes Zoster or intractable postherpetic neuralgia, acute herniated disk or worsening of lumbar radiculopathy, intractable trigeminal neuralgia, early complex regional pain syndrome, acute cluster headache or intractable headache conditions. These all require intervention by the pain specialist, and locoregional techniques could be very useful to manage and ease pain relief, reducing the side effects of several therapies, in case of their discontinuation or non-compliance, and reducing the need of close follow-up. Few experiences have been reported on the use of interfascial plane blocks in COVID-19 patients. Interfascial plane block of the abdominal and thoracic wall such as TAP Block, QLB block or Paravertebral PVB Block and ESP block can even replace paraneuroaxial and epidural thanks to the Local Anesthetic spread into paravertebral and epidural space, and above all for their simplicity of execution and safety if compared to paraneuraxial and crentroneuraxial blocks.

In conclusion, interfascial plane blocks are a simple, safe and effective technique that could be considered as a therapeutical option for the management of chronic oncologic pain, especially during the COVID-19 pandemic. The use of the ultrasound-guidance and the monitoring of the effects make these anesthesiological techniques safe and easily reproducible even in COVID-19 patients. We hope that it will be possible to implement and improve these branches of study at a time of crisis for humanity, accepting the challenges that this historical period imposes and transforming them into opportunities. Less is more, as they say, and this could be the motto for our future as anesthesiologists and pain therapists.

RECOMMENDED READING

- Olvani Martins da Silva, Danielle Bezerra Cabral, Sandra Mara Marin, Julia Valeria de Oliveira Vargas Bitencourt, Mara Ambrosina de Oliveira Vargas, William Campo Meschial, Biosafety measures to prevent COVID-19 in healthcare professionals: an integrative review, Revista Brasileira de Enfermagem, 10.1590/0034-7167-2020-1191, 75, 1, (2022).
- Steven P Cohen, MD, Zafeer B Baber, MD, Asokumar Buvanendran, MD, Brian C McLean, MD, Yian Chen, MD, W Michael Hooten, MD, Scott R Laker, MD, Ajay D Wasan, MD, MSc, David J Kennedy, MD, Friedhelm Sandbrink, MD, Scott A King, MD, Ian M Fowler, MD, Milan P Stojanovic, MD, Salim M Hayek, MD, PhD, Christopher R Phillips, MD, Pain Management Best Practices from Multispecialty Organizations During the COVID-19 Pandemic and Public Health Crises, Pain Medicine, Volume 21, Issue 7, July 2020, Pages 1331–1346, https://doi.org/10.1093/pm/pnaa127

- Canadian Anesthesiologists' Society (CAS): COVID-19 recommendations during airway manipulation (2020)
- Cook TM, El-Boghdadly K, McGuire B, McNarry AF, Patel A, Higgs A. Consensus guidelines for managing the airway in patients with COVID-19;. *Anaesthesia* in press. Available here.
- Lima RME, Reis LA, Thyrso de Lara FS, Dias LC, Matsumoto M, Mizubuti GB, Hamaji A, Cabral LW, Mathias LADST, Lima LHNE. Recommendations for local-regional anesthesia during the COVID-19 pandemic. Braz J Anesthesiol. 2020 Mar-Apr;70(2):159-164. doi: 10.1016/j.bjane.2020.06.002. Epub 2020 Jun 10. PMID: 32834193; PMCID: PMC7286225.
- M. Sorbello, K. El-Boghdadly, Di Giacinto, et al. *The Italian coronavirus disease 2019 outbreak: recommendations from clinical practice Anaesthesia*, 75 (2020), pp. 724-732
- Apfelbaum JL, Hagberg CA, Caplan RA, et al. Practice guidelines for management of the difficult airway: an updated report by the American Society of Anesthesiologists Task Force on Management of the Difficult Airway. *Anesthesiol* 2013; 118:251–270.
- Uppal V, Sondekoppam RV, Landau R, El-Boghdadly K, Narouze S, Kalagara HKP. Neuraxial anaesthesia and peripheral nerve blocks during the COVID-19 pandemic: a literature review and practice recommendations. Anaesthesia. 2020 Oct;75(10):1350-1363. doi: 10.1111/anae.15105. Epub 2020 May 14. PMID: 32344456; PMCID: PMC7267450.
- American Society of Regional Anesthesia and Pain Medicine (ASRA) and European Society of Regional Anesthesia and Pain Therapy (ESRA): Joint statement on practice recommendations on neuraxial anesthesia and peripheral nerve blocks during the COVID-19 pandemic(2020)
- Lie SA, Wong SW, Wong LT, Wong TGL, Chong SY. Practical considerations for performing regional anesthesia: lessons learned from the COVID-19 pandemic. Can J Anaesth. 2020 Jul;67(7):885-892. doi: 10.1007/s12630-020-01637-0. Epub 2020 Mar 24. PMID: 32212103; PMCID: PMC7095295.
- Aminnejad R, Shafiee H. Is Regional Anesthesia Safe Enough in Suspected or Confirmed COVID-19 Patients? ACS Chem Neurosci. 2020 May 6;11(9):1371. doi: 10.1021/acschemneuro.0c00146. Epub 2020 Apr 9. PMID: 32227844.
- Macfarlane AJR, Harrop-Griffiths W, Pawa A. Regional anaesthesia and COVID-19: first choice at last? Br J Anaesth. 2020 Sep;125(3):243-247. doi: 10.1016/j.bja.2020.05.016. Epub 2020 May 28. PMID: 32532429; PMCID: PMC7254013.
- Uppal V, Shanthanna H, Kalagara H, Sondekoppam RV, Hakim SM, Rosenblatt MA, Pawa A, Macfarlane AJR, Moka E, Narouze S. The practice of regional anesthesia during the COVID-19 pandemic: an international survey of members of three regional anesthesia societies. Can J Anaesth. 2021 Nov 18:1–13. doi: 10.1007/s12630-021-02150-8. Epub ahead of print. PMID: 34796460; PMCID: PMC8601752.
- Herman JA, Urits I, Kaye AD, Urman RD, Viswanath O. COVID-19: Recommendations for regional anesthesia. J Clin Anesth. 2020 Oct;65:109885. doi: 10.1016/j.jclinane.2020.109885. Epub 2020 May 20. PMID: 32454343; PMCID: PMC7237915.
- Lie SA, Wong SW, Wong LT, Wong TGL, Chong SY. In reply: Regional anesthesia during the COVID-19 pandemic: a time to reconsider practices? (Letters #1 and #2). Can J Anaesth. 2020 Sep;67(9):1286-1287. doi: 10.1007/s12630-020-01683-8. Epub 2020 May 1. PMID: 32358765; PMCID: PMC7194079.
- Fusco P, Petrucci E, Marinangeli F, Scimia P. Block failure or lack of efficacy? The "Double V" sign: a novel sonographic sign for a successful interfascial plane block. Minerva Anestesiol. 2019 Aug;85(8):917-918. doi: 10.23736/S0375-9393.19.13457-8. PMID: 31339030.
- Dias R, Mendes ÂB, Lages N, Machado H. Ultrasound-guided fascial plane blocks as unique anesthetic technique for total mastectomy in a covid-19 era: A case report. Rev Esp Anestesiol Reanim (Engl Ed). 2021 Aug-Sep;68(7):408-413. doi: 10.1016/j.redare.2020.09.004. Epub 2021 Feb 18. PMID: 34509278; PMCID: PMC8425180.
- Fusco P, Pizzorno L, Arcangeli V, Marinangeli F. Tube or not tube in COVID-19 positive patients: that is the question. Korean J Anesthesiol. 2021 Dec;74(6):552-554. doi: 10.4097/kja.21063. Epub 2021 May 3. PMID: 33934594; PMCID: PMC8648507.
- Guven BB, Erturk T, Güner T, Ersoy A. Abdominal wall blocks for emergency ileostomy operation in a patient with COVID-19 pneumonia: a case report. Braz J Anesthesiol. 2021 Sep-Oct;71(5):572-575. doi: 10.1016/j.bjane.2021.06.009. Epub 2021 Jun 29. PMID: 34214519; PMCID: PMC8240437.
- O. Ng, S.Y. Thong, C.S. Chia, et al. Revision of loop colostomy under regional anaesthesia and sedation Singapore Med J, 56 (2015), pp. e89-e91
- Barnett K, Mercer SW, Norbury M, Watt G, Wyke S, Guthrie B. Epidemiology of multimorbidity and implications for health care, research, and medical education: a cross-sectional study. Lancet. 2012;380(9836):37-43. doi: 10.1016/S0140-6736(12)60240-2. Epub 2012May 10.
- Mills SEE, Nicolson KP, Smith BH. Chronic pain: a review of its epidemiology and associated factors in population-based studies. Br J Anaesth. 2019;123(2):e273-e83. doi: 10.1016/j.bja.2019.03.023. Epub 2019May 10.
- Shanthanna H, Cohen SP, Strand N, Lobo CA, Eld- abe S, Bhatia A, Narouze S. American Society of Regional Anesthesiology. Recommendations on chronic pain practice during the COVID-19 pandemic. 2020. https://www.asra.com/page/2903/ recommendations-on-chronic-pain-practice-during- the-covid-19-pandemic. Accessed 31 Mar 2020.
- Fusco P, Maggiani C, Volpe D, Petroni GM, Bagaphou CT, Marinangeli F. Erector spinae plane block for the management of chronic cancer pain in the era of COVID-19. Minerva Anestesiol. 2021 Jul;87(7):836-837. doi: 10.23736/S0375-9393.21.15516-6. Epub 2021 Apr 14. PMID: 33853272.
- Celik M., Tulgar S., Ahiskalioglu A., Alper F. Is high volume lumbar erector spinae plane block an alternative to transforaminal epidural injection? Evaluation with MRI. Reg Anesth Celik M., Tulgar S., Ahiskalioglu A., Alper F. Is high volume lumbar erector spinae plane block an alternative to transforaminal epidural injection? Evaluation with MRI. Reg Anesth Pain Med. 2019 doi: 10.1136/rapm-2019-100514. In press.
- SIAARTI. Raccomandazioni per l'utilizzo dell'anestesia locoregionale (ALR) nel paziente chirurgico Covid-19 sospetto o positivo.

CLINICAL CASE 1 – EFFICACY OF ESP BLOCK FOR THORACIC ONCOLOGICAL PAIN

Clinical history and anamnesis We report a case of a 75-year-old man affected by parotid carcinoma with multiple costal and vertebral metastasis, in particular at D7-D9 level, which obliterates the bilateral recesses. The patient reported moderate neuropathic pain (six on numerical rating scale [NRS]) radiating from his spine to the middle axillary line, in a dermatomal area between T7 and T12, and poor adherence to treatment (tapentadol 100 mg three times per day and fentanyl 100 μg as needed), because of modest response and onset of side effects. In March 2020, he was admitted to the sub-intensive care unit of our hospital with bilateral COVID-19 pneumonia and respiratory failure. During this period, the pain got worse and the patient discontinued his therapy. He came to our attention in October 2020, as pain intensity had increased from six to eight on NRS.

Technique description For this patient we considered performing either a paravertebral block (PVB) or an erector spinae plane bloc (ESP block): the paravertebral injection was ruled out as being too invasive for the clinical setting. The ESP block was performed as follows: the patient was placed in a prone position and a high-frequency linear ultrasound transducer (12 MHz) was placed in a longitudinal orientation at level of T9 transverse process (**Figure A2.1 A**).

A 22-Gauge 50 mm block needle was used, and the tip of the needle was directed towards the transverse process, in the fascial plane deep to the erector spinae muscle, then 20 ml of 0.2% ropivacaine and dexamethasone 8 mg were injected (**Figure A2.1 B**).

Materials and methods The block was executed in continuous monitoring of major vital signs: SpO_2%, Heart rate (HR), Non-Invasive Blood Pressure (NIBP), End tidal CO_2 on Capnography. A good analgesia of the dermatomerical region T7-T12 was obtained, and no adverse effects were registered. Within a few minutes the patient reported a significant improvement in symptoms and, after a few hours, a complete resolution of the pain. At the 7-day follow-up visit, he reported recurrence of the pain, but lower in intensity (four on NRS). The same treatment was carried out two more times and the pain became progressively mitigated.

Conclusions ESP block is a simple, safe and effective technique that could be considered as a therapeutical option for the management of chronic ontological pain, especially during the COVID-19 pandemic.

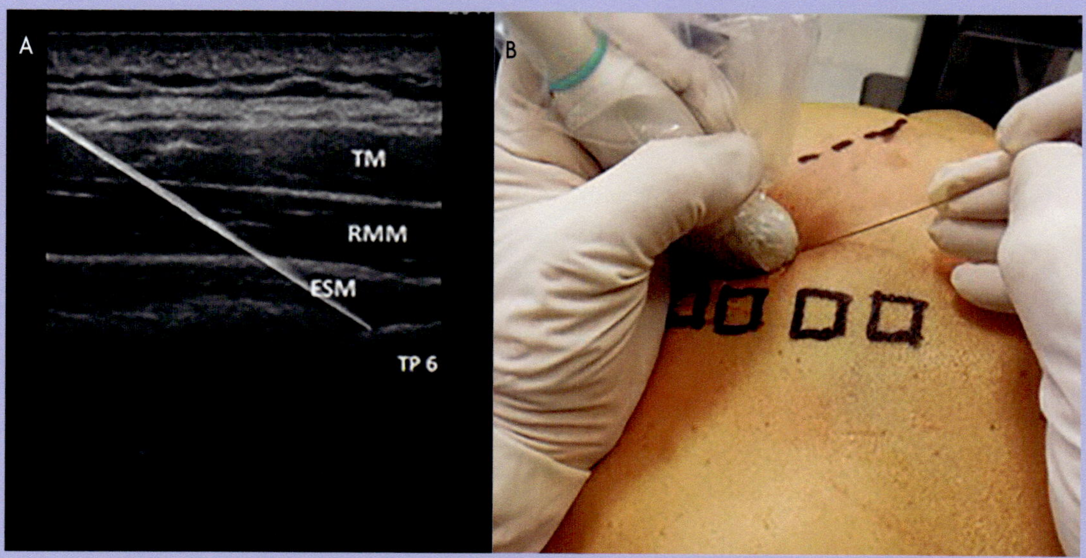

Figure A2.1 A Ultrasound image ESM: erector spinae muscle; RMM: rhomboid muscles; TM: trapezius muscle; TP: transverse process. **B** In-plane placement of a 50 mm block needle at level of the transverse process under ultrasound guidance.

Subject Index

A

Abdominal aortic surgery 104
Abdominal hernia repair 159
Abdominal wall blocks in children 165-168
  ilioinguinal and iliohypogastric nerve block 171
  thoracic paravertebral block 166
  transversus abdominis plane (TAP) block 169
Abdomino-pelvic surgeries 194
Acute pain 10
Adjuvants 20, 34, 75, 76, 199
  non-opioid(s)
    clonidine 102, 180, 181, 200, 210, 221
    dexamethasone 34, 38, 76, 200, 203, 204, 209, 210, 227
    dexmedetomidine 76, 85, 89, 102, 191, 192, 200, 209, 214, 215
    magnesium 102, 22
    midazolam 25, 37, 54, 59
  opioid(s)
    epinephrine 199
    tramadol 37, 200
Algic flare-ups 104
Alzheimer's disease 192
amputation of lower limb 199
Analgesia in hepatopathic patient 104
Anestetics, pharmacokinetics 75, 169, 209
Anesthetic technique and combined to DEX sedation 37
Ankle surgery 199
Anterior QLB (once transmuscular QLB, tQLB or QLB III) 158
Anterior scalene muscle 40, 62,
Appendicectomy 148, 172
Atelectasis 205
Axillary block 220
Axillary node dissection 199

B

Biceps 40, 62
Blind technique 94, 103, 116, 118, 120, 127, 128
Blockade of the rectus abdominis muscle and chronic pain 136
Blockade of the sheath of the rectus abdominis muscle fascia in pediatric patients 136
Blood patch 220
Blurred vision 189
Bone harvesting 104
Bowel lesions 149
Brachial plexus blocks 220
  interscalene 187, 189
  lateral cord 40, 63, 64
  posterior cord 40, 42, 63, 64
Brain ischemia 186
Breast lump excision 199
Breast reconstruction 159
Bullous emphysema 191
Buprenorphine 200

C

Cadaveric dissection 94
Cancer pain in neoplasms 104
Cardiac sternal surgery 89
Carotid endarterectomy (CEA) 183, 186, 191
Carotid stenosis 191
Carotid surgery 188
Carpal tunnel release 199
Catheter(s)
  choice of catheter exit-site 197
  drain 197
  insertion 197
  dressing 198
  infusion 198
  positioning 197
  priming 198
  related problems 201
  securement 197
  selection 197
Cervical plexus block (CPB)
  anatomy 183
  carotid endarterectomy (CEA) 183
  carotid surgery 187
  chronic pain 187
  complications 189, 187
  contraindications 187, 189
  deep 185
  dosages 188
  indication 187, 188
  intermediate 185

Cervical plexus block (CPB) (*Continued*)
neck regional anesthesia 186
neck surgery 183, 187
sonoanatomy 183
superficial 185
technique 185
intermediate cervical plexus block 185
superficial cervical plexus block 185
thyroidectomy 187
volume 188
Chest wall deformities 85
Chronic pain 105, 112, 112, 122, 136
in COVID-19 patients 225
Chronic pulmonary disease (COPD) 191
Clavipectoral fascia 3
Clonidine 200
Coagulation disorder 203
Colectomy 159
Collagen 9
fibers 9
type I 9
type III 8
Colorectal surgery 199
Colostomy 159, 171, 172, 221,
Combined spinal-epidural anesthesia (CSEA) 205
Continuous block of the rectus muscle sheath 134
Continuous lumbar spinal anesthesia (CLSA) 206
Continuous thoracic paravertebral block (PVB) 19
Continuous thoracic spinal anesthesia (CTSA) 206
Continuous wound infusion (CWI) 193
abdomino-pelvic surgery 194
anatomy 194
basic common procedures 195
basic principles 193
breast surgery 194
cardiothoracic surgery 194
complications 201
contraindications 201
dosages of local anesthetics 198
indications 199
long term analgesia
for hip fracture repair 203
sonoanatomy 194
technique 195
Coracobrachialis muscle 40, 62
COVID-19 era 219, 228
chronic pain management in COVID-19 patients 225
focus on interfascial plane blocks 220
recommendations and practical considerations
for regional anesthesia 220
regional anesthesia in the 219
Cutaneous nerves 92

D

Dalens' technique 173
Day surgery 76, 123, 124, 148, 149
Deep adipose tissue (DAT) 2
Deep and superficial serratus plane block 39-60
anatomy 39
cardiac surgery pain management 48
complications 47
contraindications 47
indications in chronic pain 48
local anesthetic indications and dosages 46
pediatric application 47
serratus anterior plane block in cardiac surgery 48
serratus plane block in thoracic
surgery and trauma 51
sonoanatomy 39
technique 43
Deep cervical fascia 1
Deltoid fascia 3
Deltoid muscle 3
Dentate muscle 40, 42, 44
Dexmedetomidine 200
Dexamethasone 76, 81, 85, 200
Dexmedetomidine (DEX) cooperative sedation 37
Diclofenac 200

E

Elderly patient 76, 104, 225
Emergency department 188
Emergency intra-abdominal surgery 104
Endothoracic fascia 6, 14, 83, 110, 154
Epidural anesthesia (EA) 205
Epidural hematoma 209
Erector spinae muscles 1
Erector Spinae Plane block (ESP block) 27-38, 210
anatomy 28
complications 35
contraindications 34
absolute 34
relative 34
dosage 33

indications 33, 34
sonoanatomy 28
technique 30
Eyelid droop 189
External oblique muscle 3
Extracellular matrix (ECM) 8, 9
fibers of the 9

F

Fascia(e) 3
anterior layer of the TLF 3
clavipectoral 3
deltoid 3
of external oblique muscle 3
of infraspinatus 3
of inferior oblique muscle 3
of intercostal muscles 3
of latissimus dorsi muscle 3
of pectoral 3
of periosteum 3
of rhomboid muscles 3
of Rizk 3
of serratus 3
of supraspinatus 3
of supraspinatus fascia 3
of transversus muscle 3
thoracolumbar 3
Fascial plane block 1, 205-216
in COVID-19 positive patients 80
innervation 2
of the neck 183-192
superficial fascia 2
vascularization 2
Fascial tissue 8
Fast-track tracheal extubation 58
Fentanyl 200
Foot surgery 199
Fusion anesthesia 210

G

Gastrectomy 199
Gastric bypass 199
Genitofemoral (GF) nerve block 111
anatomy 112
applications in the pediatric setting 120
complications 120
contraindications 120
absolute 120
relative 120
indication of chronic pain 122
indications and dosages 119
sonoanatomy 112
techniques 115
Glycosaminoglycans 9
Gluteus maximus muscle 3

H

Hand lacerations 199
Hepatectomy 172
Hepatopathic patients, analgesia in 104
Herniorrhaphy 151
Hip 194
arthroplasty 159
fracture repair 203
replacement 199
surgery 159, 160
Hydrodissection 157
Hypotension 209
Hysterectomy 199
Hoarse voice 189
Horner's syndrome 189

I

Iliac crest 40, 91, 93-95, 98, 103, 104
Iliac crest bone harvest 159, 172
Iliohypogastric (IH) nerve block 111, 112
anatomy 112
applications in the pediatric setting 120
complications 120
contraindications 120
absolute 120
relative 120
indication of chronic pain 122
indications and dosages 119
sonoanatomy 112
techniques 115
Iliolumbar ligament 153
Ilioinguinal (II) nerve block 111
anatomy 112
applications in the pediatric setting 120
complications 120

Ilioinguinal (II) nerve block (*Continued*)
  contraindications 120
    absolute 120
    relative 120
  indication of chronic pain 122
  indications and dosages 119
  sonoanatomy 112
  techniques 115
Infiltration, for local analgesia 193-202
Infraspinatus, muscle 3, 40, 63
Inguinal hernia repair 172
Inguinal hernioplasty 126
Inguinal herniorraphy 125, 151
Innervation 10
Intensive care hospitalization 89, 138, 191, 214, 215, 221
Intercostal nerve block 39-60
  anatomy 53
  complications 56
  contraindications 56
    absolute 56
    relative 56
  indication for chronic pain 57
  indications and dosages 56
  pediatric applications 57
  sonoanatomy 53
  technique 54
Intercostal muscle 3
Intercostal plexus 93
Intercostal nerve block 53
Interfascial plane blocks and COVID-19 220
Intermediate cervical plexus block and carotid endarterectomy 186
Intermediate fascia 1
Internal oblique muscle 3
Interpectoral Plane Block (IPP) 61-80
Interscalene brachial plexus block 189
Intraabdominal surgery 104
Intravascular injection 189
Ivor-Lewis surgery 212

K

Ketamine 200
Ketorolac 200
Knee 194
  amputation 159
  arthroplasty 196
  joint 195
  planes for catheter placement 194
  replacement 199

L

Laparotomic hysterectomy
  opioid (almost) free anesthesia/analgesia 204
Laparotomy 159
Laparoscopic cholecystectomy 108
Laparoscopic sigmoidectomy 214
Laparoscopy 33, 176, 171, 172, 215
Lateral pectoral nerve 40-43, 63
Lateral QLB approach (once QLB I) 157
Latissimus dorsi 1 40, 41, 42, 50, 58, 62, 67, 91, 114, 153-157, 169-170
Ligth sedation 186
Limb weakness 161
Liver surgery 199
Living donor nephrectomy 199
Local anesthetic systemic toxicity (LAST) 161, 178, 187, 189, 201
Local hematoma 189
Local infiltration analgesia (LIA) 193
  adjuvants 199
  anatomy 194
  basic common procedures 195
  basic principles 193
  complications 201
  contraindications 201
  dosages 198
  indications 198, 199
  local anesthetics 198
  periarticular 195
  sonoanatomy 194
Locoregional anesthesia/analgesia (LRA) 112
Long chest nerve 40,41
Lower extremity vascular surgery 159

M

Magnesium sulfate 200
Mammoplasty 199
Mastectomy 198
Medial cord 40,63,64
Medial cutaneous nerve of the arm 40, 43, 67
Medial cutaneous nerve of the forearm 40, 63
Medial pectoral nerve 4, 40-42, 63

Median nerve 40, 63, 64
Meloxicam 200
Meperidine 50 200
Metameric spinal anesthesia 206
Methylprednisolone 200
Midazolam 25, 37, 54, 59, 88, 115, 126
Morphine 200
Muscles
  abdominal 6
  deltoid 3
  erector spinae 1, 5, 27
  external oblique 3, 6, 7, 8
  gluteus maximus 3
  infraspinatus 3
  internal oblique 7
  large abdominal 5
  latissimus dorsi 3
  pectoralis major 3, 5
  rectus 5
  rhomboid 3
  serratus anterior 3
  serratus inferior 1
  serratus major 5
  serratus posterior 3
  subclavius and pectoralis minor 3
  supraspinatus 3
  transverse 6
  transversus abdominis 3
  trapezius 3
Musculocutaneous nerve 40, 63, 67
Musculoskeletal pain 10
Myofascial planes of the trunk 1-12, 3
  deep 1, 3
  first 3
  intermediate 1, 3
  second 4
  superficial 1-3
  third 6

N

Needle-probe alignment 73, 95, 217
Nephrectomy 160, 172
Nerve injury 189
Neuraxial analgesia 209
Neuraxial blocks 205-216
Neurolysis with alcohol or phenol 104

O

Occipital nerve 184
Oncologic pain 225
Oncologic surgery 220
Opioids 109, 115, 188, 191, 210, 214
  intrathecal 91
  systemal 91
Otoplasty 188

P

Pacemaker implantation 192
Pain therapy 33, 39, 52, 121
Pancreatic surgery 199
Paracetamol 80, 109, 181
Parasternal block 81-90
Parasternal intercostal plane (PIP) block 81-86
  cardiac sternal surgery 89
Paravertebral block (PVB) 13, 210
Patient-Control Analgesia (PCA) 221
PECS 1 and intermediate
    cervical plexus block in Alzheimer's disease 192
PECS I and PECS II blocks 9, 61-80
  anatomy 62
  complications 77
  contraindications 76, 77
  indications and dosages 74
  patients with high anesthetic risk 7
  sonoanatomy 62
  surgical indications 76
  target of the block 69
    IPP block 69
    PSP block 69
  techniques 69
    IPP Block 70
    PSP Block 72
Pectoral fascia 3
Pectoralis major muscle 3
Pectoserratus plane block (PSP) 61-80
Pediatric Anesthesia 47, 112, 115, 116, 12
  in Iliohypogastric (IH) nerve block 120
  in Ilioinguinal (II) nerve block 120
  in genitofemoral (GF) nerve block 120
Pediatric Regional Anesthesia Network (PRAN) 171
Peridural
  analgesia 127
  anesthesia 20

Peridural (*Continued*)
  block 13
  space 13, 35, 135
  technique 102
Perinervous catheter 13, 19
Perioperative pain 52
Perioperative morbidity 61
Pinnaplasty 188
Phrenic nerve paralysis 189
Pyelo-ureteroplasty 172
Pleura 16, 17, 19
Pleural drain-placement sites 48-49
Pleural puncture 22, 35, 81
Posterior QLB (once QLB II) 157
Postoperative analgesia 207
Postoperative nausea and vomiting (PONV) 39
Premedication 180
Proctosigmoidectomy 159
Prostatectomy 199
Pyloromyotomy 192
Pumps related problems 201

Q

Quadratus lumborum block (QLB) 153-164
  anatomy 153
  anterior QLB (once transmuscular QLB, tQLB or QLB III) 158
  chronic pain indication 161
  complications and contraindications 161
  description of techniques 156
  indications and local anesthetic doses 159
  lateral QLB approach (once QLB I) 157
  posterior QLB (once QLB II) 157
  sonoanatomy 155

R

Radial nerve 40, 63, 67
Radical nephrectomy 159
Radiofrequency 57, 123, 189
Reconstructive/esthetic surgery 20
Rectus sheath block 127-140, 175
  anatomy and sonoanatomy 129
  continuous block of the rectus muscle sheath 134
  description of the ultrasound-guided technique 132
  in COVID-19 221
  local anesthetic indications and dosages 127, 135
  target of the block 131
Recurrent laryngeal nerve block 189
Regional anesthesia 186
  in the COVID-19 era 219
  Pediatric Regional Anesthesia Network (PRAN) 171
Rhomboid muscle 77
Ropivacaine Readyfusor 193
Rotatory cuff repair 199

S

Scapula 3, 22, 40
Second-degree Atrioventricular Block Mobitz type 1 192
Sedation for breast cancer surgery 38
Segmental anesthesia 206
Serratus anterior plane block
  mini-thoracotomy
    and pneumothorax pain management 59
Sensation of breathlessness 189
Serratus anterior plane block in cardiac surgery 48
Serratus fasciae 3
Serratus muscles 3
Serratus plane block
  dosages 49
  technique description 49
Serratus posterior inferior muscles 1
Shamrock technique 155
Shoulder 194
  arthroscopy 199
  replacement 199
Simulate ultrasound guided fascial blocks 217
Simulator of ultrasound guided fascial block 218
Sympathetic ganglion 14, 15
Systemic analgesia 39, 221
  ERAS recommendations 48, 50, 51, 86, 204
  lidocaine 70, 33, 159, 187, 188, 201, 209
  magnesium 102, 200
  opioids 25, 37, 51, 52, 61, 75, 79, 138, 204, 210, 214
  paracetamol 81, 109, 181
Small pectoral muscle 40
Spinal anesthesia (SA) 205
Spine fusion 199
Splenectomy 58, 172
Sternotomy 199
Subarachnoid anesthesia 22, 126, 187, 189, 206
Subclavius muscle 3, 40, 62-64

Subcostal and mid-axillary tap block approach
  postoperative analgesia
    in cholecystectomy with xifo-umbilical laparo-tomy technique 109
Subcostal Tap Block
  postoperative Analgesia in laparoscopic cholecystectomy 108
Subcutaneous tissue 2, 42, 73, 85
Subscapular nerves 40, 63
Superficial adipose tissue (SAT) 2
Superficial and intermediate cervical plexus block 183
Superficial fascia 1
Superficial parasternal intercostal plane (PIP) block 81, 85
  anatomy 82
  applications to the pediatric setting 85
  complications 85
  contraindications 85
  indications and dosages 84
  technique 83
Superficial serratus plane block 39-60
Supraclavicular branches 192
Supraspinatus muscle 3

T

Thoracic oncological pain
  efficacy of esp block for 227
Thoracic spine 13
Thoracic paravertebral block 13-26
  anatomy 13
  chronic pain 22
  complications 22
    accidental peridural administration of LA 22
    accidental subarachnoid administration of LA 22
    hematomas 22
    LA toxicity 22
    pneumothorax 22
  complications 22
  continuous blocks and perinervous catheter 19
  contraindications 22
  indications 20
  local anesthetic 20
    longitudinal spread 20
  sonoanatomy 16
    longitudinal approach 17
    transverse approach 16
    ultrasonographic anatomic
      landmarks in the longitudinal approach 17
  techniques 17
    continuous blocks 19
    perinervous catheter 19
  volumes and drug dosages 20
Thoracic paravertebral space (TPVS) 13, 14, 154, 156, 158
Thoracic spinal anesthesia 206
Thoracodorsal nerve 63, 64, 68, 72, 75
Thoracodorsal nerve 63, 64, 68, 72, 75
Thoracolumbar fascia 3
Thoracotomy 20, 22, 34, 47, 49, 59, 172, 194, 199
Thoracoscopy 20, 21, 152, 166, 172, 199
Tramadol 37, 180, 204
Transitory ischemic attack (TIA) 191
Transversalis fascia plane (TFP) 8
Transversalis fascia plane block 141-152
  an alternative approach
    for anesthesia in inguinal herniorrhaphy 151
  anatomy and sonoanatomy 141
  complications 149
  contraindications 148
  description of the ultrasound-guided technique 144
  dosages 148
  indications in chronic pain 149
  sonoanatomy 143
  when tfp block is not recommended 148
Transversus abdominis plane (TAP) block 9-110
  anatomy 91
  approaches to tap block execution 97
    bilateral dual TAP block 101
    lateral QLB (before "Posterior approach") 98
    mid-axillary approach (before "Lateral TAP Block") 97
    oblique subcostal approach 99
    subcostal approach 100
  chronic pain 105
  complications 103
  continuous tap block 101
  contraindications 103
  indications and dosages of local anesthetic 102
  pediatric setting 105
  plexus 93
  sonoanatomy 91
  TAP block and adjuvant use 102
  target and timing of the block 93
  techniques 94
    blind technique 94
    echo-guided technique 95
Transversus abdominis muscle 3

Transversus thoracic muscle 82
Trapezius muscle 3, 32, 38, 67, 177, 227
Tympanomastoid surgery 188
Trunk
dissection of 1
myofascial planes 3-11

U

Ulnar nerve 40, 63, 67
Ultrasound-guided regional anesthesia simulation 217-218
Ultrasound guided Serratus Plane Block (US-SPB) in thoracic trauma patients 58
Umbilical hernia repair 172
Upper arm anesthesia 189
Ultrasound-guided Erector Spinae plane block
and cancer surgery 38
anesthetic technique and combined to DEX sedation 37
as a single anesthetic technique combined with mild sedation for breast cancer surgery 38
Ultrasound-guided ilioinguinal-iliohypogastric nerve block
and genitofemoral (GF) nerve block 126
as anesthetic technique for inguinal herniorraphy 125
associated to awake sedation for anesthesia in inguinal hernioplasty 126
associated to DEX cooperative sedation 37
for inguinal hernia correction 181
Ultrasound-guided paraverterbal block for thoracoscopic lung resection 180
US-guided trunk and abdominal wall blocks in children 165
Erector Spinae Plane (ESP) Block 176
anatomy 176
block target 176
complications 178
contraindications 178
indications 178
sonoanatomy 176
technique 177
ilioinguinal and iliohypogastric nerve block 171
anatomy 171
block target 172
complications 175
contraindications 175
indications 174
sonoanatomy 171
technique 173
rectus sheath block 175
anatomy 175
block target 175
complications 176
contraindications 176
indications 176
sonoanatomy 175
technique 175
thoracic paravertebral block 166
anatomy 166
block target 166
complications 169
indications 168
sonoanatomy 166
technique 166
transversus Abdominis Plane (TAP) block 169
anatomy 169
block target 169
complications 171
contraindications 171
indications 170
sonoanatomy 169
technique 169
Ultrasound-guided unilateral paravertebral block 24
hernia repair surgery 24
Ultrasound-guided UPB 24
undergo breast surgery 25

V

Vascularization 11
of fascial planes 11
of limbs 199
Venturi-mask 214
Video laparoscopic surgery 207

X

Xifo-umbilical laparotomy technique 109

W

Wound healing 201
Wound infection 201